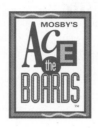

MOSBY'S

Ace the BOARDS

Anatomy

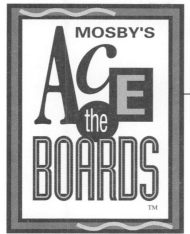

MOSBY'S
USMLE *step* 1
REVIEWS

Anatomy

N. Anthony Moore, Ph.D.

Associate Professor of Anatomy
Director, Medical Gross and Developmental Anatomy,
University of Mississippi Medical Center,
Jackson, Mississippi

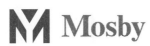 Mosby

St. Louis Baltimore Boston Carlsbad Chicago Naples New York Philadelphia Portland
London Madrid Mexico City Singapore Sydney Tokyo Toronto Wiesbaden

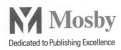

Mosby

Dedicated to Publishing Excellence

A Times Mirror
Company

Vice President and Publisher *Anne S. Patterson*
Editor *Emma D. Underdown*
Developmental Editor *Christy Wells*
Project Manager *Dana Peick*
Production Editor *Jeffrey Patterson*
Manufacturing Supervisor *Karen Boehme*
Book Designer *Amy Buxton*
Cover Design *Stacy Lanier/AKA Design*

Printed in the United States of America
Composition by Graphic World, Inc.
Printing/binding by Plus Communications

Mosby–Year Book, Inc.
11830 Westline Industrial Drive
St. Louis, Missouri 63146

Library of Congress Cataloging-in-Publication Data

Moore, N. Anthony.
    Mosby's USMLE step 1 reviews—anatomy / N. Anthony Moore.
        p.   cm.—(Ace the boards)
    1. Human anatomy—Examinations, questions, etc.   I. Title.
II. Series.
    [DNLM: 1. Anatomy—examination questions.   QS 18.2 M823m 1996]
QM32.M66   1996
611'.0076—dc20
DNLM/DLC
for Library of Congress   96-27384
                                                              CIP

ISBN 0-8151-6905-1 (IBM)
ISBN 0-8151-8671-1 (MAC)

97 98 99 00 / 9 8 7 6 5 4 3 2 1

PREFACE

Ace Anatomy offers a comprehensive review of the information covered in a modern medical gross anatomy course and tested on the USMLE Step 1 Exam. Throughout, every effort has been made to ensure that the information is complete and accurate. This essential information is presented in a bulleted, colorized format that makes the material easily accessible. Summary tables and lists are included to facilitate organization and synthesis. The text is supplemented by clear, two-color illustrations that promote recall and enhance understanding. Icons in the margins help you find information quickly. The page layout provides ample space for note taking, so you can consolidate all your review notes in one place.

Ace Anatomy includes USMLE-style questions at the end of each chapter to reinforce the key information.

Additionally, the accompanying computer diskette includes many more practice questions. These questions are categorized to enable you to determine areas for further study. Importantly, not only are you told why the right answer is correct, but also why the other answers are incorrect. The perforated answer sheets in the back of the book can be torn out and placed next to the questions as you review for immediate feedback.

A solid foundation in human anatomy is crucial to your career. It is my sincere hope that *Ace Anatomy* helps you master the material and "ace" in-class exams and the Step 1 exam.

N. Anthony Moore

ACKNOWLEDGMENTS

I thank Emma Underdown at Mosby for allowing me the opportunity to undertake this project, and Christy Wells for her persistent prodding to keep the project moving. A special thanks is due my chairman, Duane E. Haines, Ph.D., for providing much needed encouragement and support throughout the project.

I also appreciate the efforts of all the medical students throughout my career who have provided critiques and suggestions to my teaching materials. In particular, I wish to acknowledge two medical students for their feedback and insights into the manuscript:

Michelle Rawson
University of Texas School of Medicine
Yi-Meng Yen
University of California-Los Angeles School of Medicine

Test-Taking Strategies

Suzanne F. Kiewit, M.Ed.

To perform well on the USMLEs, it is imperative that you begin with a **plan.** Preparation time is at a premium, so you will want to be as efficient and effective as possible by planning well.

MONTHS AHEAD OF THE EXAM

- Sit down with a blank calendar and block in your commitments: classes, final exams, scheduled events.
- Include time for activities of daily life: eating, sleeping, exercising, socializing, banking, maintaining your home, and so forth.
- The remaining time is available for study/review.
- Determine an orderly approach to the material you need to cover that fits your particular set of needs (e.g., subject-by-subject approach, systems approach, pathologic state approach).
- Assign the remaining time to content areas. This is done in various ways: material covered freshman year first, easiest first, least comfortable material first, detailed subjects last, whatever. Your plan should reflect your goal: to maximize your score.
- Establish a warm-up, which may consist of breaking the tension in major muscle groups (neck rolls, shoulder rolls, etc.), a quick visualization of you performing successfully, or a brief meditation. Practicing this warm-up routine before each of your study sessions will make it a familiar activity that helps you learn effectively, as well as take exams effectively.
- Designate time at the end of your study period for panoramic review. Depending on your needs, that might be a week or just several days before the exam.
- Plan for feedback on your efforts. Schedule time for answering questions on the material you are reviewing and for taking at least one mock comprehensive exam.
- Do the comprehensive exam midway through your study period so that you can refine your efforts to reflect the degree of your performance.

DAYS AHEAD OF THE EXAM

- Divide each day into thirds: morning block, afternoon block, and evening block.

- Consider the time of day that is most productive for you and do the most difficult or least favorite material at that time.
- Assign more blocks of study to those areas requiring the most review to reach a comfortable knowledge level.
- A popular way to use blocks is to pair subjects or materials. For instance, pair strong content with weaker content so that you are not always in the position of not knowing material (which would invite negative feelings or ineffectiveness). Or pair a conceptual subject with a detail subject, such as physiology with anatomy, so that you are not always doing the same kind of thinking (this invites positive effort).
- Use your most productive blocks of time for actual study/review. Use the nonpeak times for reinforcement of material covered or feedback by answering questions on material that you have covered.

Planning the Blocks

- Once you determine time allocations for each content area and an orderly approach that fits your needs and goals, you want to specify what you plan to do during each block.
- Be specific as to content area, material to study, and task; for example, MICRO: review chart on viruses; PHYS: answer questions on renal; and so forth.
- Each study block will last approximately 3 to 4 hours. To be most efficient and effective, plan to take a 5- or 10-minute break every hour. If you are having difficulty getting into the study mode, plan to study for 25 minutes, then take a 5-minute break. Reserve longer breaks for switches between subjects. Get up and move around on breaks.

BEFORE THE EXAM

Knowing about the USMLEs helps demystify them. In general, the USMLE exams are a 2-day, four-book examination. Approximately 3 hours are allotted per exam book. Each day you will complete one book of about 200 items in the morning and another book in the afternoon.

In each exam book, questions are organized by question type, not content. Specific directions precede each set of questions. Only two question formats are used: one-best-answer multiple choice items (which typically come first on the exam) and matching items (toward the end of the exam). Students have reported that one-best-answer items make up the bulk of the exam (70% to 75%) and negatively stemmed items make up only 10% to 15% of the questions (Bushan, Le, and Amin). Matching sets, which make up about 15% to 20% of the items, may include short leading lists or long leading lists of up to 26 items from which to choose.

From year to year there may be variations in the organization and presentation of both content and item formats. It would be wise to read the National Board of Medical Examiners' *General Instructions* booklet, which you will receive when you register. This booklet contains descriptions of content, item format, and even a set of practice items. Be certain you read this booklet and familiarize yourself with the questions.

You can further maximize exam performance by taking control. Adults tend to perform better when they feel that they have a measure of control. For the USMLE it is easy to feel out of control. You are told what time to arrive, where to go, what writing instrument to use, when to break the seal, and so on. You want to assume control of as many aspects as possible to maximize your performance:

STUDY   Follow the sage advice of planning your work and working your plan to maintain satisfactory preparation with regard to study.

SLEEP   Get a good night's rest. Sleep needs vary, but 6 hours is usually minimum. Try to get the appropriate amount of sleep that you require.

NUTRITION   Maintain proper nutrition during both study time and exam time. Eat breakfast. Choose foods that help keep you on an even energy level. Eat light lunches on exam days. If you have a favorite food and can take it with you, treat yourself.

MEDICATION   It may be cold, flu, or allergy season. Take no medications that may make you drowsy.

CLOTHING   Heating and cooling systems are rarely balanced enough to suit everyone. Wear articles of clothing that can be added or removed as necessary. Strive for personal comfort.

READINESS   Develop physical, mental, emotional, and psychologic readiness for the exam. Keep your thoughts about the exam and your preparation efforts running positively. You must believe that *you can do this!*

ARRIVAL   Plan to arrive as close to the designated time as possible and still allow yourself sufficient time to check in. Keep to yourself so that other people's anxieties will not affect you. Take care of personal needs. Find your seat.

ACCLIMATION   Settle in and get comfortable. Take several deep breaths . . . RELAX. A relaxed mind thinks better than a tense one—it's that old "fight-or-flight" syndrome. Do your warm-up routine to help you relax.

ATTENTION   Pay attention to the proctor. Complete all identification material as required. Read all instructions carefully. Ask for clarification as needed. Do not open your booklet until told to do so. After you are told to break the seal, quickly glance through the whole test to see how it is set up and how questions are organized. Again, you want to take control of the situation. A quick purview eliminates surprises and allows you to develop a plan.

DURING THE EXAM

Plan Your Approach

There are numerous approaches to answering questions. Answer questions in the order that appeals to you. Doing the easier ones first may give a psychologic boost; however, the ones you skip may stay on your mind and cloud your thinking.

Another approach is to answer each question in sequence. Start with the first one in the section with which you begin and fill in an answer for each question. Do not leave any blanks! The theory behind this is that if you spend any time at all on an item, you should mark your best response at that time and go on. If you are not certain of your choice, mark "R" in the test booklet for review and return to it later as you have time.

Some students plan to do the matching items first. Matching items are the last set of questions in the booklets. If you prefer matching items, this is a reasonable plan because it helps you get started with items about which you feel confident. It is also reasonable because matching items are not good items on which to guess if you run short of time. **You** must decide the order in which you want to do the questions.

Complete the Bubble Sheet or Answer Card Carefully

There are two schools of thought on this matter. One is to fill in the bubble sheet **item by item** as you go. This method minimizes transcription errors. The other method is **block transfer.** Complete a logical chunk of questions in the test booklet (one or two pages) and then transfer responses to the bubble sheet. Be sure that the last question number on the page is the last numeral you blacken. This method saves time and offers a mini–mental break at the end of each block. Such minibreaks help decrease fatigue during a long exam. Choose the method that will work for you and *practice* it as you take prep questions.

Budget Your Time

If only the allotted time and the number of questions were considered, you would have approximately 54 seconds per question. Obviously, some questions may go more quickly and balance out the ones that take longer. To keep track, you need a pacing strategy. A good strategy is to establish checkpoints at 30-minute intervals. When you overview the booklet, circle the numerals corresponding to where you should be at 30 minutes, 60, 90, 120, and so on. For example, if you have 200 questions on a 3-hour exam, you should be at question number 33 at 30 minutes. As you complete the exam, check your time at the circled items. This technique keeps you from watching the clock too much, yet permits multiple opportunities to adjust your pacing.

If you find yourself spending too much time on any one question, select your best choice at that time, mark an answer, and "R" it for later review. The point is to keep going. Laboring too long on one question limits you from responding to other items you may know well. Remember, controlling your time helps you maximize your points.

ANSWERING THE QUESTIONS

- **Read and *understand* the stems and alternatives.**
  The most frequent error made on exams is misreading or misinterpreting the various aspects of a question. The **stem** is the introductory question or statement. The **alternatives** are the options from which you select the one best response. To encourage reading and understanding, use a process.
- **Follow a process to answer questions.**
  1. Quickly read the stem.
  2. Quickly read the options. (Combined, the first two steps create a preview of the item.)
  3. Carefully read, underline, and mark the stem in a timely fashion.
     - Selectively underline key words and phrases.
     - Pay attention to nouns, verbs, and modifiers.

- Circle age and gender.
- Note data in telescopic form (e.g., $\uparrow$ BP).
- Graphically represent material if it helps you to understand (e.g., diagram the renal tubule to answer a question about reabsorption).

4. Carefully read each alternative. Mark as appropriate.

- **Consider each alternative as one in a series of true, false, or not sure (?) statements.**
  Read each alternative. Rather than slashing out the ones you eliminate, work with each one and designate it as **true, false,** or varying degrees of **true/false/?.** This marking strategy requires you to make judicious decisions about alternatives relative to the stem. It also provides a record of your original thinking, which will save you re-thinking time if you need to reconsider a question. Practice this strategy on preparation questions so it becomes second nature.
- **Avoid premature closure.**
  Sometimes you may read a question and anticipate a response. Such a reaction helps focus your attention. However, be sure to read *all* the options so that you are selecting the *best* response. In one-best-answer multiple choice questions, there is one *best* and several *likely* responses. Avoid being misled; consider all the alternatives.
- **Be leery of negative stems.**
  Negative stems require shifting to a negative thinking mode to determine which alternatives are not correct. You can avoid this shift by using this strategy:
  - Circle such words as *except, least, false, incorrect, not true* to raise your awareness of them.
  - Cross out the negative and read the stem as though it were a positive.
  - Mark each option as T/F/?. The F option will then be the appropriate choice.
- **Keep your original answers.**
  To change or not to change answers is a difficult decision. The answer depends on a person's previous history. If you are the kind of student who, if you change answers, changes them from wrong to right, then selectively changing answers may be worthwhile. If, on the other hand, your past experience has been to change right answers to wrong answers, selectively changing answers is probably not a good idea. Good performers change answers, but only if they have reason, such as acquired insight or discovery of misreading or misinterpretation.

- **Maintain an even emotional keel.**
  If a question upsets you, calm yourself. Take several deep breaths. Tell yourself, "I can do this!" Give yourself a mental or physical break. Pay special attention to the next two or three questions after a bout of emotional uneasiness. It is possible to miss items when attention is diffused.

THINKING THROUGH QUESTIONS

- **Use logical reasoning and sound thinking.**
  - Read the item carefully. After careful reading, ask "What is this question really asking?" Restate it so that you know what is being asked.
  - Engage in a mental dialogue with the question. Talk to yourself about what you do know. Always start with what **you** know. Verbalize your thinking.
  - If a diagram or graphic representation is included, orient yourself to it **first** so that the options do not lead your thinking.
- **Use information found within the questions themselves to help you answer others.**
  There will not be "gimmes" on a nationally standardized exam. However, there may be items or graphics that trigger remembrances.
- **Create a diagram, chart, map, or graphic representation of given information.**
  Material that is visually presented usually helps clarify thinking. Use selective, quick sketching as warranted.
- **Reason through information like a detective.**
  - Sift through the details (preview).
  - Determine the relevant information (selectively mark).
  - Put the clues together as in solving a puzzle (reason).
- **Read carefully and note key descriptors.**
  - Note words such as *chronic, acute, greater than, less than, adult, child.*
  - Attend to prefixes such as *hyper-, hypo-, non-, un-, pre-, post-.*
- **Analyze base words and affixes.**
  Studying a question at the word level may help you remember salient information. Look for base words or related words. Determine Latin or Greek word parts and use their meanings to assist you.
- **Consider similar options equally.**
  If you mark one alternative as "false" for a particular reason and another option is qualified for the same reason, it's probably "false" as well.
- **Trust the questions.**
  The questions are designed to determine if you

have a working knowledge of the material. They are not written to trick you. You need to believe that your medical school curriculum and your study efforts prepared you for most of the questions.

- **Meet the challenge of clinical vignettes.**
  Longer, vignette items challenge you to discern the relevant from the irrelevant material. In doing so, you are given multiple clues to consider. To effectively handle the vignette item, follow this strategy:
  - Scan the stem and read the first several lines.
  - Skip to the end of the stem and read the last several lines.
  - Check the alternatives to narrow your focus.
  - Now that you know what the question is about, go back to the stem; read and mark what's important to your informed decision making.
  - Make good T/F/? decisions.
- **Reread your underlines and markings when you are down to two choices, at 50/50.**
  By the time you work through a stem and numerous alternatives, it is easy to lose the gist of the question. Checking your focus by rereading only the underlines ensures that you are answering the question being posed.

ANSWERING MATCHING ITEM SETS

Matching items are used to measure your ability to distinguish among closely related items. They require knowledge of specific sets of information. As you study, be alert to potential material that could be tested in this way.

Matching items can be formatted in two ways. **Short leading list matching** items include a set of five, lettered options followed by a lead-in statement and then several numbered stems. **Long leading list matching** items include a set of up to 26 lettered options, followed by a lead-in statement and then several numbered stems.

To efficiently deal with a short leading list item, consider it as an upside-down multiple choice item with the same repeated options. To handle it effectively, do the following:

- Scan the list; determine the topic.
- Read the lead-in statement; determine the focus.
- Quickly read the stem; then read and mark key words.
- In the left margin, create a grid with A, B, C, D, E at the top.

- Make good T/F/? decisions about each stem, marking them in the grid. In this way you can see the pattern of your responses. Similarly, a grid with the item numbers can be drawn beside the leading list and responses marked there.

Handling long leading list matching items effectively requires some modifications in the process. It is not efficient to make T/F/? decisions about each option, so follow this strategy:

- Scan the list; determine the topic.
- Read the lead-in; determine the focus.
- Read a stem and generate your own response.
- Narrow the focus. Put a check mark by those related options in the long list.
- Read and mark specifics in the stem to differentiate among those alternatives you marked.
- Make good T/F/? decisions.

For each stem, mark the narrowed-list options with a different symbol (star, dash, etc.). Items are listed in logical order, alphabetically or numerically. When looking for an option such as "xanthinuria," do not start at the beginning of the list. Looking in the appropriate place saves valuable seconds.

TEST WISENESS

How a question is worded can often influence your response to it. Most clues about "test psychology" are a function of the way in which a question is worded—test constructors cannot rename body parts, drugs, diseases, and so forth. Being aware of the psychology behind the wording can often help you answer the test question.

Using techniques of test psychology to arrive at a correct answer has limited value on standardized exams because those who construct the exams are well aware of the use of these techniques. Nonetheless, being wise to these techniques of test psychology may add another point or two to your score, and they can also enhance your sense of control. Knowing these techniques provides additional strategies to employ should the question temporarily stump you.

The best way to take any exam is to be totally prepared with a strong knowledge base and personal test confidence. The following techniques should be used only if you have exhausted your knowledge base, eliminated all distractors, and cannot come up with the answer even with logical thinking and sound reasoning. Such techniques are **not** a substitute for knowledge, nor are they foolproof.

- **Identify common ideas or themes within the options and between the stem and options.**

- Circle repeated words in the options.
- Select the option with the most repeated words or phrases.
- Circle words repeated in both stem and options.
- Select the option that contains key words or related words from the stem. This is a stem/option repetition.
- **Beware of words that narrow the focus or are too extreme because they tend to be incorrect.**
  Circle such words as *all, always, every, exclusively, never, no, not, none.*
- **Options that are look-alikes are good candidates for exclusion.**
- **Note qualifiers that broaden the focus because they may be correct.**
  Circle words such as *generally, probably, most, often, some, usually.*
- **Identify antonyms or two opposing statements as potentially correct options.**
  Test constructors may use pairs of opposites, so this tip may lose its effectiveness.
- **Select the most familiar-looking option.**
  Always go from what you know. Alternatives with unknown terms may be likely distractors.
- **Select the longest, most inclusive answer.**
  This would include "All of the above" as a strong potential response.
- **In numerical items, knock out the high and low alternatives and select one in the middle that seems most plausible.**
- **In negatively stemmed questions, categorize responses; the one that falls out of the category is a likely candidate.**
- **Mark the same alternative consistently throughout the test if you have no best guess and cannot eliminate distractors.**
  Before the test, decide which letter (A, B, C, D, E) will be your choice. In this way, if you have given a question your best effort and cannot decide, mark your favorite response and move to questions that cover more comfortable material.

AFTER THE EXAM
- **Between sessions and overnight:**
  - Take a well-deserved break. Eat nutritionally.
  - If you feel the urge to study, study material that is comfortable, from a source with which you are familiar (e.g., personally developed study cards or your annotated review book).
  - If you discovered a recurring "theme," you might desire to consult that set of information.

- Do something pleasurable. Relax. Get a good night's rest.
- **After the final booklet:**
  - Recognize that this exam is a measure of what you know on a given day for a given set of information at a given point in time. Keep a reasonable perspective.
  - **Celebrate!**

References

Bushan V, Le T, Amin C: *First aid for the USMLE Step 1,* ed 5, Norwalk, Conn., 1995, Appleton & Lange.

MONEY-BACK GUARANTEE

We are confident that ACE THE BOARDS will prepare you for passing the USMLEs. We are so sure of this, that we'll offer you a money-back guarantee should you fail the USMLE. To receive your refund, simply mail us a copy of your failed USMLE report, plus the original receipt for this product. Mail these materials to:

Marketing Manager, medical textbooks
Mosby–Year Book, Inc.
11830 Westline Industrial Drive
St. Louis, MO 63146

Contents

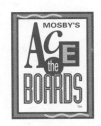

Anatomy

Chapter 1

Basic Structures and Concepts

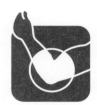

- ■ **Skeletal System**
  - Is typically composed of 206 individual bones with some normal variation in number
  - Consists of an **axial skeleton** and an **appendicular skeleton**
  - Has many functions, including
    - — **Support** of soft tissues
    - — **Attachment** for skeletal muscle, facilitating movement of body parts
    - — **Protection** of the body organs
    - — **Storage** of calcium and phosphorus
    - — **Hemopoiesis** in the marrow cavities
  - ● **Axial skeleton**
    - **Skull**—composed of **cranial bones** and **facial bones**
    - **Vertebral column**—composed of the individual **vertebrae,** the **sacrum** (the fused sacral vertebra), and the **coccyx**
    - **Rib cage**—composed of the 12 pairs of **ribs,** the **sternum,** and the **costal cartilages**
    - **Hyoid bone**
    - **Auditory ossicles**—malleus, incus, and stapes
  - ● **Appendicular skeleton**
    - **Pectoral girdle** (includes the paired **clavicles** and **scapulae**)
    - Bones of the **upper extremity** (including the humerus, radius, ulna, carpals, metacarpals, and phalanges)
    - **Pelvic girdle** (paired **hip bones** composed of the fused ilium, ischium, and pubis)
    - Bones of the **lower extremity** (including the femur, tibia, fibula, patella, tarsals, metatarsals, and phalanges)
  - ● **Bones**
    - Consist of both **cancellous** (spongy) and **compact** bone; considerable variation in proportion and distribution
    - — *Long bones*
      - Include the clavicle and the bones of the extremities (excluding the carpals and tarsals)
      - Have a tubular shaft, the **diaphysis,** and two expanded ends, the **epiphyses**

- Have **epiphyseal plates** of hyaline cartilage, which separate the diaphysis from the epiphyses
- Grow **circumferentially** by **appositional growth**
- Grow in **length** by **endochondral ossification** at the epiphyseal plates
- **Diaphysis**

    — Consists of a thick collar of **compact bone** surrounding a **medullary**, or marrow, **cavity**
    — Is covered by **periosteum** and lined by **endosteum**

- **Epiphysis**

    — Consists **mostly** of **spongy bone** surrounded by a thin shell of compact bone
    — Has an **articular** surface covered by a layer of **hyaline cartilage**

- **Metaphysis**

    — Is the part of the diaphysis adjacent to the epiphyseal plate

— *Short bones*

- Include the **carpal bones** of the hand and the **tarsal bones** of the foot
- Are roughly **cuboidal** in **shape**
- Consist of spongy bone and marrow enclosed by a thin layer of compact bone
- Are covered with periosteum except for the articular surface, which has hyaline cartilage

— *Flat bones*

- Include the ribs, sternum, scapula, and calvaria
- Consist of two thick layers of compact bone separated by a layer of spongy bone, the diploe

— *Irregular bones*

- Are of **mixed shapes** and do not conform to the other classifications
- Include the **vertebrae,** the **hip bones** (os coxae), and bones of the **skull** base and face
- Usually have a thin layer of compact bone surrounding a core of spongy bone
- In the skull may **contain** air-filled spaces or **sinuses**

— *Sesamoid bones*

- Are **short bones** that develop in certain **tendons**
- Are found primarily in the hands and feet
- Develop in **response to friction** on the tendon
- May function to **alter** the direction of **pull of the tendon**
- Include the **patella** and relatively constant bones in the tendons of the flexor pollicis brevis and flexor hallucis brevis

● **Joints**

- Form wherever two or more skeletal elements meet (either bone or cartilage)

- Do **not** necessarily facilitate movement
- Are **innervated** according to **Hilton's law** (the nerves that supply the muscles that move a joint also supply the joint and the overlying skin)
- Are commonly classified according to the **material that joins them**

— *Fibrous joints*

- Are joined by a thin layer of **fibrous connective tissue**
- Allow for **little movement**

Sutures

- Join irregular and interlocking bony surfaces
- Are found only in the **skull**

Syndesmoses

- Join bony surfaces without marked irregularities
- Contain considerably more connective tissue than sutures
- Include the tibiofibular and tympanostapedial joints

— *Cartilaginous joints*

Primary cartilaginous joints (synchondroses)

- Are joined by a plate of **hyaline cartilage**
- Allow no movement
- Serve as **growth zones** for the adjoining bone
- Include the **epiphyseal plates** of growing long bone and the **sphenooccipital synchondroses** of the skull base

Secondary cartilaginous joints (symphysis)

- Are joined by **fibrocartilage**
- Have hyaline cartilage interposed between the fibrocartilage and bone
- Allow only **limited movement**
- Include the **pubic symphysis** and the joints between the **bodies of vertebrae**

— *Synovial joints (Fig. 1.1)*

- Allow a great deal of movement
- Are classified according to the **shape** of the articular surfaces and the **movement** taking place at the joint
- Have **articular hyaline cartilage** covering the ends of the opposing bones
- Have an **articular capsule** lined by **synovial membrane** that produces **synovial fluid**
- May be separated into two cavities by a fibrocartilaginous **articular disc**

Plane joints (see Fig. 1.1, *F*)

- Are also called **gliding** joints
- Allow only a **sliding movement** between the apposed surfaces
- Include the intercarpal, sternoclavicular, and acromioclavicular joints

Hinge joints (see Fig. 1.1, *A*)

- Are also called **ginglymus** joints
- Allow only **flexion** and **extension** of the joint

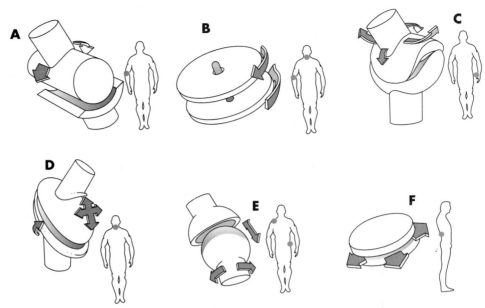

Fig. 1.1 Types of synovial joints. **A,** Hinge joint; **B,** pivot joint; **C,** saddle joint; **D,** condyloid joint; **E,** ball and socket joint; **F,** plane joint.

- Include the **elbow, knee, and ankle joints**

Pivot joints (see Fig. 1.1, *B*)

- Are also called **trochoid** joints
- Only allow movement around a single axis that is parallel to the long axis (i.e., **rotation**)
- Include the **atlantoaxial joint** and the **superior and inferior radioulnar joints**

Condyloid joints (see Fig. 1.1, *D*)

- Have two distinct concave surfaces that articulate with two distinct convex surfaces
- Allow **flexion, extension, abduction,** and **adduction,** *but little rotation*
- Include the **metacarpophalangeal, metatarsophalangeal,** and **atlantooccipital** joints

Ellipsoid joints

- Are a variation of the condyloid joint
- Have an elliptical concave surface that articulates with an elliptical convex surface
- Allow **flexion, extension, abduction,** and **adduction,** *but no rotation*
- Include the radiocarpal (wrist) joint

Saddle joints (see Fig. 1.1, *C*)

- Have reciprocal concave and convex surfaces resembling saddles joining at right angles
- Allow **flexion, extension, abduction, adduction,** and **rotation**

- Allow somewhat more restricted movement than ball-and-socket joints
- Include the **carpometacarpal joint of the thumb**

Ball-and-socket joints (see Fig. 1.1, *E*)

- Have a ball-shaped head of one bone articulating with a concavity of a second bone
- Allow **flexion, extension, abduction, adduction, rotation, and circumduction**
- Include the **shoulder** and **hip** joints

■ **Muscle** Muscle occurs in three forms: **smooth, cardiac,** and **skeletal.**

● **Smooth muscle**

- Is **involuntary** and **nonstriated**
- Forms the muscular wall of **viscera** (except the heart) and **blood vessels**
- On contraction thickens the wall and narrows the lumen of a hollow organ
- In the walls of hollow organs is usually arranged in **two layers,** circular and longitudinal
- May serve to **propel the contents** through the lumen (as in the gut) or to **reduce** the caliber of the **lumen** (as in the blood vessels)
- Is modulated by the action of **autonomic nerves, hormones,** or **mechanical stimulation** (stretching)

● **Cardiac muscle**

- Is **involuntary** and **striated**
- Comprises the **myocardium** of the heart
- Consists of branching cells that have end-to-end connections with neighboring cells, allowing the spread of **electrical activity** from cell to cell
- Contracts spontaneously
- Does not receive direct innervation (rate of **contraction** is **modulated by** the action of **autonomic nerves** at the sinoatrial node)

● **Skeletal muscle**

- Is **voluntary** and **striated**
- Is approximately 40% of the body mass
- Consists of **bundles** of multinucleated muscle **fibers**
- Receives direct innervation from the **somatic nervous system**
- Brings about movement by acting across a joint
- Has an **origin,** typically the more fixed and proximal attachment
- Has an **insertion,** usually the distal end where the greater movement occurs
- Functions to produce **movement** of the body, generate **body heat,** and maintain body **posture**

— *Other structures related to the musculoskeletal system*

Tendon

- Is a long cord of dense connective tissue (collagen) that connects muscle to bone (or cartilage)

Aponeurosis

- Is a broad, flattened tendon that provides attachment for a flat muscle

Synovial tendon sheath

- Occurs where a tendon runs in an osseofibrous tunnel
- Consists of an inner layer covering the tendon and an outer layer lining the osseofibrous tunnel
- Contains synovial fluid, which facilitates movement by reducing friction

Bursa

- Is a flattened synovial sac
- Resembles a synovial tendon sheath except that the tendon is not bound in an osseofibrous tunnel
- Occurs where tendons lie against bone, ligaments, or other tendons or where the skin moves over bony prominences
- May communicate with an adjacent joint cavity providing a pathway for the spread of infection into the joint

Ligament

- Is a connective tissue band that crosses a joint binding together articulating bones
- Stabilizes joints and limits their movement

Raphe

- Is an interdigitation of the tendinous ends of flat muscles
- Allows stretching and elongation at the union
- Include the pterygomandibular, mylohyoid, pharyngeal, and anococcygeal raphes

Superficial fascia

- Invests the entire body, lying immediately deep to the skin
- Is also called the **tela subcutanea** or **panniculus adiposus**
- Is a mixture of **loose connective tissue** (areolar tissue) and **adipose tissue**
- Contains the superficial nerves, arteries, veins, and lymphatics
- Contains hair follicles, sebaceous glands, sweat glands, mammary glands, and the muscles of facial expression
- Consists of a fatty superficial layer and a membranous deep layer (in the lower abdominal wall these are Camper's and Scarpa's fascias)
- Functions to bind the skin to the underlying deep fascia, round out the body contours, absorb pressure (as on the palm of the hand and the sole of the foot), and conserve body heat

Deep fascia

- Invests the entire body lying immediately deep to the superficial fascia
- Forms a fascial covering for muscles and muscle groups

Retinaculum

- Is a localized thickening of deep fascia in the region of joints

- Binds down tendons and their synovial tendon sheaths functioning as a pulley around which the tendons move

■ Vascular Systems

● **Blood vascular system**

- Consists of the **heart** and the **arteries, capillaries,** and **veins**
- Distributes blood to the various parts of the body
- Carries **oxygen** from the lungs to the tissues and **carbon dioxide** produced by cellular respiration in the tissues back to the lungs for elimination in exhaled air
- Carries **absorbed nutrients** from the intestines through the liver to the tissues
- Carries metabolic **waste products** from the tissues to the kidneys for excretion in the urine
- Distributes blood-borne chemical messengers (**hormones**) to their target organ
- Carries cells that **promote healing** in response to injury and the cells of the immune system, which **combat infection**

— *Heart*

- Is a hollow four-chambered muscular organ
- Is located in the **middle mediastinum** of the thoracic cavity
- Pumps blood to two separate circulatory loops, the **pulmonary circulation** and the **systemic circulation**

Pulmonary circulation

- Transports blood from the right side of the heart to the lungs and back to the left side of the heart
- Facilitates the exchange of oxygen and carbon dioxide in the lungs
- Includes the right ventricle; the pulmonary arteries, capillaries, and veins; and the left atrium

Systemic circulation

- Transports blood from the left side of the heart to all areas of the body except the lungs and back to the right side of the heart
- Facilitates the exchange of oxygen and carbon dioxide in the tissues
- Includes the left ventricle, the right atrium, and all arteries, capillaries, and veins except those of the pulmonary circulation

— *Arteries*

- Carry blood from the heart to all areas of the body
- Consist of a network of tubules with **progressively smaller** diameters

Elastic arteries

- Are the **largest** arteries and include the aorta, the pulmonary trunk and arteries, the common carotid arteries, and the subclavian arteries
- Are also called **conducting arteries** because they carry blood from the heart to the distributing arteries

- Contain numerous layers of **elastic fibers** between **smooth muscle** cells
- Expand and recoil with contraction of the heart

Muscular arteries

- Are **medium-sized** and include the majority of the arteries in the body
- Are also called **distributing arteries** because they control the distribution of blood to the various parts of the body
- Contain **fewer** elastic fibers and **more** smooth muscle
- Do **not** expand and recoil with contraction of the heart
- Range widely in size from about 10 mm to 0.1 mm

Arterioles

- Are the **smallest** of the arterial blood vessels, with a diameter of less than 0.1 mm
- Contain no elastic fibers and only one to three layers of smooth muscle
- Have a terminal component known as a **precapillary sphincter,** which regulates the flow of blood into the capillary bed

— *Capillaries*

- Are the **smallest** of blood vessels and are microscopic in size
- Consist only of an **endothelium** and its **basement membrane**
- Form a continuous anastomosing network called a **capillary bed**
- Are the site for the **exchange** of carbon dioxide, oxygen, nutrients, and waste products between the tissues and the blood
- Are **not** present in the **epidermis** of the skin, the **cornea,** or in **hyaline cartilage**
- In other areas may be completely lacking or may be bypassed by an **arteriovenous anastomosis**

— *Veins*

- Carry blood back to the heart from the peripheral tissues
- Consist of a converging network of tubules with **progressively larger** diameters
- Generally **accompany** the corresponding **artery** but have a larger diameter and a thinner wall
- Are much more variable in structure than arteries
- In the extremities frequently accompany muscular arteries as paired veins, the **venae comitantes**
- Except for the largest, have **valves,** which aid in the return of blood to the heart

Venules

- Are the **smallest** veins
- Arise by the **confluence** of several **capillaries**
- Are generally less than 0.1 mm in diameter

Small veins

- Are generally less than 1.0 mm in diameter

- Contain a small amount of circularly arranged smooth muscle in their wall

Medium veins

- Include most of the veins of the **extremities** and all but the largest of the **visceral branches**
- Have a diameter of 1 to 10 mm
- Have predominately **longitudinally arranged** connective tissue and smooth muscle

Large veins

- Are veins with a diameter larger than 10 mm
- Include the superior and inferior venae cava, the portal vein, the renal veins, the brachiocephalic veins, and the internal jugular veins
- Have abundant **longitudinally arranged** elastic fibers and smooth muscle
- Do not have valves

— *Other features of the blood vascular system*

Sinusoids

- Are **discontinuous capillaries** that are much (five to ten times) larger than ordinary capillaries
- Are not cylinders but rather take the **shape of spaces** between epithelial cell cords or plates
- Are found in the adrenal and pituitary glands, liver, spleen, and bone marrow

Portal system

- Consists of a system of vessels interposed between **two capillary beds**
- Includes the **hepatic-portal system,** which drains blood from the intestinal capillaries through the portal vein to the hepatic capillary sinusoids
- Includes the **hypophyseal-portal system,** which drains blood from the median eminence of the hypothalamus to the capillary sinusoids of the anterior pituitary gland

● Lymph vascular system (Fig. 1.2)

- Consists of **lymph vessels** and **lymph nodes**
- Returns **tissue fluids** to the venous system
- Provides **immunologic defense** against disease-causing agents
- Provides a route for **lymphocytes** from the lymphatic tissues to reach the blood vascular system
- Provides a route for **absorbed fat** to be transported from the intestine to the blood vascular system
- May provide an important route for the **spread of malignant tumor cells** (metastasis)

— *Lymph vessels*

- Begin in the interstitial connective tissues as blindly ending

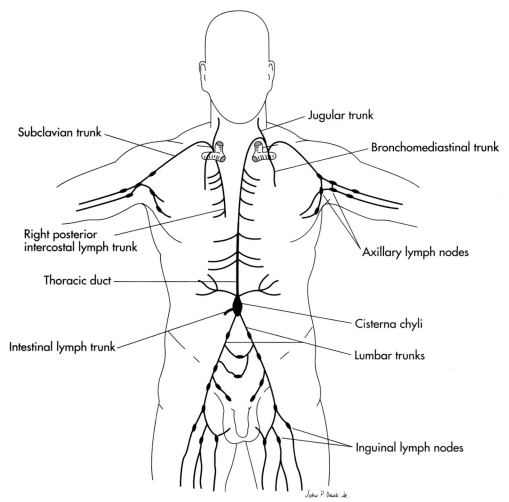

Fig. 1.2 Major lymphatic vessels of the body.

lymph capillaries, which are greater in diameter than blood capillaries

- Coalesce to form collecting vessels, which

  — Are interrupted in their course by regionally located lymph nodes
  — Enter lymph nodes as afferent lymph vessels
  — Leave lymph nodes as efferent lymph vessels
  — Join to form regional lymph trunks, which converge to form the right lymphatic duct and the thoracic duct

Right lymphatic duct

- Receives lymph from

  — Right side of the head and neck through the right jugular lymph trunk
  — Right upper extremity through the right subclavian lymph trunk

— Right side of the thoracic cavity through the right **bron-chomediastinal lymph trunk**

- Ends by opening into the junction of the right **internal jugular** and right **subclavian veins** in the root of the neck

Thoracic duct

- Begins in the **abdomen** behind the right crus of the diaphragm as the **cisterna chyli**
- Is formed by the convergence of the

    — Right and left **lumbar lymph trunks**
    — **Intestinal lymph trunk**

- Terminates by opening near the union of the left **internal jugular** and **left subclavian veins**
- Receives lymph from

    — Most of the body **below** the **respiratory diaphragm**
    — The left and lower right **posterior intercostal spaces**

- Near its termination **receives lymph from the**

    — Left side of the head and neck through the **left internal jugular lymph trunk**
    — Left upper extremity through the **left subclavian lymph trunk**
    — Left side of the thoracic cavity through the **left broncho-mediastinal lymph trunk**

— *Lymph nodes*

- Are small flattened or bean-shaped lymphoid organs that lie along the course of the collecting lymph vessels
- Filter the lymph passing through the node
- Vary in size from a few millimeters to 2 cm
- Occur in groups that have a consistent location in a particular region
- Commonly occur in the neck, axilla, and groin and along the course of the large vessels of the mediastinum and abdomen
- When activated in response to infection or malignant disease may enlarge and become tender

■ **Nervous System**

- Is **conceptionally** divided into the

    — **Central nervous system** (CNS) consisting of the brain and spinal cord
    — **Peripheral nervous system** (PNS) consisting of the cranial nerves, the spinal nerves, and their associated ganglia

- Is **functionally** divided into the

    — **Somatic nervous system,** which controls voluntary activities
    — **Visceral nervous system,** which controls visceral activities

- **Neuron**
  - Is the nerve cell, consisting of the cell body, axon, and dendrites
  - Is the functional unit of the nervous system
  - Is specialized for the purpose of communication

- **Central nervous system**
  - Consists of the **brain** and **spinal cord**
  - Is composed of **neurons** and specialized supporting cells called **neuroglia** arranged as **gray matter** and **white matter**
  - **White matter:** largely myelinated axons and their supporting neuroglia
  - **Gray matter:** largely neuron cell bodies and dendrites and their supporting neuroglia
  - **Nucleus:** a collection of **neuron cell bodies** within the substance of the **CNS**
  - *Spinal cord*
    - Begins at the **foramen magnum** where it is continuous with the medulla of the brain stem
    - Ends at the level of the **lower border of the first lumbar vertebra** in the adult
    - Is only about **two thirds** as long as the vertebral canal
    - Has a **cervical enlargement** related to the **brachial plexus** and innervation of the **upper extremity**
    - Has a **lumbosacral enlargement** related to the **lumbosacral plexus** and innervation of the **lower extremity**
    - Has a tapered lower end known as the **conus medullaris**
    - Has a centrally located **gray matter** and a peripherally located **white matter**

- **Peripheral nervous system**
  - Consists of **afferent neurons** and **efferent neurons**
  - *Afferent neurons*
    - Conduct impulses from **sensory receptors** to synapses in the CNS
    - Sense changes in the **external** or **internal** environment
    - Are sensitive to **various modalities,** including touch, pressure, pain, position, muscle tension, chemical concentration, light, and other mechanical stimuli
    - Form the **afferent limb** of the important **reflex arc** controlling the activity of the end organ
    - With only a few exceptions are **pseudounipolar neurons** with an **axon** consisting of
      - A **central process,** which conducts the impulse from the receptor to the cell body
      - A **peripheral process,** which conducts the impulse from the cell body into the CNS

- In spinal nerves
  — Have **cell bodies** located in the **dorsal root ganglion**
  — Have **axons**, which reach the spinal cord through the **dorsal root** of the spinal nerve
- In cranial nerves
  — Have **cell bodies** located in the associated **sensory ganglion** of the **cranial nerve**
  — Have **axons**, which reach the brain through the root of the **cranial nerve**
- **Ganglion:** collection of **neuron cell bodies** outside the CNS

— *Efferent neurons*
  - Conduct impulses away from the CNS to the peripheral **end organ**
  - Are also called **motor neurons**
  - Have cell bodies located in the **nuclei** of the brain or spinal cord
  - Innervate **skeletal muscle** or visceral structures such as **cardiac muscle, smooth muscle, or glands**
  - Form the **efferent limb** of the important **reflex arc** controlling the activity of the end organ

— *Functional components of peripheral nerves*
General somatic afferent (GSA) neurons (Fig. 1.3)
  - Extend from the receptor organ to the CNS
  - Convey sensations such as pain, temperature, touch, and proprioception from the skin, skeletal muscles, tendons, and joints
  - Have cell bodies located in the **dorsal root ganglia** or in the **sensory ganglia** of cranial nerves V, VII, IX, or X

General visceral afferent (GVA) neurons (Fig. 1.4)
  - Extend from **cardiac muscle, smooth muscle, or glands** to the CNS
  - Are concerned with **subconscious reflex activity** and also convey the sensations of **pain** and **fullness**
  - Have cell bodies located in the **dorsal root ganglia** or in the **sensory ganglia** of cranial nerves VII, IX, or X

General somatic efferent (GSE) neurons (see Fig. 1.3)
  - Extend from the CNS to activate **skeletal muscle** derived from somites
  - Have cell bodies located in the **ventral horn** of the spinal cord or in the **motor nuclei** of cranial nerves III, IV, VI, XI, or XII

General visceral efferent (GVE) neurons (see Fig. 1.4)
  - Are motor to **cardiac muscle, smooth muscle,** and **glands**
  - Are the sole component of the **autonomic nervous system**
  - Include the **sympathetic** and **sacral parasympathetic** components of **spinal nerves** and the **parasympathetic** components of **cranial nerves**

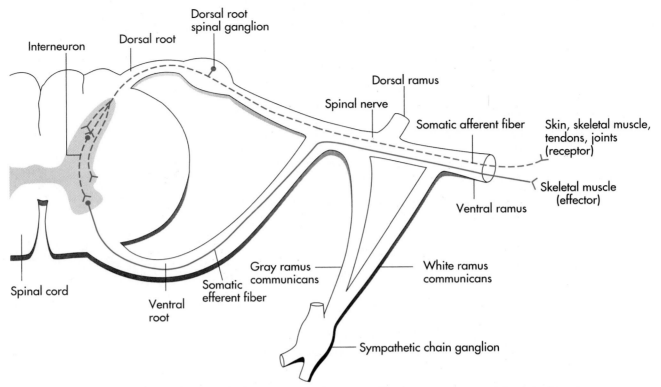

Fig. 1.3 General somatic efferent and general somatic afferent components of the spinal nerve.

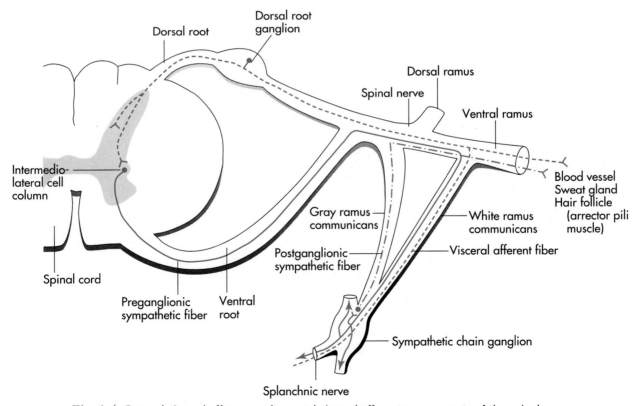

Fig. 1.4 General visceral efferent and general visceral afferent components of the spinal nerve.

- Consist of **preganglionic** and **postganglionic** neurons

Special visceral efferent (SVE) neurons

- Extend from the CNS to activate **skeletal muscle** derived from branchial arch mesoderm
- Are found only in cranial nerves
- Have cell bodies located in the **motor nuclei** of cranial nerves V, VII, IX, X, and XI

Special visceral afferent (SVA) neurons

- Are associated with the "special" senses of **taste** and **smell**
- Include cell bodies relaying **smell,** which are located in the **olfactory mucosa** and are associated with cranial nerve I
- Include cell bodies relaying taste from the mucosa of the tongue and palate, which are located in the sensory ganglia of cranial nerves VII, IX, and X

Special somatic afferent (SSA) neurons

- Provide the "special" sensory function from the **eye** and the **ear**
- Are found in the **optic nerve** (CN II) with cell bodies in the ganglion cell layer of the **retina**
- Are found in the **vestibulocochlear nerve** (CN VIII) with cell bodies in the **spiral ganglion** and the **vestibular ganglion**

— *Cranial nerves*

- Consist of **12 pairs** of nerves, which arise from the brain stem
- Like the spinal nerves, are part of the **peripheral nervous system**
- Are limited in distribution to the head and neck with the exception of the vagus nerve (CN X), which extends into the thorax and abdomen
- Are **named** and also **numbered** sequentially with Roman numerals progressing rostrally to caudally
- Contain **efferent neurons** with cell bodies in nuclei of the brain stem and **afferent neurons** with cell bodies in the associated sensory ganglia
- Contain all seven **functional components** in varying combinations

— *Spinal nerves (Fig. 1.5)*

- Consist of **31 pairs** of segmentally arranged nerves: 8 cervical, 12 thoracic, 5 lumbar, 5 sacral, and 1 coccygeal
- Are formed by the union of a **dorsal root** and a **ventral root** at the intervertebral foramen
- Exit the vertebral canal through the **intervertebral foramen**
- Outside the intervertebral foramen terminate by dividing into a **dorsal ramus** and a **ventral ramus**
- Each receives a **gray ramus communicans** from the sympathetic trunk, which conveys **postganglionic sympathetic fibers** to the spinal nerve
- Are **mixed nerves** containing all of the **general functional components**

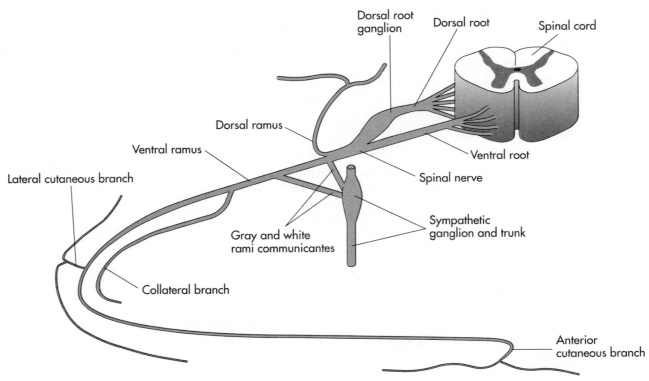

Fig. 1.5 The typical spinal nerve.

- **Dorsal root**

    — Contains the axons of **afferent** neuron cell bodies located in the **dorsal root ganglion**

- **Ventral root**

    — Contains the axons of **efferent** neuron cell bodies located in the **ventral horn** of the spinal cord

    — At the T1-L2 level contains the axons of **efferent** preganglionic sympathetic neuron cell bodies located in the **intermediolateral cell column (IMLCC)** of the spinal cord

- **Dorsal rami**

    — Supply the intrinsic back muscles and the overlying skin

- **Ventral rami**

    — Supply the muscles and skin of the anterolateral neck and trunk and all of the muscles and skin of the upper and lower extremities

Components of the mixed spinal nerve (see Figs. 1.3 and 1.4)

- GSA fibers from cell bodies in the dorsal root ganglion
- GVA fibers from cell bodies in the dorsal root ganglion
- GSE fibers from cell bodies in the ventral horn of the spinal cord
- GVE fibers (**postganglionic sympathetic**) from cell bodies in the sympathetic chain ganglia

Other components

- At the **T1-L2** levels, the **trunk** of the spinal nerve (and not the dorsal or ventral ramus) contains **preganglionic sympathetic fibers (GVE)** from cell bodies in the intermediolateral cell column of the spinal cord.
- At the **S2-S4** levels, the **trunk and proximal ventral rami** contain **preganglionic parasympathetic fibers (GVE)** from cell bodies in the sacral parasympathetic nucleus of the spinal cord. These leave the ventral rami as **pelvic splanchnic nerves** (nervi erigentes).

● Autonomic nervous system

- Is divided into two parts: the **sympathetic nervous system** and the **parasympathetic nervous system**
- Innervates the **visceral organs**, including the vascular and glandular systems
- Is motor to **cardiac muscle, smooth muscle,** and **glands**
- Generally acts below the level of consciousness and is said to be **involuntary**
- Functions to maintain the **homeostasis** of the internal environment
- By traditional definition is purely **efferent** and contains only GVE components
- Always consists of **two motor neurons in a circuit,** which transmits impulses from the brain or spinal cord to the peripheral effector organ
- **Preganglionic neurons**

  — Are the **first** neurons in the circuit
  — Have cell bodies in **nuclei** of the brain stem or spinal cord
  — Synapse with **postganglionic neuron** cell bodies in **autonomic ganglia**

- **Postganglionic neurons**

  — Are the **second** neurons in the circuit
  — Have cell bodies in the peripheral **autonomic ganglia** located at varying distances from the CNS
  — Synapse with the axon of the **preganglionic neuron**
  — Have an axon that extends to the **peripheral effector organ**

— *Sympathetic nervous system (Fig. 1.6)*

- Activates the body's response to **stress,** including the **fight-or-flight** response
- **Preganglionic neurons**

  — Have cell bodies located in the IMLCC of the lateral horn of the thoraci and upper lumbar spinal cord (T1-L2)

- **Postganglionic neurons**

  — Have cell bodies located in a **prevertebral ganglion** or a **paravertebral** (sympathetic chain) **ganglion**

- **Preganglionic fibers**

  — Leave the spinal cord through the **ventral roots** of the T1-L2 spinal nerves

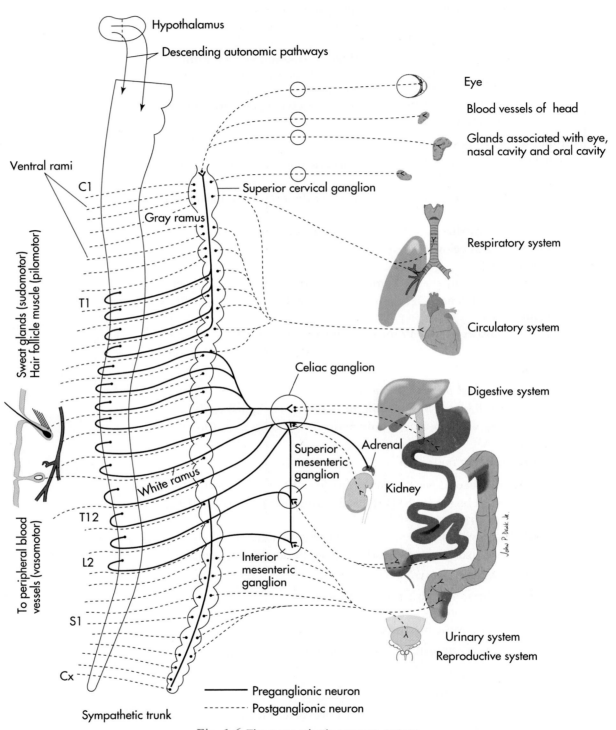

Fig. 1.6 The sympathetic nervous system.

Hypothalamus

Descending autonomic pathways

Eye

Blood vessels of head

Glands associated with eye, nasal cavity and oral cavity

Ventral rami

C1

Superior cervical ganglion

Gray ramus

Respiratory system

Sweat glands (sudomotor) Hair follicle muscle (pilomotor)

T1

Circulatory system

Celiac ganglion

Digestive system

Superior mesenteric ganglion

Adrenal

Kidney

White ramus

To peripheral blood vessels (vasomotor)

T12

L2

Interior mesenteric ganglion

Urinary system

S1

Reproductive system

Cx

—— Preganglionic neuron

------ Postganglionic neuron

Sympathetic trunk

— Leave the spinal nerve through a **white ramus communicans** to join a **paravertebral ganglion**

— May synapse with the **postganglionic neuron** cell body in the sympathetic ganglion at the level of its entrance to the sympathetic trunk

— May course through their own ganglion to **ascend or descend** in the sympathetic chain before synapsing in another ganglion in the chain

— May course through their own paravertebral ganglion to emerge into a **splanchnic nerve** to reach a **prevertebral ganglion** for synapse with postganglionic neurons

- **Postganglionic fibers**

    — Do **not** travel up or down the sympathetic chain

    — Leave the sympathetic chain at the level at which the synapse occurs

    — May rejoin the spinal nerve through a **gray ramus communicans** to supply arrector pili muscles and glands of the skin and vascular smooth muscle

    — May emerge as a **visceral branch** of the sympathetic chain to join one of the visceral plexuses (cardiac, aortic, hypogastric)

White ramus communicans

- Connects each **spinal nerve** from **T1 to L2** to a corresponding **paravertebral ganglion**

- Occurs **only** between T1 and L2 because this represents the craniocaudal extent of the **IMLCC**

- Contains **preganglionic sympathetic fibers** and **general visceral afferent** fibers

Gray ramus communicans

- Connects **every** spinal nerve to a **paravertebral ganglion**

- Contains **postganglionic sympathetic fibers,** which end on sweat glands, vascular smooth muscle, and arrector pili muscles

— *Parasympathetic nervous system (Fig. 1.7)*

- Is also called the **craniosacral outflow** because of its origin from the brain stem and the second through fourth sacral spinal cord segments

- Is part of cranial nerves III, VII, IX, and X

- Supplies cardiac muscle, visceral smooth muscle, and glands but **does not** innervate blood vessels (except for the erectile tissue of the external genitalia)

- Is distributed only to the visceral structures and not to the carcass of the body

- **Preganglionic neurons**

    — Have cell bodies in the **parasympathetic nuclei** of the brain stem or in the **sacral parasympathetic nucleus** of the spinal cord

    — Have long axons

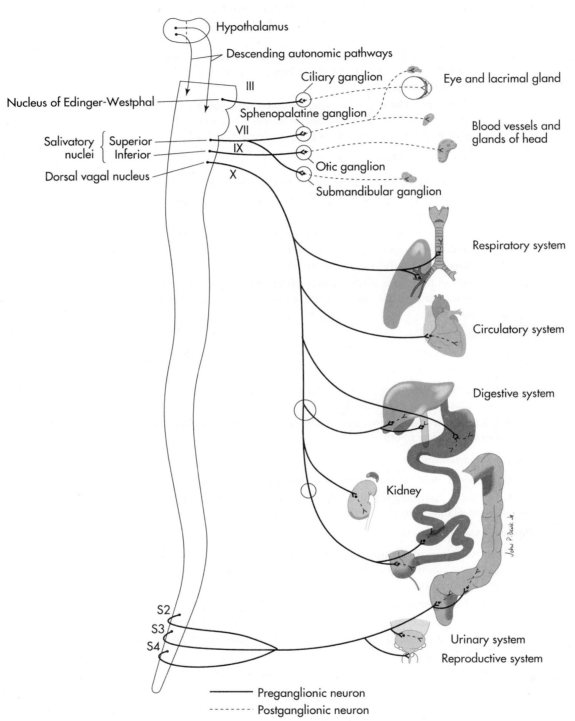

Fig. 1.7 The parasympathetic nervous system.

- **Postganglionic neurons**
  - — Have cell bodies located in **terminal ganglia** lying close to or in the wall of the organ to be innervated
  - — Have short axons

General visceral afferent fibers

- Are the axons of pseudounipolar neurons located in the dorsal root ganglia or cranial nerve ganglia
- Are **not** a part of the autonomic nervous system or its components, the sympathetic and parasympathetic systems
- Are **complementary** to the general visceral efferent fibers and "hitch hike" along with sympathetic and parasympathetic fibers
- Represent the afferent side of the autonomic reflex arc
- Except for cranial nerve III are generally present wherever sympathetic and parasympathetic fibers are present and follow the same pathway back to the CNS
- Are contained in the dorsal and ventral rami, which are distributed to the "somatic" areas of the body
- Are contained in the white ramus communicans but not the gray ramus communicans
- Accompany sympathetic preganglionic fibers that ascend or descend in the sympathetic trunk
- Accompany sympathetic fibers that leave the sympathetic trunk in visceral branches (e.g., cardiac or splanchnic nerves)

MULTIPLE CHOICE
REVIEW QUESTIONS

1. A mixed spinal nerve typically contains all *except* which of the following functional components?

    a. GSA
    b. GSE
    c. SVE
    d. GVE

2. Which of the following describes the gray ramus communicans?

    a. It contains only preganglionic sympathetic fibers.
    b. It is found only above T1 and below L2.
    c. It contains the axons of neuron cell bodies located in the dorsal horn.
    d. It contains GVE fibers.
    e. It contains GVA fibers.

3. Movement of a body part away from the main axis of the body is which of the following?

    a. Adduction
    b. Abduction
    c. Pronation
    d. Flexion
    e. Extension

4. Which of the following is a connective tissue band that crosses a joint binding together articulating bones?

    a. Tendon
    b. Aponeurosis
    c. Raphe
    d. Ligament
    e. Retinaculum

5. The thoracic duct typically receives lymph from which of the following?

    a. Most of the body below the diaphragm
    b. All of the body above the diaphragm
    c. All of the body except the head and neck
    d. The thorax and abdomen only
    e. The thorax only

6. The cell bodies of the general somatic efferent (GSE) neurons in spinal nerves are located in which of the following?

    a. Dorsal root ganglion
    b. Sympathetic chain ganglion
    c. Ventral horn of the spinal cord
    d. Dorsal horn of the spinal cord
    e. Intermediolateral cell column

7. Which of the following describes elastic arteries?

    a. They are composed mostly of smooth muscle with a few layers of elastic fibers.
    b. They are also called distributing arteries.
    c. They regulate the flow of blood into the capillary bed.
    d. They include most of the arteries of the body.
    e. They expand and recoil with the contraction of the heart.

8. Synchondroses are described by which of the following?

    a. They allow a great deal of movement.
    b. They are found only in the skull.
    c. They serve as growth zones for the adjoining bone.
    d. They are a type of synovial joint.
    e. They are joined by fibrocartilage.

9. Cardiac muscle is described by which of the following?

    a. It is involuntary and nonstriated.
    b. It consists of bundles of multinucleated muscle fibers.
    c. It receives direct innervation from the autonomic nervous system.
    d. It undergoes spontaneous and rhythmic contraction.
    e. It forms the muscular wall of the blood vessels of the heart.

10. The patella is best classified as which of the following?

    a. Sesamoid bone
    b. Flat bone
    c. Irregular bone
    d. Short bone
    e. Long bone

Chapter 2

The Upper Extremity

■ **Bones of the Upper Extremity**

● **Pectoral girdle and proximal humerus**

- The pectoral girdle and proximal humerus are the bones of the shoulder.
- The pectoral girdle consists of the **clavicle** and the **scapula**.

— *Clavicle*

- Is commonly called the **collarbone**
- Is **S**-shaped with the **medial two thirds convex anteriorly** and the **lateral one third concave anteriorly**
- Articulates medially with the **sternum** and laterally with the **acromion**
- Is **subcutaneous** and readily palpable throughout its length
- Is commonly **fractured** at the **junction** of its **middle and lateral third** as a result of a fall onto the shoulder

- Forms by both intramembranous and cartilaginous ossification and notably is the **only long bone to undergo intramembranous ossification**
- Is the **first** bone to **begin ossification**, but growth is not complete until 18 to 20 years of age
- Has a **conoid tubercle** and a **trapezoid line** on its lateral inferior surface for attachment of the **coracoclavicular ligament**
- Has a roughened area on its medial inferior surface for attachment of the **costoclavicular ligament**
- Provides attachments for the **deltoid, pectoralis major, trapezius, sternocleidomastoid,** and **subclavius** muscle

— *Scapula (Fig. 2.1)*

- Is commonly called the **shoulder blade**
- Is large, flattened, and roughly triangular in shape
- Articulates laterally with the **clavicle** and the **humerus**
- Overlies the **second to seventh ribs**
- Consists of a **body,** a **spine,** and a **coracoid** process
- **Body**

— Anterior and posterior **surfaces**
— Medial, lateral, and superior **borders**
— Superior and inferior **angles**

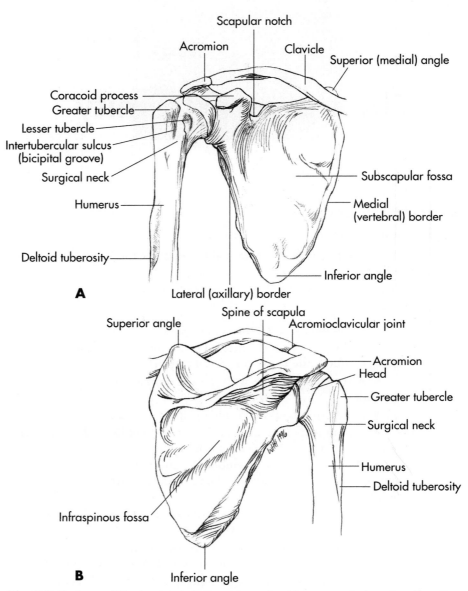

Fig. 2.1 Features of the pectoral girdle and proximal humerus. **A,** Anterior view. **B,** Posterior view.

- Spine
  - Divides the posterior surface into a **supraspinous fossa** for the supraspinatus muscle and an **infraspinous fossa** for the infraspinatus muscle
  - Typically lies at the level of the **third spinous process**
  - Continues laterally as the **acromion**

- **Acromion**
  - Is the lateral expanded end of the spine; articulates with the **clavicle**
  - Overhangs the **glenoid cavity**
  - Provides attachment for the **deltoid** and **trapezius** muscles

- Coracoid process

  — Projects anteriorly and laterally in front of the glenoid cavity
  — Provides attachment for the **pectoralis minor,** short head of the **biceps brachii,** and **coracobrachialis** muscles
  — Can be palpated below the clavicle under the anterior margin of the deltoid
  — Provides attachment for the coracoclavicular, coracoacromial, and coracohumeral ligaments and the costocoracoid membrane

- Glenoid cavity

  — Lies at the union of the superior and lateral borders
  — Is a shallow cavity that is deepened by the fibrocartilaginous **glenoid labrum**
  — Articulates with the **head of the humerus**

- Other features

  — **Supraglenoid tubercle** (marks the attachment of the **long head of the biceps** brachii muscle)
  — **Infraglenoid tubercle** (marks the attachment of the **long head of the triceps** brachii muscle)
  — **Spinoglenoid notch** (allows communication between the **supraspinous and infraspinous fossae** around the lateral margin of the spine and transmits the **suprascapular nerve and artery**)
  — **Scapular notch** on the superior border (bridged by the **superior transverse scapular ligament** and traversed by the **suprascapular nerve**)

— *Features of the proximal humerus (see Fig. 2.1)*

  - Head

    — Is the smooth hemispherical surface that articulates with the glenoid cavity of the scapula

  - Anatomical neck

    — Is the constriction surrounding the head to which the fibrous capsule attaches
    — Separates the head from the tubercles

  - Greater tubercle

    — Is a large projection on the upper and lateral surface just distal to the anatomical neck
    — Provides attachments for the **supraspinatus, infraspinatus,** and **teres minor** muscles

  - Lesser tubercle

    — Is a smaller projection on the anterior and medial surface just distal to the anatomical neck
    — Provides attachment for the **subscapularis** muscle

- Intertubercular sulcus (bicipital groove)

  — Separates the greater and lesser tuberosities
  — Contains the **tendon of the long head of the biceps brachii** muscle
  — Has a **lateral lip** that is continuous with the **crest of the greater tubercle** and provides attachment for the **pectoralis major** muscle
  — Has a **floor** that provides attachment for the **latissimus dorsi** muscle
  — Has a **medial lip** that is continuous with the **crest of the lesser tubercle** and provides attachment for the **teres major** muscle
  — Is bridged by the **transverse humeral ligament**

- Surgical neck

  — Joins the proximal end of the humerus to the **shaft**
  — Is a **common site for fractures** of the humerus
  — Is related to the course of the **axillary nerve** and **posterior humeral circumflex artery**, which are **vulnerable in fractures**

- Spiral groove

  — Is a broad, shallow depression on the **posterior** aspect of the **shaft**
  — Contains the **radial nerve** and **profunda brachii artery**, which are **vulnerable in fractures** of the shaft
  — **Separates** the origin of the **lateral head** of the triceps above from the origin of the **medial head** of the triceps below

- Deltoid tuberosity

  — Is a roughened prominence about halfway down the lateral border of the **shaft**
  — Marks the attachment of the **deltoid** muscle

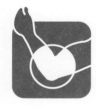

● Skeleton at the elbow (Fig. 2.2)

  — *Features of the distal humerus*

    • The lower end of the humerus consists of the **condyle** and the **medial and lateral epicondyles.**

    • The **condyle** includes the **trochlea,** the **capitulum,** the **coronoid fossa,** the **olecranon fossa,** and the **radial fossa.**

    • The **medial epicondyle** gives **origin** to the **flexor muscles** of the forearm; is easily palpable on the **medial** side of the elbow; extends upward as the **medial supracondylar ridge,** which gives attachment to the **medial intermuscular septum;** and is **grooved posteriorly** by the **ulnar nerve,** which can be palpated there.

    • The lateral epicondyle gives **origin** to the **extensor muscles** of the forearm and the **supinator** and **anconeus** muscles; is easily palpable on the **lateral** side of the elbow; is **less prominent** than the medial epicondyle; and extends upward as the **lateral supracondylar ridge,** which gives attachment to the **lateral intermuscular septum.**

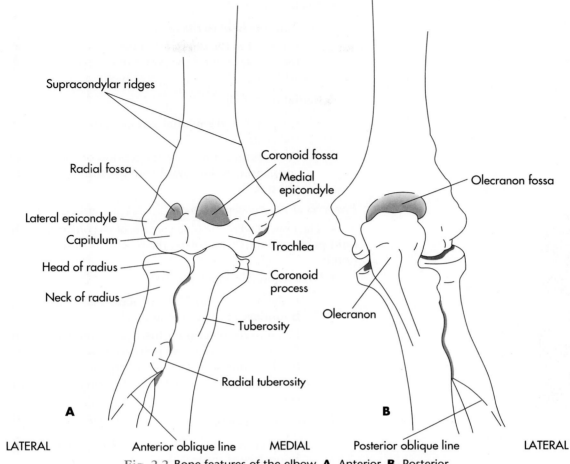

Fig. 2.2 Bone features of the elbow. **A,** Anterior. **B,** Posterior.

- The **trochlea** is the **articular surface** for the **trochlear notch** of the ulna. It **spirals** from anterior to posterior, which accounts for the "**carrying angle**" at the elbow in anatomic position.
- The **capitulum** is the **articular surface** lateral to the trochlea for the **head of the radius.**
- The **coronoid fossa** is the **depression** above the trochlea anteriorly that **accommodates** the **coronoid process** of the ulna in extreme flexion.
- The **olecranon fossa** is the **depression** above the trochlea posteriorly that **accommodates** the **olecranon process** of the ulna in extreme extension.
- The **radial fossa** is the shallow **depression** above the capitulum that **accommodates** the **head of the radius** in flexion.

— *Features of the proximal radius*

- The upper end of the radius consists of the **head, neck,** and **tuberosity.**
- **Head**

   — Is the concave expansion that **articulates** with the **capitulum** of the radius and the **radial notch** of the ulna
   — Is **encircled** by the strong **annular ligament** and is easily palpated **posteriorly** just **below the lateral epicondyle**

- **Neck**
  - Joins the head to the body
  - Is related to the **deep radial nerve** as it pierces the supinator muscle to enter the posterior compartment of the forearm

- **Radial tuberosity**
  - Is located on the **medial** surface at the junction of the neck and shaft
  - Provides attachment for the **tendon of the biceps brachii** and continues downward onto the shaft as the **anterior oblique line**

— *Features of the proximal ulna*

- The upper end of the ulna consists of the **olecranon**, the **coronoid process** and its **tuberosity**, the **trochlear notch,** and the **radial notch.**

  - **Olecranon** (olecranon process)
    - Is the posterior **hooklike process** that forms the **upper boundary** of the trochlear notch
    - Fits into the **olecranon fossa** of the humerus when the forearm is extended and posteriorly provides attachment for the **tendon of the triceps brachii** muscle
    - At its point is separated from the skin by an **olecranon bursa**

  - **Coronoid process**
    - Is the anterior **hooklike process** that forms the **lower boundary** of the trochlear notch
    - Fits into the coronoid fossa of the humerus when the forearm is flexed and provides attachment for the **brachialis** muscle at its lower part, the **ulnar tuberosity**

  - **Trochlear notch**
    - Is the facet for articulation with the **trochlea** of the humerus
    - Is formed anteriorly by the **coronoid process** and posteriorly by the **olecranon**

  - **Radial notch**
    - Is the **facet** on the lateral side of the coronoid process **for** articulation with the **head of the radius**

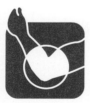

- ● Skeleton of the wrist and hand
  - — *Features of the distal radius*
    - The lower end is its **largest part.**
    - The most distal surface is the concave **facet for the wrist joint.**
    - The **ulnar notch** is the concave **facet** on its medial surface for articulation with the **head of the ulna.**
    - The **styloid process** is the prolonged lower end. It is **grooved** anterior to the base by the tendons of the **abductor pollicis longus**

and the **extensor pollicis brevis** and can be palpated in the anatomical snuffbox.

• The dorsal surface is **grooved** from medial to lateral by the tendons of the **extensor indicis**, the **extensor pollicis longus**, and the **extensors carpi radialis longus and brevis.**

• The **dorsal tubercle** (of Lister) lies near the middle of the dorsal surface interposed **between** the groove for the **extensor pollicis longus** and the groove for the **extensors carpi radialis longus and brevis.**

— *Features of the distal ulna*

• The lower end is its **smallest part.**

• The most distal surface is for **articulation** with the **articular disc,** which separates it from the carpal bones.

• The **head** is the expanded lower end. It has a medial and posterior projection, the **styloid process,** and a **facet** on its medial half for **articulation** with the **ulnar notch** of the radius. It can be readily **palpated** when the forearm is **pronated.**

— *Carpal bones (Fig. 2.3)*

• Are the **eight bones** of the **wrist**

• Form the **transition between** the bones of the **forearm** and the bones of the **hand**

• Are arranged in **two rows** of four

• Except for the capitate, hamate, and pisiform, **begin ossification at 3 to 5 years** of age

• **Proximal row**

— Contains from lateral to medial the **scaphoid, lunate, triquetral,** and **pisiform,** which lies in front of the triquetral

— Except for the pisiform, **articulates** with the **radius** and **articular disc**

— Is **bound** together by **interosseus ligaments** so they move **as a unit** at the wrist and midcarpal joints

• **Distal row**

— Contains from lateral to medial the **trapezium, trapezoid, capitate,** and **hamate**

— **Articulates** with the **proximal row** of carpal bones and with the **metacarpals**

• **Pisiform**

— Is commonly included in the proximal row of carpal bones but **is in fact a** constant **sesamoid bone** in the tendon of the flexor carpi ulnaris

— Does **not** participate in the wrist joint

— Is the **last** carpal bone to **ossify** beginning at **10 to 12 years** of age

• **Scaphoid**

— Has a large facet for **articulation** with the distal end of the **radius**

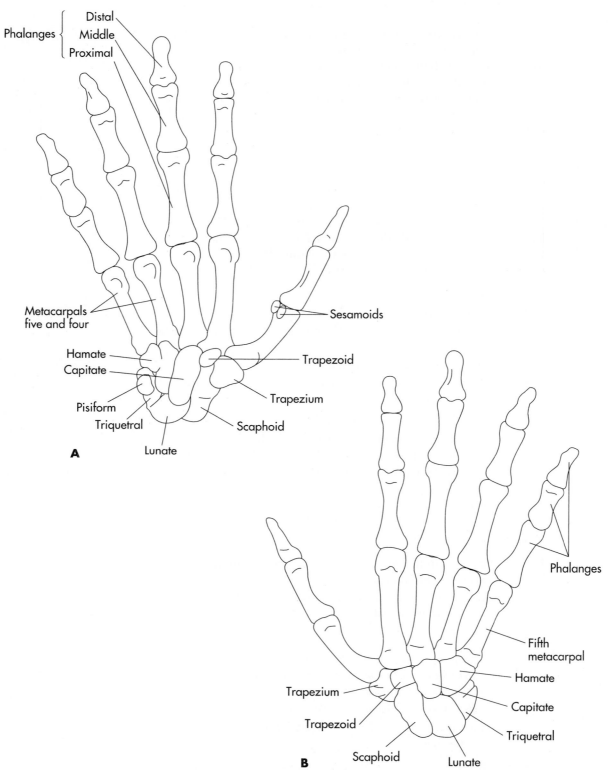

Fig. 2.3 Bones of the wrist and hand. **A,** Palmar view. **B,** Dorsal view.

— Has a prominent **tubercle**, which can be **palpated** at the base of the thenar eminence
— Lies in the distal floor of the **anatomic snuffbox**
— Is the **most commonly fractured** carpal bone

- Lunate

    — Is the middle bone of the proximal row
    — **Articulates** with the **radius** and the **articular disc**
    — Lies approximately **between** the two major **skin creases** at the wrist

- Triquetral

    — Is the medial bone of the proximal row
    — Has a prominent **tubercle**, which can be **palpated** at thebase of the thenar eminence with the tubercle of the scaphoid
    — Articulates with the **articular disc** of the wrist joint

- Trapezium

    — Has a prominent **tubercle** on its palmar surface
    — Lies between the **scaphoid** and the **first metacarpal**
    — Is **grooved** medially by the **tendon** of the **flexor carpi radialis**

- Trapezoid

    — Lies between the **scaphoid** and the **second metacarpal**

- Capitate

    — Is the **largest** of the carpal bones
    — Is the **first** carpal bone to begin ossification at 2 to 3 months of age
    — Has a large rounded **head,** which **articulates with** the concavity formed by the **scaphoid and lunate**
    — Distally **articulates** largely with the **third metacarpal**

- Hamate

    — Is **triangular** with the base lying distally
    — Articulates **proximally** with the **lunate and triquetral**
    — Articulates **distally** with the **fourth and fifth metacarpals**
    — On its palmar surface has a prominent hook, the **hook of the hamate**
    — Begins ossification shortly after the capitate at 3 to 4 months of age

— *Metacarpal bones (see Fig. 2.3)*
- Are the **five** miniature long bones of the **hand**
- Are numbered **1 to 5** from the **thumb to the little finger**
- Have a proximal **base**, a **shaft**, and a distal **head**
- Articulate at their **base** with the distal row of **carpal bones**
- Articulate at their **head** with the **proximal phalanges** forming the knuckles

- Have **facets** at their bases **for** articulation with the **adjacent metacarpal** (except for the thumb)
- Begin **ossification** at the shaft in the **third month** in utero
- **First metacarpal**
  — Articulates with the **trapezium**
  — Is **concave** toward the palm
- **Second metacarpal**
  — Articulates with the **trapezium,** the **trapezoid,** and the **hamate**
  — Is the **longest** metacarpal
- **Third metacarpal**
  — Articulates with the **capitate**
- **Fourth and fifth metacarpals**
  — Articulate with the **hamate**

— *Phalanges*

- Are the miniature long bones of the **fingers**
- Are 2 **for the thumb** and 3 **for the fingers**
- Have a proximal **base,** a **shaft,** and a distal **head**
- Begin **ossification** at the shaft in the **third month** in utero
- Form the **knuckles** of the fingers at the heads of the proximal and distal phalanges

■ **Joints of the Upper Extremity**

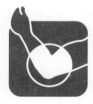

● Sternoclavicular joint

- Is the only joint between the **pectoral girdle** and the **axial skeleton**
- Is the joint between the expanded medial end of the **clavicle,** the **manubrium,** and the **first costal cartilage**
- Is a **synovial joint** divided into two cavities by an **intraarticular disc**
- **Functions** as a **ball-and-socket joint** although **structurally** it resembles a **saddle joint**
- Has a fibrous **capsule,** which is reinforced by **anterior and posterior sternoclavicular ligaments** and an **interclavicular ligament**
- Is further stabilized by the strong **costoclavicular ligament,** which anchors the medial end of the **clavicle to the first rib** and costal cartilage

● Acromioclavicular joint

- Is the joint between the **acromion** and the **lateral end of the clavicle**
- Is an **atypical synovial joint** in that the joint surfaces are covered by fibrocartilage
- Has a **fibrous capsule** reinforced by the **acromioclavicular ligament**
- Is reinforced by the **coracoclavicular ligament,** which limits joint movement
- Is often **dislocated** in a fall on the outstretched hand with the **acromion** being driven **under the clavicle**

● **Shoulder (glenohumeral) joint** (see Fig. 2.1)

   • Is a **synovial ball-and-socket joint** between the head of the humerus and the glenoid cavity of the scapula

   • Joins the **upper extremity** to the **pectoral girdle**

   • Has a fibrocartilage rim, the **glenoid labrum,** which deepens the glenoid cavity

   • Is surrounded by a **fibrous capsule,** which

     — Is relatively **loose** and permits **free movement**

     — Is attached to the outside of the **glenoid fossa** and to the **anatomical neck** of the humerus except on the medial side where it reaches the surgical neck

     — Is **reinforced anteriorly** by three capsule thickenings, the superior, middle, and inferior **glenohumeral ligaments**

     — Is **reinforced superiorly** by the **coracohumeral ligament**

     — Bridges the bicipital groove as the **transverse humeral ligament**

   • Depends largely on the **surrounding muscles and tendons** for its stability, particularly the **rotator cuff**

   • Is most often **dislocated inferiorly** because the inferior aspect of the capsule is weak and there is little muscular support

   • Has a **wider range** of movement **than any other joint,** allowing flexion and extension, abduction and adduction, and rotation and circumduction

   • Is supplied by the axillary, suprascapular, and lateral pectoral nerves

● **Elbow joint** (see Fig. 2.2)

   • Is a **synovial hinge joint**

   • Consists of

     — A humeroradial joint between the **capitulum of the humerus** and the **head of the radius**

     — A humeroulnar joint between the **trochlea of the humerus** and the **trochlear notch of the ulna**

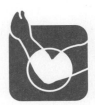

   • Is limited in movement to **flexion** and **extension**

   • Shares a **common cavity** with the **proximal radioulnar joint**

   • Has a **capsule,** which is thin and **loose anteriorly and posteriorly** to accommodate flexion and extension

   • Is supplied by the **median, musculocutaneous, radial,** and **ulnar** nerves

   • Is **strengthened medially and laterally** by strong **collateral ligaments** and is very stable

   • Ulnar (medial) **collateral ligament**

     — Is **triangular**

     — Has **anterior** and **posterior bands** that run from the **medial epicondyle** to the **coronoid process** and **olecranon,** respectively, and an **oblique band** that connects the **olecranon** and **coronoid process**

   • Radial (lateral) **collateral ligament**

     — Is **not directly** attached to the radius

— Is **triangular** in shape
— Is attached at its apex to the **lateral epicondyle** and at its base to the **annular ligament** and to the **ulna** at the margins of the radial notch

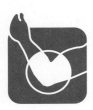

● Radioulnar joints

  • **Are necessary for the movements of pronation and supination of the forearm and hand because the elbow joint allows only for flexion and extension**

  — *Proximal radioulnar joint*

    • Is a synovial joint and shares a **common cavity** with the **elbow joint**
    • Allows the **head of the radius to rotate** in the ring formed by the **radial notch** of the ulna and the **annular ligament**
    • **Annular ligament**

      — Is the **chief ligament** of the proximal radioulnar joint
      — Surrounds the head of the radius down to the neck, thus **resisting downward dislocation**
      — Attaches to the ulna at the **margins** of the **radial notch**
      — Is lined by synovial membrane

  — *Distal radioulnar joint*

    • Is a **synovial pivot type of joint** between the **head of the ulna** and the **ulnar notch of the radius**
    • Has a **triangular articular disk** of fibrocartilage, which

      — At its **base** is attached to the edges of the **ulnar notch** of the radius
      — At its **apex** is attached to the inner base of the **styloid process** of the ulna
      — **Moves with the radius** about its ulnar attachment
      — Provides the **strongest attachment** between the radius and ulna at this joint

    • Allows the lower end of the radius to **rotate** around the ulnar head
    • Is **separated** from the **wrist** (radiocarpal) **joint** by the articular disc

  — *Interosseus membrane*

    • Is a sometimes said to form the **middle radioulnar joint**
    • **Connects** the interosseus borders of the **radius and ulna**
    • Consists of **fibers** that run obliquely **downward from lateral to medial**
    • Provides a surface for **attachment** of the **deep muscles** of the forearm
    • Is **taut in pronation** and **lax in supination**
    • Allows **force** applied at the hand and wrist to be **transferred** from the radius **to the ulna** because the ulna is more substantial proximally and has a more stable articulation with the humerus

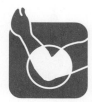

● Joints of the wrist and hand

— *Radiocarpal (wrist) joint*

• Is the **synovial condyloid joint** between the radius and articular disc proximally and the scaphoid, lunate, and triquetral bones distally (see Fig. 2.3)

• Does **not** include the ulna or pisiform bones

• Has a **synovial cavity,** which does **not** communicate with the distal radioulnar joint

• Has a **capsule,** which is **strengthened by** the

— **Radial collateral ligament,** which runs from the styloid process of the radius to the scaphoid

— **Ulnar collateral ligament,** which runs from the styloid process of the ulna to the triquetral and pisiform

— **Palmar and dorsal radiocarpal ligaments**

• Functioning with the midcarpal joint allows **flexion, extension, abduction,** and **adduction** of the hand

— *Midcarpal joint*

• Is a **synovial** joint between the proximal and distal rows of carpal bones (see Fig. 2.3)

• Is a **plane joint** except for the joint between the capitate and the lunate and scaphoid, which is an **ellipsoid joint**

• Extends proximally and distally into the gaps between adjacent carpal bones

• Functioning with the radiocarpal joint allows **flexion, extension, abduction,** and **adduction** of the hand

— *Carpometacarpal joints*

• The carpometacarpal joints are between the **distal row of carpals** and the **metacarpals** (see Fig. 2.3).

• The joint between the medial four metacarpals and the carpals is the **plane synovial** joint. It allows for little movement.

• The joint of the thumb between the first metacarpal and the trapezium is a **saddle synovial** joint. It is highly moveable, allowing **flexion, extension, abduction, adduction,** and **rotation,** and allows the **important** composite movement of **opposition.**

— *Metacarpophalangeal joints*

• Join the convex heads of the metacarpals and the concave bases of the proximal phalanges (see Fig. 2.3)

• Are **condyloid synovial** joints

• Allow **flexion, extension, abduction, adduction,** and some **rotation**

• Allow some **opposition** at the **fifth** metacarpophalangeal joint

• Have a capsule that is reinforced by a **palmar ligament** and **two collateral ligaments**

— *Interphalangeal joints*

• Are **synovial hinge** joints

• Allow only **flexion** and **extension**

• Have strong **collateral ligaments** that prevent abduction and adduction

■ Blood Vessels of the Upper Extremity

● Superficial veins of the upper extremity

- **Dorsal venous arch**

  — Is an irregular venous network on the **back of the hand**
  — Forms from the veins of the palm and fingers
  — Is drained on the lateral side by the **cephalic vein** and on the medial side by the **basilic vein**

- **Cephalic vein**

  — Arises from the **lateral** side of the **dorsal venous arch**
  — At the wrist consistently lies in the **anatomical snuffbox,** where it is accessible for intravenous cannulation
  — Courses upward on the **lateral side of the forearm**
  — At the cubital fossa lies lateral to the **biceps tendon**
  — Passes upward on the lateral side of the biceps muscle to enter the **deltopectoral groove**
  — Pierces the **clavipectoral fascia** to end in the **axillary vein**

- **Basilic vein**

  — Arises from the **medial** side of the **dorsal venous arch**
  — Courses upward on the **medial side of the forearm**
  — In the arm lies along the **medial border of the biceps**
  — Pierces the deep fascia to lie **alongside** the **brachial artery** in the upper arm
  — At the lower border of the teres major joins the **venae comitantes** of the brachial artery to form the **axillary vein**

- **Median cubital vein**

  — Passes over the **cubital fossa** in front of the elbow
  — Connects the **basilic** and **cephalic** veins
  — Is separated by the **bicipital aponeurosis** from the **brachial artery,** which can be inappropriately punctured during phlebotomy or intravenous injection

- **Median antebrachial vein**

  — Arises in the **palm** and ascends in the **middle of the forearm**
  — Joins the median cubital or the basilic vein or splits to join both the basilic and cephalic veins

● Deep veins of the upper extremity

- **Venae comitantes**

  — Are deep veins, usually **paired,** which run alongside arteries

- **Axillary vein**

  — Is the **main venous structure** draining the **upper extremity**
  — Is formed at the lower border of the teres major muscle as a **continuation of the basilic vein** and is **joined by the venae comitantes** of the brachial artery
  — **Receives** the **cephalic vein** and **deep veins** corresponding to the branches of the axillary artery

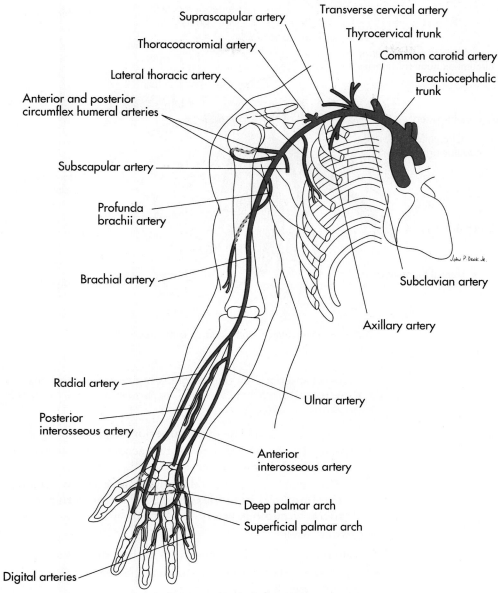

Fig. 2.4 Main arteries of the upper extremity.

— In the axilla lies **medial** to the **axillary artery**

— **Becomes** the **subclavian vein** at the outer border of the first rib

● **Arteries of the upper extremity**

  • The arterial supply to the upper extremity is summarized in Fig. 2.4.

— *Axillary artery (Fig. 2.5)*

  • Is a continuation of the **subclavian artery** and becomes the **brachial artery**

  • Extends from the outer border of the **first rib** to the lower border of the **teres major muscle**

  • Is enclosed in the axillary sheath along with the axillary vein and components of the brachial plexus

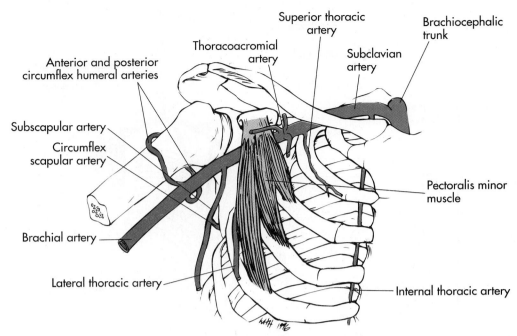

Fig. 2.5 The axillary artery and its branches.

- Is crossed anteriorly by the pectoralis minor muscle dividing it into three parts (*note that the number of the part corresponds to the number of branches arising from that part*)

    — First part—gives rise to the **superior thoracic artery**
    — Second part—gives rise to the **thoracoacromial artery** and the **lateral thoracic artery**
    — Third part—gives rise to the **subscapular artery**, the **anterior humeral circumflex artery**, and the **posterior humeral circumflex artery**

Superior thoracic artery

- Is alternatively called the supreme or highest thoracic artery
- Passes on the chest wall along the medial border of the pectoralis minor muscle
- Supplies the upper intercostal spaces, the pectoralis muscle, and the breast

Thoracoacromial artery

- Arises as a short trunk or multiple branches that pierce the clavipectoral fascia
- Supplies the pectoral and shoulder regions
- Has pectoral, clavicular, acromial, and deltoid branches

Lateral thoracic artery

- Passes on the chest wall along the lower border of the pectoralis minor muscle
- Supplies the serratus anterior and the mammary gland

Subscapular artery

- Is the largest branch of the axillary artery

- Descends along the axillary border of the scapula
- Supplies the scapular region and the lateral thoracic wall
- Anastomoses with branches of the subclavian artery forming an **important collateral channel** to bypass obstruction of the distal sub-clavian or proximal axillary arteries
  - Has two named branches, the **scapular circumflex artery** and the **thoracodorsal artery**

    — **Scapular circumflex artery** passes through the **triangular space** to reach the posterior scapula

    — **Thoracodorsal artery** passes with the **thoracodorsal nerve** on the surface of the latissimus dorsi muscle

Anterior humeral circumflex artery

- **Anastomoses** with the posterior humeral circumflex artery around the **surgical neck** of the humerus
- Is considerably smaller than the posterior humeral circumflex artery

Posterior humeral circumflex artery

- Passes with the **axillary nerve** through the **quadrangular space**
- **Anastomoses** with the anterior humeral circumflex artery and with the ascending branch of the profunda brachii artery
- Often arises from or in common with the subscapular artery

— *Other arteries of the shoulder*

Suprascapular artery

- Arises in the neck from the **thyrocervical trunk,** a branch of the first part of the subclavian artery
- Passes across the posterior triangle of the neck parallel to and behind the clavicle
- Passes **above the superior transverse scapular ligament** to reach the supraspinous fossa

- Descends through the great scapular notch to reach the infraspinous fossa
- Participates in the **anastomosis** around the scapula
- Supplies the scapular muscles and the glenohumeral and acromioclavicular joints

Transverse cervical artery

- Arises in the neck from the **thyrocervical trunk,** a branch of the first part of the subclavian artery
- Passes across the posterior triangle of the neck to reach the shoulder
- At the anterior border of the levator scapulae, divides into **superficial** and **deep** branches
- **Superficial branch of the transverse cervical artery**

  — Passes **deep to** and supplies the **trapezius** muscle

  — Runs with the accessory nerve

- **Deep branch of the transverse cervical artery**

  — Descends on the medial border of the scapula deep to rhomboid muscles

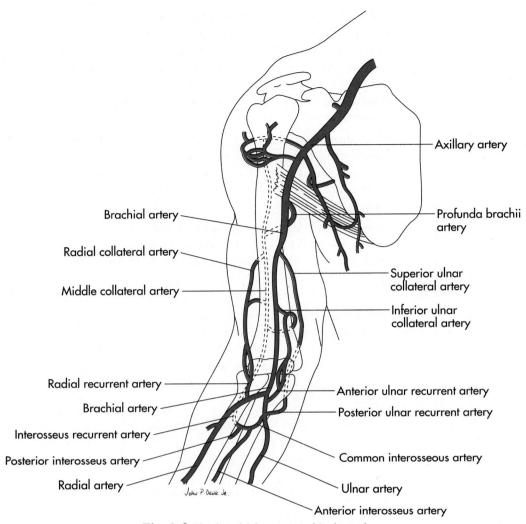

Fig. 2.6 The brachial artery and its branches.

    — Runs with the **dorsal scapular nerve**

    — Participates in the anastomosis around the scapula

Dorsal scapular artery

- Replaces the **deep branch of the transverse cervical artery**
- Arises as a **direct branch of** the second or third part of the **subclavian artery**
- Runs with the **dorsal scapular nerve**
- Participates in the anastomosis around the scapula

● **Arteries of the arm**

    — *Brachial artery (Fig. 2.6)*

- Is a continuation of the **axillary artery**
- Descends the length of the flexor compartment of the arm covered only by skin and fascia

- Ends in the cubital fossa at the level of the neck of the radius by dividing into **radial** and **ulnar** arteries
- In the cubital fossa, lies deep to the **bicipital aponeurosis** and between the **biceps tendon** laterally and the **median nerve** medially
- Branches include the **profunda brachii** artery, the **superior ulnar collateral** artery, and the **inferior ulnar collateral** artery

Profunda brachii artery

- Lies with the **radial nerve** in the **spiral groove** between the lateral and medial heads of the triceps
- Supplies the posterior (extensor) compartment of the arm
- Gives rise to the

  — **Nutrient artery** to the humerus
  — **Ascending branch,** which anastomoses with the posterior humeral circumflex artery
  — **Radial collateral artery,** which accompanies the radial nerve into the forearm and anastomoses with the radial recurrent artery (see Fig. 2.6)
  — **Middle collateral artery,** which passes posterior to the lateral condyle to anastomose with the interosseus recurrent artery deep to the anconeus muscle

Superior ulnar collateral artery

- Arises near the middle of the arm
- Often arises from or in common with the profunda brachii artery
- Pierces the medial intermuscular septum to accompany the **ulnar nerve** behind the medial epicondyle
- Travels with the **ulnar collateral nerve** (nerve to the medial head of the triceps)
- Takes part in the arterial anastomosis around the elbow communicating with the **posterior ulnar recurrent artery**

Inferior ulnar collateral artery

- Arises from the brachial artery just above the elbow
- Descends in front of the medial epicondyle
- Takes part in the arterial anastomosis around the elbow communicating with the **anterior ulnar recurrent artery**

- **Arteries of the forearm**
  — *Radial artery (see Fig. 2.6)*
    - Is the smaller of the terminal branches of the brachial artery
    - Begins in the cubital fossa opposite the neck of the radius
    - In the proximal and middle forearm lies under cover of the brachioradialis
    - In the distal forearm lies **superficially** between the tendons of the **brachioradialis** and **flexor carpi radialis** and is covered only by skin and fascia
    - At the wrist winds dorsally through the **anatomical snuffbox** to reach the back of the hand

- Branches include the **radial recurrent** artery, the **palmar carpal** branch, the **dorsal carpal** branch, and a **superficial palmar** branch

Radial recurrent artery

- Arises from the radial artery shortly after its origin
- Ascends deep to the brachioradialis to accompany the radial nerve and anastomose with the **radial collateral branch of the profunda brachii**

Palmar carpal branch

- Passes across the distal end of the radius deep to the flexor tendons
- Anastomoses with the **palmar carpal branch of the ulnar artery**

Dorsal carpal branch

- Arises in the **anatomical snuffbox** and runs medially and deep to the extensor tendons
- Anastomoses with the **dorsal carpal branch of the ulnar artery** and the **posterior branch of the anterior interosseus artery** to form the **dorsal carpal arch**

Superficial palmar branch

- Is variable in size and often absent
- Arises in the distal forearm before the radial artery passes dorsally
- Passes superficial to (or through) the thenar muscles to contribute to the **superficial palmar arterial arch**

— *Ulnar artery (see Fig. 2.6)*

- Is the larger of the terminal branches of the brachial artery
- Begins in the cubital fossa opposite the neck of the radius
- In the middle third of the forearm is joined by the ulnar nerve and lies under cover of the flexor carpi ulnaris.
- In the distal third of the forearm lies **superficially** and is **lateral** to the tendon of the **flexor carpi ulnaris** (see Fig. 2.6)
- In the middle and distal forearm lies **adjacent and lateral** to the ulnar nerve
- Branches pass anterior to the flexor retinaculum and lateral to the pisiform to reach the hand
- Branches include the **anterior and posterior ulnar recurrent** arteries, the **common, anterior, and posterior interosseus** arteries, and the **palmar and dorsal carpal** branches

Anterior ulnar recurrent artery

- Arises from the ulnar artery shortly after its origin
- Passes anterior to the medial epicondyle to anastomose with the **inferior ulnar collateral artery**

Posterior ulnar recurrent artery

- May arise independently or in common with anterior ulnar recurrent artery
- Passes posterior to the medial epicondyle to join the ulnar nerve and anastomose with the **superior ulnar collateral artery**

Common interosseus artery

- Is a short trunk that arises from the ulnar artery shortly after its origin
- Divides into **anterior and posterior interosseus arteries**

ANTERIOR INTEROSSEUS ARTERY

- Descends on the front of the interosseus membrane with the anterior interosseus nerve (from the median nerve)
- Supplies the deep muscles of the flexor compartment of the forearm
- Terminates at the proximal part of the pronator quadratus by dividing into **anterior and posterior branches**

  — **Anterior branch** passes deep to the pronator quadratus to **anastomose** with the **palmar carpal branches** of the radial and ulnar arteries
  — **Posterior branch** pierces the interosseus membrane to reach the posterior compartment of the forearm and **anastomose** with the **dorsal carpal arch**

- Near its origin gives rise to the **median artery,** which accompanies the median nerve and at times is large enough to reach the hand to contribute to the superficial palmar arch

POSTERIOR INTEROSSEUS ARTERY

- Passes posteriorly above the proximal border of the interosseus membrane and descends behind the interosseus membrane with the **posterior interosseus nerve** (from the radial nerve)
- Supplies the posterior compartment of the forearm
- Ends by anastomosing with the dorsal carpal arch
- Near its origin gives rise to the **interosseus recurrent artery,** which ascends under cover of the anconeus muscle to anastomose with the **middle collateral branch of the profunda brachii artery**

Palmar carpal branch

- Arises near the proximal border of the flexor retinaculum and passes deep to the flexor tendons
- Anastomoses with the **palmar carpal branch of the radial artery**

Dorsal carpal branch

- Arises near the proximal border of the flexor retinaculum and winds dorsally deep to the tendons of the flexor and extensor carpi ulnaris
- Anastomoses with the **dorsal carpal branch of the radial artery** and the **posterior branch of the anterior interosseus artery** to form the **dorsal carpal arch**

Brachial Plexus and Its Branches

- Brachial plexus (Fig. 2.7)

  - Is formed in the neck from the **ventral rami** of spinal nerves **C5 to T1** and extends into the axilla
  - Gives rise to the nerves supplying the upper extremity
  - Is said to be **prefixed** when it receives a large **contribution from C4**

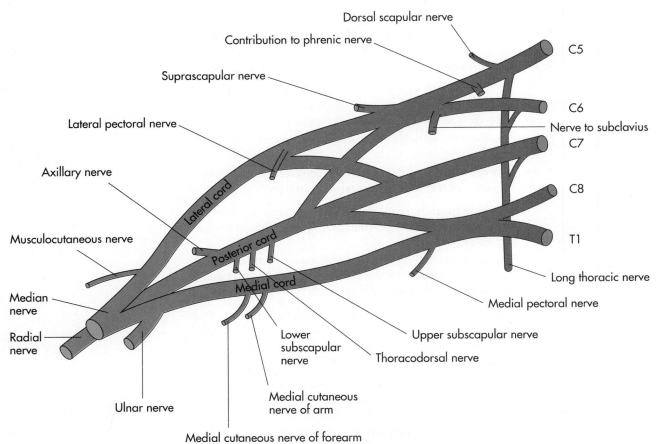

Fig. 2.7 The brachial plexus and its branches.

- Is said to be **postfixed** when it receives a large **contribution from T2**
- Is described as having **roots, trunks, divisions, and cords**
- Roots

    — Are the **ventral rami** of the five spinal nerves involved
    — Emerge in the neck between the scalenus anterior and scalenus medius muscles

- Trunks

    — Are three in number, an **upper,** a **middle,** and a **lower**
    — Pass from the neck to the axilla behind the middle third of the clavicle
    — **Upper** forms by union of the **C5 and C6 roots**
    — **Middle** is a continuation of the **C7 root**
    — **Lower** forms by union of the **C8 and T1 roots**

- Divisions

    — Arise from each trunk as **anterior** and **posterior** divisions.
    — Lie at the apex of the axilla

- Cords

    — Are three in number, a **medial,** a **lateral,** and a **posterior**

    — Are named from their **positions** relative to the **second part of the axillary artery**

    — Are enclosed with axillary artery and vein within the **axillary sheath**

    — **Posterior cord** forms from the **posterior divisions of all three trunks**

    — **Lateral cord** forms from the **anterior divisions of the upper and middle trunk**

    — **Medial cord** is a continuation of the **anterior division of the lower trunk**

● **Branches of the roots**

  — *Dorsal scapular nerve*

    - Arises in the neck from the **C5 root**
    - Passes through the **scalenus medius** and deep to the levator scapulae muscle
    - Runs on the deep surface of the rhomboid muscles with the **deep branch of the transverse cervical artery** (or the dorsal scapular artery)
    - Supplies the **rhomboid major** and **rhomboid minor** muscles

  — *Long thoracic nerve*

    - Arises in the neck from the **roots of C5, C6, and C7**
    - Descends behind the brachial plexus and the first part of the axillary artery
    - Passes inferiorly on the surface of the **serratus anterior** muscle, which it supplies

● **Branches of the trunks**

  — *Suprascapular nerve (C5 and C6)*

    - Arises in the neck from the **upper trunk**
    - Passes across the neck deep to the trapezius
    - Passes through the **scapular notch** deep to the **superior transverse scapular ligament**
    - Runs with the **suprascapular artery** through the spinoglenoid notch to the infraspinous fossa
    - Supplies the **supraspinatus and infraspinatus muscles** and the glenohumeral and acromioclavicular joints

● **Branches of the divisions** The divisions have no branches.

● **Branches of the cords**

  — *Lateral cord*

    - Gives rise to the **lateral pectoral nerve** and terminates as the **musculocutaneous nerve**

    Lateral pectoral nerve (C5, C6, C7)

    - Is named according to its origin from the **lateral cord**
    - Lies medial to the medial pectoral nerve

- Passes anterior to the axillary artery and vein to pierce the **clavi-pectoral fascia**
- Primarily supplies the **pectoralis major** muscle
- By way of a **loop** formed with the medial pectoral nerve also supplies the **pectoralis minor** muscle
- Is accompanied by the **pectoral branch of the thoracoacromial artery**

— *Medial cord*

- Gives rise to the **medial pectoral, medial brachial cutaneous,** and **medial antebrachial cutaneous** nerves
- Terminates as the **ulnar nerve** and the **medial head of the median nerve**

Medial pectoral nerve (C8, T1)

- Is named according to its origin from the **medial cord**
- Lies lateral to the lateral pectoral nerve
- Passes **between the axillary artery and vein** to form a **loop** with the lateral pectoral nerve
- Branches pass through or around the pectoralis minor to end in the pectoralis major muscle
- Supplies the **pectoralis major** and **pectoralis minor** muscles

Medial brachial cutaneous nerve (C8, T1)

- Runs on the medial side of the axillary and brachial veins
- Supplies skin on the **medial aspect of the arm**
- Communicates with the **intercostobrachial nerve**

Medial antebrachial cutaneous nerve (C8, T1)

- Arises from the medial cord to lie between the axillary artery and vein
- Descends in the arm **medial to the brachial artery**
- Becomes cutaneous in the lower arm and supplies the skin of the forearm along the course of the **basilic vein**

— *Posterior cord*

- Gives rise to the **upper subscapular, thoracodorsal,** and **lower subscapular nerves**
- Terminates as the **axillary nerve** and the **radial nerve**

Upper subscapular nerve (C5, C6)

- Arises from the proximal part of the posterior cord as it lies on the subscapularis muscle
- Supplies the upper part of the **subscapularis** muscle

Thoracodorsal nerve (C6, C7, C8)

- Arises between the upper and lower subscapular nerves and is **sometimes called the middle subscapular nerve**
- Descends on the posterior wall of the axilla with the **subscapular artery**
- Continues on the deep surface of the **latissimus dorsi** with the **thoracodorsal artery**
- Supplies the **latissimus dorsi** muscle

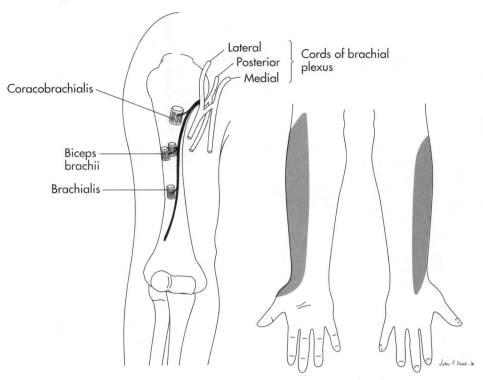

Fig. 2.8 Muscular and cutaneous distribution of the musculocutaneous nerve.

Lower subscapular nerve (C5, C6)

- Arises from the distal part of the posterior cord often in common with the **axillary nerve**
- Supplies the lower part of the **subscapularis** muscle and the teres major muscle

● **Terminal branches of the brachial plexus**

— *Musculocutaneous nerve (C5, C6, C7) (Fig. 2.8)*

- Arises from the **lateral cord** at the lower border of the pectoralis minor muscle
- Pierces the coracobrachialis to lie in the arm between the brachialis and biceps brachii muscles
- **Supplies** all three muscles of the flexor compartment of the arm, the **coracobrachialis,** the **brachialis,** and the **biceps brachii**
- Emerges on the lateral side of the biceps tendon in the distal arm and continues as the **lateral antebrachial cutaneous nerve**

— *Axillary nerve (C5, C6) (Fig. 2.9)*

- Is a terminal branch of the posterior cord
- Leaves the axilla by passing posteriorly through the **quadrangular space** with the **posterior humeral circumflex artery**
- **Anterior branch**

— Winds laterally around the **surgical neck** of the humerus

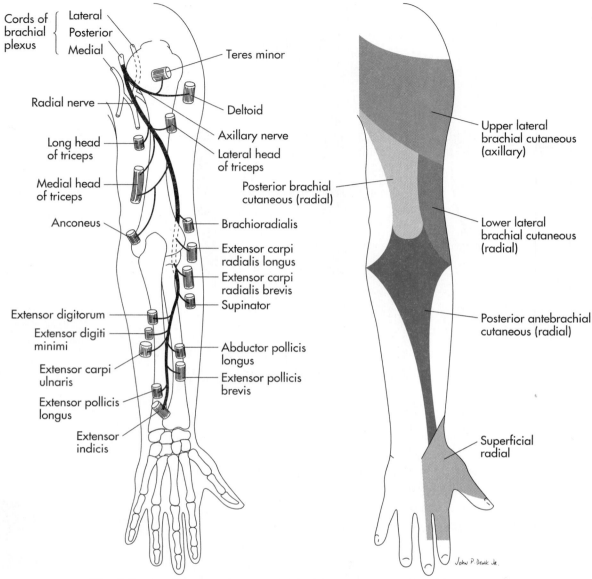

Cords of brachial plexus {
Lateral
Posterior
Medial

Radial nerve

Long head of triceps

Medial head of triceps

Anconeus

Extensor digitorum

Extensor digiti minimi

Extensor carpi ulnaris

Extensor pollicis longus

Extensor indicis

Teres minor

Deltoid

Axillary nerve

Lateral head of triceps

Posterior brachial cutaneous (radial)

Brachioradialis

Extensor carpi radialis longus

Extensor carpi radialis brevis

Supinator

Abductor pollicis longus

Extensor pollicis brevis

Upper lateral brachial cutaneous (axillary)

Lower lateral brachial cutaneous (radial)

Posterior antebrachial cutaneous (radial)

Superficial radial

Fig. 2.9 Muscular and cutaneous distribution of the axillary and radial nerves.

— Supplies the **deltoid** muscle

• **Posterior branch**

— Supplies the **teres minor** and **deltoid** muscles

— Becomes cutaneous around the posterior border of the deltoid as the **upper lateral brachial cutaneous nerve**

— *Radial nerve (C5, C6, C7, C8, T1) (see Fig. 2.9)*

• Is a **terminal branch** of the posterior cord

• Is the **largest branch** of the brachial plexus

• Is the **sole innervation to the extensor compartments** of the arm and forearm and supplies **most of the cutaneous innervation** to the back of the arm, forearm, and hand

- In the arm lies in the **spiral groove** of the humerus **between** the **lateral and medial heads** of the triceps
- Is accompanied in the **spiral groove** by the **profunda brachii** artery
- In the lower arm pierces the lateral intermuscular septum to lie in the anterior compartment **between** the **brachialis** and **brachioradialis** muscles
- Passes in front of the **lateral epicondyle** to enter the **cubital fossa**, where it divides into its two **terminal branches,** the **superficial branch** and the **deep branch**
  - In the **axilla** gives rise to the

    — Nerve to the **long head of the triceps**
    — Nerve to the **medial head of the triceps** (ulnar collateral nerve)
    — Posterior brachial cutaneous nerve

  - In the **spiral groove** of the arm gives rise to the

    — Nerve to the **lateral head of the triceps**
    — Nerve to the **anconeus**
    — Lower lateral brachial cutaneous nerve
    — Posterior antebrachial cutaneous nerve

  - In the **anterior compartment of the arm** gives rise to nerves to the

    — **Brachioradialis**
    — **Extensor carpi radialis longus**
    — **Brachialis**

  - Superficial branch

    — Is **cutaneous** in its distribution and **supplies no muscles**
    — Arises in the cubital fossa and descends in the forearm deep to the **brachioradialis** muscle
    — In its proximal extent **accompanies the radial artery**
    — Emerges from beneath the brachioradialis in the lower anterior forearm
    — Becomes **superficial** as it winds around the lateral forearm to the **dorsum of the hand**
    — Supplies the lateral half of the dorsum of the hand and gives rise to dorsal digital nerves supplying the thumb, index, middle, and half of the ring fingers

  - Deep branch

    — Arises in the **cubital fossa** deep to the **brachioradialis** muscle
    — Winds laterally around the **radius** between the superficial and deep layers of the **supinator** muscle
    — Reaches the back of the forearm to lie **between the superficial** and **deep extensor** muscles
    — **In the extensor compartment** is called the **posterior in-**

terosseus nerve and runs with the **posterior interosseus artery**

— As the **deep radial nerve** in the cubital fossa supplies the **extensor carpi radialis brevis** and the **supinator** muscles

— As the **posterior interosseus nerve** in the posterior forearm supplies the **extensors of the fingers and thumb, the abductor pollicis longus, and the extensor carpi ulnaris**

— In the distal forearm lies on the **interosseus membrane** with the **posterior branch of the anterior interosseus artery**

— Terminates as articular branches to the wrist joint

— *Ulnar nerve (C8, T1) (Fig. 2.10)*

  • Is a **terminal branch** of the medial cord

  • Lies **medial** to the **brachial artery** in the **upper arm**

  • At the middle of the arm pierces the **medial intermuscular septum** to enter the **extensor compartment**

  • Runs **behind the medial epicondyle,** where it is superficial and easily palpated

  • Enters the forearm by passing **between the two heads of the flexor carpi ulnaris**

  • Descends in the forearm **deep** to the flexor carpi ulnaris

  • At the **wrist** lies **lateral** to the tendon of the **flexor carpi ulnaris** and to the **pisiform**

  • Is the main nerve to the small **muscles of the hand** (see Tables 2.8 and 2.9 on pp. 61 and 62 and the section on nerves of the hand on p. 61)

— *Median nerve (C5, C6, C7, C8, T1) (Fig. 2.11)*

  • Is formed by union of the **medial root** from the **medial cord** and the **lateral root** from the **lateral cord**

  • Close to its origin often receives a **communicating branch** from the **ulnar nerve**

  • At its **origin** lies **lateral** to the **brachial artery**

  • In the **middle to lower arm** lies on the brachialis muscle **medial** to the **brachial artery**

  • In the **cubital fossa** lies **medial** to the **brachial artery**

  • Leaving the cubital fossa passes between the two heads of the **pronator teres** and then between the two heads of the **flexor digitorum superficialis**

  • Descends in the forearm **deep** to the flexor digitorum superficialis

  • At the **wrist** lies **between** the tendons of the **flexor digitorum superficialis** and the **flexor carpi radialis**

  • Enters the hand through the **carpal tunnel** deep to the flexor retinaculum

  • Has no distribution in the arm

  • In the forearm

    — Supplies **all** of the muscles of the **anterior forearm** except

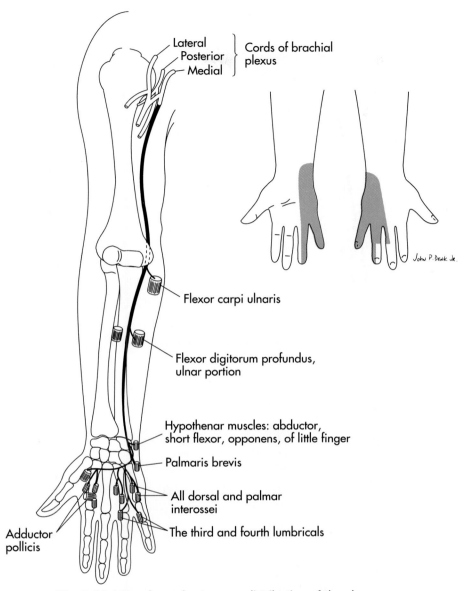

Lateral
Posterior   } Cords of brachial
Medial   plexus

John P. Denk Jr.

Flexor carpi ulnaris

Flexor digitorum profundus, ulnar portion

Hypothenar muscles: abductor, short flexor, opponens, of little finger

Palmaris brevis

All dorsal and palmar interossei

Adductor pollicis

The third and fourth lumbricals

Fig. 2.10 Muscular and cutaneous distribution of the ulnar nerve.

the **flexor carpi ulnaris** and the **ulnar half of the flexor digitorum profundus**

— Gives articular branches to the elbow and proximal radioulnar joints

— Gives rise to the **anterior interosseus nerve** and the **palmar cutaneous branch**

• In the hand

— Supplies the **thenar muscles** (excluding the adductor pollicis) and the **lateral two lumbricals** (see the section on nerves of the hand on p. 61)

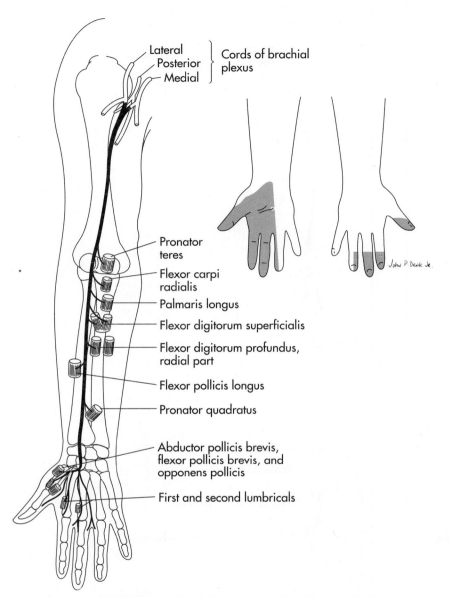

Fig. 2.11 Muscular and cutaneous distribution of the median nerve.

- **Anterior interosseus nerve**
  - Arises from the median nerve in the **cubital fossa**
  - Lies with the **anterior interosseus artery** on the interosseus membrane **between the flexor pollicis longus** and the **flexor digitorum profundus**
  - **Supplies** the flexor pollicis longus, the lateral half of the flexor digitorum profundus, and the **pronator quadratus**
  - Ends as **articular branches** to the inferior radioulnar, wrist, and carpal joints

- Cutaneous innervation of the upper extremity
  - **Supraclavicular nerves** (from the **cervical plexus**)
    - Become cutaneous over the acromion and clavicle
    - Supply the skin over the point of the **shoulder and the pectoral region** to the midline
  - **Upper lateral brachial cutaneous nerve** (from the **axillary** nerve)
    - Becomes cutaneous at the posterior border of the deltoid
    - Is distributed over the **lower half of the deltoid**
  - **Lower lateral brachial cutaneous nerve** (from the **radial** nerve)
    - Arises in the spiral groove
    - Is distributed over the **lateral and anterolateral** aspects of the **arm**
  - **Medial brachial cutaneous nerve** (from the **medial cord** of the brachial plexus)
    - Supplies skin on the **medial aspect of the arm**
    - Communicates with the **intercostobrachial nerve**
  - **Medial antebrachial cutaneous nerve** (from the **medial cord** of the brachial plexus)
    - Descends in the arm **medial to the brachial artery**
    - Becomes cutaneous in the lower arm and supplies the skin of the **forearm along the** course of the **basilic vein**
  - **Intercostobrachial nerve**
    - Is the lateral cutaneous branch of the second intercostal nerve
    - Communicates with the **medial brachial cutaneous nerve**
  - **Lateral antebrachial cutaneous nerve** (from the **musculocutaneous nerve**)
    - Is a **direct continuation** of the **musculocutaneous nerve**
    - Emerges on the lateral side of the biceps tendon in the distal arm
    - Is distributed over the **lateral and anterolateral forearm** to the base of the thumb
  - **Posterior brachial cutaneous nerve** (from the **radial** nerve)
    - Arises from the radial nerve in the **axilla**
    - Is distributed to the **back of the arm below the deltoid**
  - **Posterior antebrachial cutaneous nerve** (from the **radial** nerve)
    - Arises from the radial nerve in the **spiral groove**
    - Is distributed to the **back of the forearm to the wrist**

Axilla, Pectoral Region, and Shoulder

- Axilla
  - Is the pyramidal space between the chest wall and the arm
  - Contains

— The **axillary artery and vein**
— Parts of the **brachial plexus** and its branches
— The axillary **lymph nodes**
— The **lateral cutaneous branches** of the upper intercostal nerves
— The termination of the **cephalic vein**
— An abundance of **fat and connective tissue**

— *Boundaries of the axilla*

- Base: the axillary fascia and skin of the armpit
- Apex: the triangular interval between the **clavicle** anteriorly, the **first rib** medially, and the **superior border of the scapula** posteriorly
- Medial wall: the upper **rib cage** covered by the serratus anterior muscle
- Lateral wall: the **intertubercular groove** of the humerus
- Anterior wall: the **pectoralis major and minor** muscles
- Posterior wall: the **subscapularis, teres major,** and **latissimus dorsi** muscles

— *Axillary and pectoral fascias*

- Axillary sheath

    — Is an extension of the **prevertebral layer of deep cervical fascia** covering the posterior triangle of the neck
    — Encloses the **axillary vessels** and the **brachial plexus**

- Pectoral fascia

    — Invests the pectoralis major muscle
    — Is continuous posteriorly with the axillary fascia

- Axillary fascia

    — Forms the **base (floor) of the axilla**
    — Is continuous **anteriorly** with the **pectoral fascia**
    — Projects anteriorly and **invests** the **pectoralis minor** as the so-called **suspensory ligament of the axilla**
    — Is continuous **posteriorly** with the fascia over the **latissimus dorsi**

- Clavipectoral fascia

    — Is a **thickening** of the deep fascia **between** the **subclavius** and **pectoralis minor** muscles
    — Is attached to the chest wall, the clavicle, and the coracoid process
    — Is thickened between the **first rib** and the **coracoid process** to form the **costocoracoid membrane,** which is penetrated by the cephalic vein, the thoracoacromial artery, and the lateral pectoral nerve
    — Communicates with the **axillary fascia** via the **suspensory ligament of the axilla**
    — Is pierced by the **thoracoacromial artery,** the **cephalic vein,** and the **lateral pectoral nerve**

Table 2.1   *Muscles That Move the Shoulder Girdle*

Name	Origin	Insertion	Action	Innervation
Trapezius	Occipital bone, ligamentum nuchae, and spines of all thoracic vertebrae	Spine of scapula, acromion, and lateral one third of clavicle	Elevates and rotates scapula	Spinal portion accessory nerve (motor) and C3 and C4 (sensory)
Rhomboid major	Spines of second to fifth thoracic vertebrae	Medial border of scapula	Stabilizes shoulder girdle; medially rotates inferior angle of scapula	Dorsal scapular nerve
Rhomboid minor	Ligamentum nuchae and spines of seventh cervical and first thoracic vertebrae	Medial border of scapula	Stabilizes shoulder girdle; medially rotates inferior angle of scapula	Dorsal scapular nerve
Levator scapulae	Transverse processes of first four cervical vertebrae	Superior angle and medial border of scapula	Elevates and rotates the scapula; depresses the acromion and glenoid cavity	C3 and C4 and the dorsal scapular nerve
Serratus anterior	Upper eight ribs	Inferior angle and medial border of scapula	Draws scapula forward against chest wall; rotates scapula turning glenoid cavity upward	Long thoracic nerve
Pectoralis minor	Third to fifth ribs near their costal cartilages	Coracoid process of scapula	Draws scapula forward and downward	Medial pectoral nerve
Subclavius	First costal cartilage	Inferior surface of clavicle	Steadies the clavicle during movement of the shoulder girdle	Nerve to the subclavius (from upper trunk of brachial plexus)

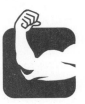

- ● Muscles of the pectoral girdle and shoulder
    - • The **muscles that move the shoulder girdle** are shown in **Table 2.1**.
    - • The **muscles of the rotator cuff** are shown in **Table 2.2**.
    - • The **other muscles that move the humerus** are shown in **Table 2.3**.
  - — *Rotator (musculotendinous) cuff (see Table 2.2)*
      - • Is the **major stabilizing factor for the shoulder joint** holding the head of the humerus firmly in the glenoid fossa
      - • Is formed by the tendons of the **supraspinatus, infraspinatus, teres minor,** and **subscapularis** muscles as they fuse with the capsule
      - • **Reinforces the joint** on all sides **except inferiorly** where dislocation is most likely
      - • Has several **bursae,** which provide a **lubricating** mechanism for tendons during movements of the shoulder
          - — **Subdeltoid bursa** lies between the tendon of the supraspinatus below and the deltoid muscle and coracoacromial arch above

Table 2.2 *Rotator Cuff Muscles*

NAME	ORIGIN	INSERTION	ACTION	INNERVATION
Supraspinatus	Supraspinous fossa of scapula	Highest facet of greater tubercle of humerus	Abducts arm; stabilizes shoulder joint	Suprascapular nerve
Infraspinatus	Infraspinous fossa	Middle facet of greater tubercle of humerus	Rotates arm laterally; stabilizes shoulder joint	Suprascapular nerve
Teres minor	Upper two thirds of lateral border of scapula	Lowest facet of the greater tubercle of humerus	Rotates arm laterally; stabilizes shoulder joint	Axillary nerve
Subscapularis	Subscapular fossa	Lesser tubercle of humerus	Rotates arm medially; stabilizes shoulder joint	Upper and lower subscapular nerves

Table 2.3 *Other Muscles That Move the Humerus*

NAME	ORIGIN	INSERTION	ACTION	INNERVATION
Pectoralis major	Sternum and upper six costal cartilages	Lateral lip of intertubercular groove of humerus	Adducts arm; rotates arm medially	Medial and lateral pectoral nerves
Pectoralis major (clavicular head)	Medial one third of clavicle	Lateral lip of intertubercular groove of humerus	Flexes arm	Medial and lateral pectoral nerves
Deltoid	Lateral one third of clavicle, acromion, and spine of scapula	Deltoid tuberosity of humerus	Abducts arm; anterior fibers flex arm; posterior fibers extend arm	Axillary nerve
Latissimus dorsi	Inferior angle of scapula, lower four ribs, lower six thoracic spinous processes, lumbar and sacral spinous processes, and iliac crest	Floor of the intertubercular groove of humerus	Adducts, medially rotates, and extends arm	Thoracodorsal nerve
Teres major	Lower one third lateral border of scapula	Medial lip of intertubercular groove of humerus	Adducts arm; rotates arm medially	Lower subscapular nerve

— **Subacromial bursa** is a continuation of the subdeltoid bursa deep to the acromion

— **Subscapular bursa** lies between the subscapularis tendon and the neck of the scapula and commonly communicates with the joint cavity through an anterior defect in the capsule

— *Quadrangular and triangular spaces*

  • Quadrangular space

    — Is bounded by the **surgical neck of the humerus** laterally, the **long head of the triceps brachii** medially, the **teres** minor and subscapularis superiorly, and the **teres major** inferiorly

— Transmits the **axillary nerve** and the **posterior humeral circumflex artery**

- **Triangular space**

  — Lies adjacent to the scapula

  — Is bounded by the **long head of the triceps brachii** laterally, the **teres minor and subscapularis** superiorly, and the **teres major** inferiorly

  — Transmits the **scapular circumflex artery**

- Second **triangular space** (or interval)

  — Lies adjacent to the humerus

  — Is bounded by the **long head of the triceps brachii** medially, the **shaft of the humerus** laterally, and the **teres major** superiorly

  — Transmits the **radial nerve** and the **profunda brachii artery**

— *Axillary lymph nodes*

- Drain the **upper extremity,** much of the **breast,** and the **upper trunk** along the tributaries of the axillary artery and vein

- Consist of **20 to 30 nodes** somewhat arbitrarily divided into **five groups**

- Ultimately drain to the **subclavian lymph trunk,** which empties into the systemic venous system near the **junction** of the **internal jugular** and **subclavian veins**

  - Lateral nodes

    — Are also called **brachial** nodes

    — Drain the **upper extremity** except for the vessels following the cephalic vein

    — Lie along the **axillary vein**

  - Posterior nodes

    — Are also called **subscapular** nodes

    — Drain the posterior **shoulder, trunk,** and **lower neck**

    — Lie **along** the **subscapular vessels** at the lateral border of the scapula

  - Pectoral nodes

    — Are also called **anterior** nodes

    — Drain the **breast** and **anterior chest wall**

    — Lie **along** the **lateral thoracic vessels** at the lower border of the pectoralis minor

  - Central nodes

    — Receive lymph from the **lateral, posterior,** and **pectoral** nodes

    — Directly receive the **vessels following the cephalic vein**

— Are embedded in the fat at the **base of the axilla**

- Apical nodes

    — Receive lymph from **all other groups**
    — Lie in front of the axillary vein **above** the upper border of the **pectoralis minor**
    — Give rise to the **subclavian lymph trunk**

● **Breast**

- Consists of the **mammary gland** embedded in the **fatty superficial fascia**
- Has **15 to 20 lobes,** each drained by a single **lactiferous duct** which opens onto the **nipple**
- Remains rudimentary in the male throughout life and in the female before puberty
- In the young adult female **extends** from the **second to the sixth rib** and from the margin of the **sternum to the midaxillary line**
- May extend into the axilla as the **axillary tail** (of Spence)
- On its deep surface overlies the **deep fascia** of the **pectoralis major, serratus anterior,** and **external oblique** muscles
- Is supported by the **suspensory ligaments** (of Cooper) connecting the **deep fascia** with the **overlying skin**
- **Nipple**

    — Is said to lie at the level of the **fourth intercostal space,** although this is highly variable
    — Is surrounded by a ring of pigmented skin, the **areola**

- **Blood supply** is from the

    — Perforating branches of the **internal thoracic** artery
    — **Anterior intercostal** arteries
    — **Lateral thoracic** artery
    — **Thoracoacromial** artery

- **Lymphatic drainage**

    — Is of importance because of its role in the **spread of malignant tumors** of the breast
    — Is predominantly (75%) to the **axillary nodes**
    — Is also (approximately 20%) to the **parasternal nodes** along the internal thoracic artery
    — To a lesser degree is to mediastinal nodes and nodes around the clavicle
    — May **communicate** across the midline to the **opposite breast**

■ **Arm and Forearm**

● **Muscles of the arm and forearm**

- The **muscles of the arm** are shown in **Table 2.4.**
- The **muscles of the flexor compartment of the forearm** are shown in **Table 2.5.**
- The **muscles of the extensor compartment of the forearm** are shown in **Table 2.6.**

Table 2.4   *Muscles of the Arm*

NAME	ORIGIN	INSERTION	ACTION	INNERVATION
Coracobrachialis	Coracoid process of scapula	Middle portion of the medial surface of humerus	Flexes and adducts arm	Musculocutaneous nerve
Brachialis	Anterior surface of lower half of humerus	Coronoid process and tuberosity of ulna	Flexes the elbow joint	Musculocutaneous nerve
Biceps brachii	*Short head:* coracoid process *Long head:* supraglenoid tubercle	Radial tuberosity and by the bicipital aponeurosis into deep fascia of forearm	Flexes the elbow joint, supinates the forearm, and weakly flexes the shoulder joint	Musculocutaneous nerve
Triceps brachii	*Long head:* infraglenoid tubercle *Lateral head:* posterior humerus above spiral groove *Medial head:* posterior humerus below spiral groove	Olecranon process of ulna	Extends the elbow joint	Radial nerve
Anconeous	Lateral epicondyle of humerus	Upper posterior surface of ulna	Extends the elbow joint	Radial nerve

Table 2.5   *Muscles of the Flexor Compartment of the Forearm*

NAME*	ORIGIN	INSERTION	ACTION
Superficial Group			
Pronator teres	*Humeral head:* medial epicondyle *Ulnar head:* coronoid process	Middle one third of the lateral border of radius	Pronates forearm
Flexor carpi radialis	Medial epicondyle of humerus	Bases of the second and third metacarpals	Flexes and abducts the hand at the wrist joint
Palmaris longus (often missing)	Medial epicondyle of humerus	Palmar aponeurosis	Flexes the hand at the wrist joint
Flexor digitorum superficialis	*Humeral head:* medial epicondyle *Radial head:* coronoid process and oblique line	Middle phalanx of medial four fingers	Flexes the proximal interphalangeal joint and wrist joint
Flexor carpi ulnaris	*Humeral head:* medial epicondyle *Ulnar head:* olecranon and posterior border	Pisiform bone, hook of the hamate bone, and base of the fifth metacarpal bone	Flexes and adducts the hand at the wrist joint
Deep Group			
Flexor digitorum profundus	Upper two thirds of anterior ulna and interosseus membrane	Distal phalanx of medial four fingers	Flexes the distal interphalangeal joint and wrist joint
Flexor pollicis longus	Anterior ulna and interosseus membrane	Base of distal phalanx of thumb	Flexes interphalangeal joint of thumb
Pronator quadratus	Anterior surface distal ulna	Anterior surface distal radius	Pronates the forearm

*Innervation: all are supplied by the **median nerve** except the flexor carpi ulnaris and ulnar half of the flexor digitorum profundus, which are supplied by the **ulnar nerve**.

Table 2.6   *Muscles of the Extensor Compartment of the Forearm*

NAME*	ORIGIN	INSERTION	ACTION
Superficial Group			
Brachioradialis	Lateral supracondylar ridge of humerus	Base of styloid process of radius	Flexes elbow joint
Extensor carpi radialis longus	Lateral supracondylar ridge of humerus	Base of second metacarpal bone	Extends and abducts the hand at the wrist joint
Extensor carpi radialis brevis	Lateral epicondyle of humerus	Base of third metacarpal bone	Extends and abducts the hand at the wrist joint
Extensor digitorum	Lateral epicondyle of humerus	Extensor expansion, bases of the middle and distal phalanges of the medial four fingers	Extends phalanges and wrist joint
Extensor digiti minimi	Lateral epicondyle of humerus	Extensor expansion of fifth finger	Extends fifth finger
Extensor carpi ulnaris	Lateral epicondyle of humerus and posterior border of ulna	Base of fifth metacarpal	Extends and adducts the hand at the wrist joint
Deep Group			
Supinator	Lateral epicondyle, supinator fossa, and crest of ulna	Upper shaft of radius	Supinates the forearm
Abductor pollicis longus	Posterior middle third of radius, ulna, and interosseus membrane	Base of first metacarpal	Abducts the thumb
Extensor pollicis brevis	Posterior middle third of radius and interosseus membrane	Base of proximal phalanx of thumb	Extends the thumb
Extensor pollicis longus	Posterior middle third of ulna and interosseus membrane	Base of distal phalanx of thumb	Extends the thumb
Extensor indicis	Posterior ulna and interosseus membrane	Tendon of extensor digitorum to index finger	Extends the index finger

*Innervation: all of the muscles of the extensor forearm are supplied by the **radial nerve**.

- **Cubital fossa**
  - Is the triangular interval lying anterior to the elbow
  - Is bounded by the **brachioradialis laterally** and the **pronator teres medially**
  - Is limited **proximally** by a line connecting the **epicondyles** of the humerus
  - Has a **floor** formed largely by the **brachialis** muscle but also by the **supinator**
  - Has a **roof** formed by the **skin and fascia** including the **bicipital aponeurosis**
  - From **medial to lateral** contains the **median nerve, brachial artery,** and the **biceps tendon**
  - At its lower end contains the **division of the brachial artery** into radial and ulnar arteries
  - Is crossed superficially by the **median cubital vein**

Table 2.7   *The Thenar Muscles*

NAME*	ORIGIN	INSERTION	ACTION
Abductor pollicis brevis	Flexor retinaculum, scaphoid, and trapezium	Base of proximal phalanx of thumb	Abducts the thumb
Flexor pollicis brevis	Flexor retinaculum and trapezium	Base of proximal phalanx of thumb	Flexes the metacarpophalangeal joint of thumb
Opponens pollicis	Flexor retinaculum and trapezium	Lateral side of first metacarpal	Opposes thumb to other digits
Adductor pollicis†	*Oblique head:* capitate and bases of second and third metacarpals *Transverse head:* palmar side of third metacarpal	Base of proximal phalanx of thumb	Adducts thumb

*Innervation: all are supplied by the **median nerve** except the adductor pollicis, which is supplied by the **ulnar nerve.**
†Although the adductor pollicis is not strictly a thenar muscle, it is often included with this group for descriptive purposes.

Table 2.8   *The Hypothenar Muscles*

NAME*	ORIGIN	INSERTION	ACTION
Abductor digiti minimi	Pisiform	Base of proximal phalanx of little finger	Abducts little finger
Flexor digiti minimi brevis	Flexor retinaculum and hook of hamate	With abductor into base of proximal phalanx of little finger	Flexes metacarpophalangeal joint of little finger
Opponens digiti minimi	Flexor retinaculum and hook of hamate	Ulnar side of fifth metacarpal	Opposes little finger to the thumb; helps in cupping the palm
Palmaris brevis	Flexor retinaculum and palmar aponeurosis	Skin on medial side of palm	Tenses skin on medial palm

*Innervation: all of the hypothenar muscles are supplied by the **ulnar nerve.**

■ Wrist and Hand

- ● Muscles of the hand
  - The **thenar muscles** are shown in Table 2.7.
  - The **hypothenar muscles** are shown in Table 2.8.
  - The **interosseus and lumbrical muscles** are shown in Table 2.9.
- ● Nerves of the hand
  - **Motor innervation** to the intrinsic muscles of the hand is derived from the **T1** spinal cord segment via the **median and ulnar nerves.**
  - **Cutaneous innervation** is from the **median, ulnar, and radial nerves.**
  - Typically, the **C6 dermatome** covers the **thumb** and the **C8 dermatome** covers the **little finger.**
  - — *Median nerve (see Fig. 2.11)*
    - At the wrist lies between the tendons of the flexor digitorum superficialis and the flexor carpi radialis

Table 2.9   *Interosseus and Lumbrical Muscles*

NAME*	ORIGIN	INSERTION	ACTION
Palmar interossei (3)†	Palmar surface of second, fourth, and fifth metacarpals	Extensor expansion	Adduct the fingers, flex metacarpophalangeal joints, extend interphalangeal joints
Dorsal interossei (4)	Sides of adjacent metacarpals	Bases of proximal phalanges and their extensor expansions	Abduct the fingers, flex metacarpophalangeal joints, extend interphalangeal joints
Lumbricals (4)	Tendons of the flexor digitorum profundus	Extensor expansion	Flex metacarpophalangeal joints, extend interphalangeal joints

*Innervation: all are supplied by the **ulnar nerve** except the lateral two lumbricals, which are supplied by the **median nerve.**

†Some authors consider a small and variable part of the flexor pollicis brevis to be a fourth palmar interosseus. Remember that the adductor pollicis serves this function for the thumb.

- Enters the hand by passing through the **carpal tunnel** deep to the flexor retinaculum and anterior to the long flexor tendons
- Divides into terminal branches at the distal end of the carpal tunnel
- Immediately gives rise to the **recurrent branch**, which takes a **superficial** course over the thenar eminence to supply the **flexor pollicis brevis, abductor pollicis brevis, and opponens pollicis**
- Gives rise to **three proper digital nerves** supplying each side of the thumb and the lateral side of the index finger and **two common palmar digital nerves,** which supply adjacent sides of the index and middle and middle and ring fingers
- Supplies the **lateral two lumbrical muscles** via twigs from the digital nerves
- Digital nerves give **dorsal branches** to supply the **nail bed** of the lateral 3½ fingers

— *Ulnar nerve (see Fig. 2.10)*

- Enters the hand by passing **anterior** to the flexor retinaculum, **lateral** to the pisiform, and **medial** to the hook of the hamate
- Lies **medial to the ulnar artery** as it enters the hand
- And ulnar artery may both be covered by superficial fibers of the flexor retinaculum
- Terminates by dividing into **superficial and deep branches**
- **Superficial branch**

   — Supplies the **palmaris brevis** muscle

   — Divides into **palmar digital nerves** supplying the medial side of the little finger and adjacent sides of the little and ring fingers

- **Deep branch**

   — Passes through the hypothenar muscles and around the hook of the hamate

— Runs with the **deep palmar arch** deep to the long flexor tendons
— Supplies the **hypothenar muscles, the adductor pollicis, all interosseus muscles, and the lateral two lumbricals**

- Digital nerves give **dorsal branches** to supply the **nail bed** of the medial 1½ fingers

— *Cutaneous innervation of the dorsum of the hand*

- Is primarily by the **superficial branch of the radial nerve** and the **dorsal branch of the ulnar nerve**
- Dorsal branches of the palmar digital nerves supply the distal fingers (including the nail beds)
- **Superficial branch of the radial nerve**

    — Emerges from beneath the brachioradialis in the lower anterior forearm
    — Becomes superficial as it winds around the lateral forearm to the dorsum of the hand
    — Supplies the lateral half of the dorsum of the hand and gives rise to dorsal digital nerves supplying the thumb, index, middle, and half of the ring fingers

- **Dorsal branch of the ulnar nerve**

    — Arises in the lower anterior forearm and passes around the medial border of the wrist to the dorsum of the hand
    — Supplies the medial half of the dorsum of the hand and gives rise to dorsal digital nerves supplying the little finger and the medial side of the ring finger

— *Cutaneous innervation of the palm of the hand*

- Cutaneous innervation of the palm of the hand is by the **palmar cutaneous branches of the median and ulnar nerves** and the **palmar digital branches of the median and ulnar nerves.**
- The **palmar digital branches of the ulnar nerve** arise in the hand from the superficial branch of the ulnar nerve.
- The **palmar digital branches of the median nerve** arise in the hand as terminal branches of the median nerve.
- The **palmar cutaneous branch of the median nerve** arises in the lower forearm and descends across the wrist to supply the lateral palm.
- The **palmar cutaneous branch of the ulnar nerve** arises in the lower forearm and descends across the wrist to supply the medial palm.

● Arteries of the hand

— *Radial artery (Fig. 2.12)*

- Winds dorsally through the **anatomical snuffbox** deep to the tendons of the abductor pollicis longus, extensor pollicis longus, and extensor pollicis brevis
- From the dorsum of the hand enters the palm by passing between the heads of the **first dorsal interosseus muscle**

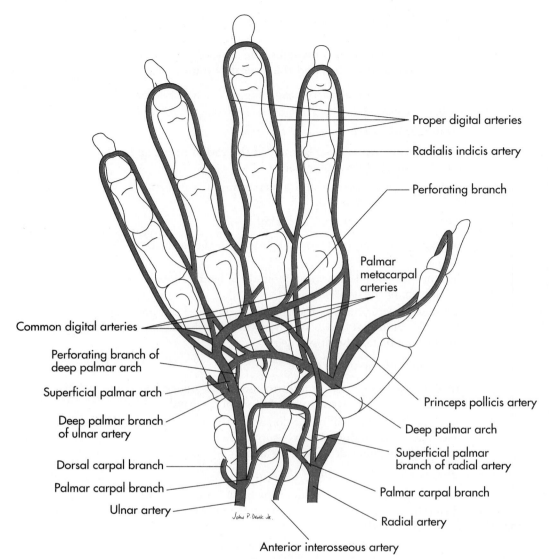

Fig. 2.12 Arteries of the palm.

- In the palm passes medially between the heads of the **adductor pollicis**
- Anastomoses with the **deep branch of the ulnar artery** to form the **deep palmar arch**
- Includes **dorsal digital arteries** for the thumb and index finger, the **princeps pollicis artery,** and the **radialis indicis artery**

Dorsal digital arteries (for the thumb and index finger)

- Arise as the radial artery lies on the first dorsal interosseus
- Typically are **two for the thumb** and **one for the radial side of the index finger**

Princeps pollicis artery

- Arises as the radial artery enters the palm and descends along the medial border of the first metacarpal

- Divides into **proper palmar digital arteries** for each side of the thumb
- May arise in common with the radialis indicis as the **first palmar metacarpal artery**

Radialis indicis artery

- Arises as the radial artery enters the palm and descends along the medial border of the first metacarpal
- Is the last named branch of the radial artery
- May arise in common with the princeps pollicis as the **first palmar metacarpal artery**

Deep palmar arch

- Is the direct continuation of the **radial artery**
- Is formed by the anastomosis of the **radial artery** and the **deep branch of the ulnar artery**
- Lies on the **interosseus muscles** deep to the flexor tendons
- Gives rise to **three palmar metacarpal arteries,** which join the three common palmar digital arteries at the web of the fingers

— *Ulnar artery (see Fig. 2.12)*

- Enters the hand by passing **anterior** to the flexor retinaculum, **lateral** to the pisiform and **medial** to the hook of the hamate
- Lies **lateral to the ulnar nerve** as it enters the hand
- And ulnar nerve may be covered by superficial fibers of the flexor retinaculum
- Terminates by giving a **deep palmar branch** and continuing as the **superficial palmar arch**

Deep palmar branch

- Anastomoses with the termination of the radial artery to form the **deep palmar arch**
- Passes through the hypothenar muscles with the deep branch of the ulnar nerve

Superficial palmar arch

- Is the main continuation of the **ulnar artery**
- Is formed by the anastomosis of the **ulnar artery** and the **superficial palmar branch of the radial artery**
- Lies immediately beneath the **palmar aponeurosis**
- Not uncommonly **may be incomplete** on the radial side
- Gives rise to **three common palmar digital arteries** and a **proper palmar digital artery** to the medial side of the little finger; each common palmar digital artery **bifurcates** into **proper palmar digital arteries,** which supply the adjacent sides of the fingers

— *Dorsal carpal arch*

- Is formed by the anastomosis of the dorsal carpal branches of the **ulnar and radial arteries**
- Receives the terminations of the posterior interosseus artery and posterior branch of the anterior interosseus artery
- Gives rise to **three dorsal metacarpal arteries** and a **dorsal digital artery** to the medial side of the little finger; each dorsal meta-

carpal artery **bifurcates** into **dorsal digital arteries,** which supply the adjacent sides of the fingers

● **Other significant features of the wrist and hand**

— *Palmar aponeurosis*

- Is a triangular layer of thickened, fibrous **deep fascia** covering the palm between the thenar and hypothenar eminences
- Provides **protection** for the superficial palmar arterial arch, the digital nerves, and the underlying tendons
- Is continuous proximally with the tendon of the **palmaris longus,** when present
- Is anchored to the **skin** and to the **flexor retinaculum**
- Splits into **four slips,** which blend with the **fibrous flexor sheaths** of the fingers

— *Flexor retinaculum*

- Is a band of tough, fibrous connective tissue that **converts** the **carpal arch** into the **carpal tunnel**
- Is attached to the tubercles of the **scaphoid and trapezium laterally** and to the hook of the **hamate and pisiform medially**
- **Binds** the long **flexor tendons** into position at the wrist so that they will not "bowstring" when the wrist is flexed

— *Carpal tunnel*

- Is formed by the **carpal arch** and the **flexor retinaculum**
- Is a rigid and confining space that contains the **long flexor tendons** and the **median nerve**

— *Flexor synovial sheaths*

- The flexor synovial sheaths **facilitate movement** of the long flexor tendons in the hand.
- They consist of **three** separate sheaths at the wrist.
- The **common synovial sheath** is formed by an **invagination** of the common sheath from the lateral side. It surrounds the **tendons of the flexor digitorum superficialis and profundus** to the fingers and ends at midpalm **except** for an extension along the tendons to the **little finger.**
- A **separate sheath** surrounds the **tendon of the flexor pollicis longus** from the wrist to its termination.
- A **separate sheath** surrounds the **flexor carpi radialis tendon** at its termination.
- The tendons to the **index, middle,** and **ring fingers** are surrounded by separate **digital synovial sheaths** as they pass onto the fingers.

— *Long flexor tendons in the fingers*

- Are surrounded by a **synovial sheath** to facilitate movement
- Are connected near their termination to the dorsal part of their synovial sheath by synovial folds called **vincula longus and brevis,** which carry the **important blood supply** to the tendons
- Are bound firmly to the phalanges by **fibrous flexor sheaths,** which prevent bowstringing of the tendons.

- Tendon of the **flexor digitorum superficialis**

  — **Splits** around the tendon of the flexor digitorum profundus

  — **Attaches** to the lateral sides of the **middle phalanx**

- Tendon of the **flexor digitorum profundus**

  — Passes **between** the slips of the **flexor digitorum superficialis** tendon

  — **Attaches** to the base of the **distal phalanx**

— *Fascial spaces of the palm*

  - Are **potential spaces** deep to the palmar aponeurosis
  - Are filled with loose connective tissue
  - Are separated by a **midpalmar (oblique) fascial septum** into **thenar** and **midpalmar** spaces
  - **Thenar space**

    — Lies between the first and third metacarpals medial to the thenar muscles

    — Lies anterior to the adductor pollicis

    — Contains the first lumbrical and the long flexor tendons to the thumb and index finger

  - **Midpalmar space**

    — Lies between the third and fifth metacarpals lateral to the hypothenar muscles

    — Lies anterior to the lateral three metacarpals and the intervening interosseus muscles

    — Contains the lumbricals and long flexor tendons to the medial three fingers

— *Extensor retinaculum*

  - Is a thickening of the antebrachial fascia at the distal forearm and wrist
  - Binds the extensor tendons into place
  - Attaches laterally to the distal end of the radius and medially to the styloid process of the ulna and to the triquetral and pisiform bones

— *Extensor aponeurosis (expansion) (Fig. 2.13)*

  - Is a triangular expansion of extensor digitorum tendon beginning over the metacarpophalangeal joint
  - Is often referred to as the extensor hood
  - Receives the insertions of the lumbrical and interossei muscles
  - On the index finger also receives the insertion of the extensor indicis
  - On the ring finger also receives the insertion of the extensor digiti minimi
  - Over the **proximal phalanx** splits into a **central slip** and two **lateral slips**
  - Inserts via the **central slip** into the base of the **middle phalanx**

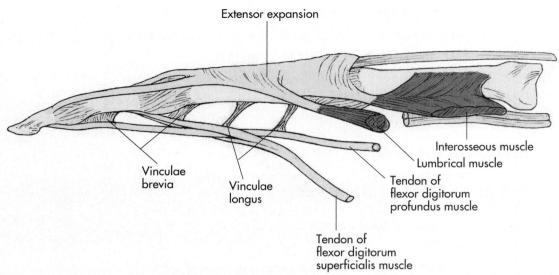

Fig. 2.13 Extensor expansion and flexor tendons.

- Inserts via the united **lateral slips** into the base of the **distal phalanx**

— *Anatomical snuffbox*

- Is seen as a **depression** on the lateral surface of the wrist when the thumb is extended
- Is bordered **anteriorly** by the **tendons** of the **abductor pollicis longus** and the **extensor pollicis brevis**
- Is bordered **posteriorly** by the **tendon** of the **extensor pollicis longus**
- Has a **floor** formed by the **scaphoid** and **trapezium**
- **Contains** the **radial artery** as it passes to the dorsum of the hand

■ **Movements of the Upper Extremity**

● **Movements of the shoulder girdle (scapula)**

- Elevation: trapezius (upper fibers), levator scapulae
- Depression: gravity, trapezius (lower fibers), serratus anterior (lower fibers)
- Superior rotation: serratus anterior, trapezius
- Inferior rotation: levator scapulae, rhomboid major and minor
- Protraction: serratus anterior, pectoralis minor
- Retraction: trapezius, rhomboid major and minor

● **Movements of the shoulder (glenohumeral) joint**

- Flexion: pectoralis major (clavicular head), deltoid (anterior fibers), coracobrachialis
- Extension: latissimus dorsi, deltoid (posterior fibers), triceps brachii
- Abduction: deltoid, supraspinatus
- Adduction: pectoralis major, latissimus dorsi

- Medial rotation: subscapularis, pectoralis major, deltoid (anterior fibers), latissimus dorsi, teres major
- Lateral rotation: infraspinatus, teres minor, deltoid (posterior fibers)

● **Movements of the elbow joint**
- Flexion: brachialis, biceps brachii, brachioradialis
- Extension: triceps brachii, anconeus

● **Movements of the radioulnar joints**
- Pronation: pronator teres, pronator quadratus
- Supination: supinator, biceps brachii

● **Movements of the radiocarpal (wrist) and midcarpal joints**
- Flexion: flexor carpi ulnaris, flexor carpi radialis, palmaris longus
- Extension: extensor carpi ulnaris, extensor carpi radialis longus and brevis
- Abduction: flexor carpi radialis, extensor carpi radialis longus and brevis
- Adduction: flexor carpi ulnaris, extensor carpi ulnaris

● **Movements of the carpometacarpal joints (of the second to fifth fingers)** Only limited movement is permitted.

● **Movements of the metacarpophalangeal joints (of the second to fifth fingers)**
- Flexion: lumbricals, interossei
- Extension: extensor digitorum
- Abduction: dorsal interossei
- Adduction: palmar interossei

● **Movements of the interphalangeal joints (of the second to fifth fingers)**
- Flexion: flexor digitorum superficialis, flexor digitorum profundus
- Extension: extensor digitorum, lumbricals, interossei

● **Movements of the thumb (including the first carpometacarpal joint)**
- Flexion: flexor pollicis longus, flexor pollicis brevis
- Extension: extensor pollicis longus and brevis, abductor pollicis longus
- Abduction: abductor pollicis longus, abductor pollicis brevis
- Adduction: adductor pollicis
- Opposition: opponens pollicis

■ **Summary of the Innervation of the Upper Extremity**

● Summary of motor innervation by nerve
- Musculocutaneous nerve: flexor compartment of the arm
- Median nerve
  — Flexor compartment of the forearm except the flexor carpi ulnaris and the ulnar half of the flexor digitorum profundus
  — Thenar muscles (excluding the adductor pollicis) and the lateral two lumbricals

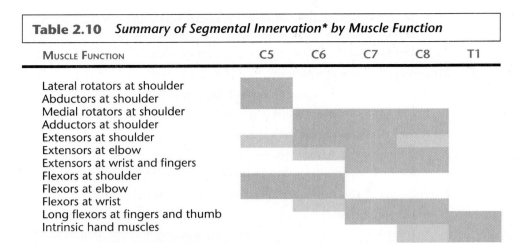

Table 2.10 *Summary of Segmental Innervation* by Muscle Function*

Muscle Function	C5	C6	C7	C8	T1
Lateral rotators at shoulder					
Abductors at shoulder					
Medial rotators at shoulder					
Adductors at shoulder					
Extensors at shoulder					
Extensors at elbow					
Extensors at wrist and fingers					
Flexors at shoulder					
Flexors at elbow					
Flexors at wrist					
Long flexors at fingers and thumb					
Intrinsic hand muscles					

*Location of motor neurons by spinal cord segments for each function listed. The dark shading depicts the usual distribution of segmental innervation and the light shading depicts the less common segmental innervation.

- Ulnar nerve:

    — Flexor carpi ulnaris and the ulnar half of the flexor digitorum profundus

    — Hypothenar muscles

    — Adductor pollicis

    — Interossei and the lateral two lumbricals

- Radial nerve

    — Extensor compartment of the arm

    — Extensor compartment of the forearm

● Summary of segmental innervation by muscle function (Table 2.10)

● Dermatomes of the upper extremity (Fig. 2.14)

■ **Nerve Injuries of the Upper Extremity**

● Injuries of the brachial plexus

    — *Injury of the upper roots and trunk (Erb-Duchenne palsy)*

        • Involves damage to the **C5 and C6** spinal nerves

        • Is produced when the **shoulder** is wrenched **downward** and the **head and neck** are forced to the **opposite side**

        • Is commonly caused by a **violent fall** such as in a **motorcycle accident**

        • Also occurs as a **birth injury** resulting from forceful pulling on the head during a **difficult delivery**

        • Results in a loss of abduction, flexion, and lateral rotation of the shoulder and of supination of the forearm

        • Produces a condition known as **waiter's-tip hand** in which the arm hangs at the side medially rotated at the shoulder and extended at the elbow with the forearm pronated

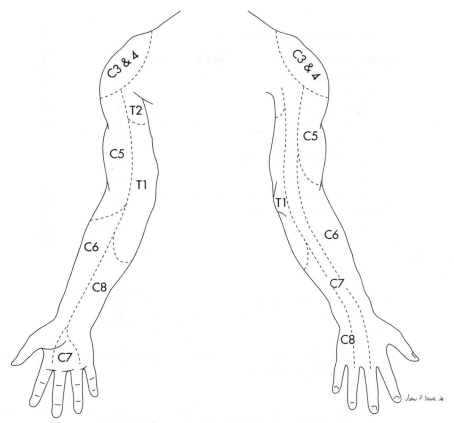

Fig. 2.14 Dermatones of the upper extremity.

— *Injury of the lower roots and trunk (Klumpke's paralysis)*
  - Involves damage to the **C8 and T1** spinal nerves
  - Is produced by forcibly abducting the **arm above the head**
  - Is commonly caused by a grabbing a support during a **fall from a height**
  - Also occurs as a **birth injury** during a **breech delivery** when the arm remains above the head
  - Affects the **intrinsic muscles of the hand** and the **long flexors of the fingers**
  - Results in a **clawhand** deformity

— *Injury of the posterior cord*

  • Results in varying degrees of **paralysis of the extensor muscles** producing variable flexion at the shoulder, elbow, wrist, and fingers

  • Is commonly caused by pressure from prolonged or **improper use of a crutch** resulting in **transient paralysis** called **crutch palsy**

  • May occur from pressure to the axilla caused by **draping the arm over the back of a chair** while in a state of diminished consciousness resulting in **transient paralysis** called **Saturday night palsy**

● Injuries of individual nerves

— *Injury to the long thoracic nerve*

• Results in **paralysis of the serratus anterior** muscle and a corresponding **inability to elevate the arm** above the horizontal position

• Is characterized by a **winged scapula** in which the medial border and inferior angle of the scapula stand out from the posterior thoracic wall

— *Injury to the musculocutaneous nerve*

• Is uncommon

• Will affect **flexion of the elbow** (biceps and brachialis) and **supination of the forearm** (brachialis)

• May be accompanied by **anesthesia** over the **lateral** aspect of the **forearm**

— *Injury to the axillary nerve*

• May result from a **fracture of the surgical neck** of the humerus or an **inferior dislocation** of the shoulder joint

• Results in an **inability to abduct the arm** beyond the first few degrees because of paralysis of the **deltoid**

• Will also result in a loss of cutaneous sensation **over the lower deltoid** above its insertion

— *Injury to the radial nerve*

• Injury to the radial nerve results in the characteristic **wristdrop** caused by **paralysis of extensors** of the wrist and fingers.

• Radial nerve injury produces a **variable degree of paralysis** of the extensor muscles of the arm and forearm **dependent on the level** at which the nerve is injured.

• Because of overlap, **sensory loss** is small and may be confined to a small area **over the first dorsal interosseus.**

• Injury in the arm commonly results from a **fracture of the humerus** as the nerve lies in the **spiral groove.** It will likely **not affect extension at the elbow** because branches to the triceps arise proximal to this point.

• Injury in the cubital fossa may result from compression caused by **hypertrophy of the supinator** muscle or from **fracture of the neck of the radius.** It **may not result in wristdrop** because branches to the extensor carpi radialis longus and brevis, the extensor carpi ulnaris, and the brachioradialis arise proximal to this point.

• **Remember** that with radial nerve injury the **interphalangeal joints** can still be **extended** because of the action of the **interossei and lumbricals. Paralysis of the supinator** can in part be **compensated for by the biceps brachii** except in full extension of the elbow.

— *Injury to the median nerve*

• Is commonly caused by a **supracondylar fracture** of the humerus, accidental or self-inflicted **sectioning at the wrist,** or **compression in the carpal tunnel**

- At the wrist results in

  — Paralysis of the thenar muscles with an **inability to oppose the thumb** and a **weakened flexion of the thumb** at the first metacarpophalangeal joint

  — Impaired movement of the **lateral two fingers** caused by paralysis of the **lumbricals**

  — A debilitating **sensory loss** over the **lateral palm** and the lateral 3½ **fingers**

  — A **wasting** of the **thenar eminence**

- At higher levels will also result in

  — A loss of **pronation**

  — An inability to flex the **thumb** and **lateral two fingers** at the interphalangeal joints

  — An impaired ability to flex the **medial two fingers** at the interphalangeal joints

  — Weakened **wrist flexion** and **abduction**

  — A **wasting** of the flexor **forearm**

— *Injury to the ulnar nerve*

  - Is commonly caused by a **fracture of the medial epicondyle** of the humerus or by accidental or self-inflicted **sectioning at the wrist**

  - At the wrist results in

    — Paralysis of the **intrinsic muscles** of the hand **except** those of the **thenar eminence** (but including the adductor pollicis)

    — An inability to **abduct or adduct the fingers** or to **adduct the thumb**

    — An inability to simultaneously **flex the metacarpophalangeal joints** and **extend the interphalangeal joints**

    — **Clawhand** characterized by a wasted palm and hypothenar eminence, hyperextended metacarpophalangeal joints, and flexed interphalangeal joints

  - At higher levels will also result in

    — An impaired **ulnar deviation** (adduction) **at the wrist** caused by loss of the flexor carpi ulnaris

    — An impaired ability to **flex the medial two fingers** because of loss of the ulnar head of the flexor digitorum profundus

MULTIPLE CHOICE REVIEW QUESTIONS

1. A penetrating wound to the axilla that severs the posterior cord of the brachial plexus would denervate which of the following?

    a. Serratus anterior
    b. Pronator teres
    c. Deltoid
    d. Biceps brachii
    e. Infraspinatus

2. Injury to which of the following nerves would most likely be associated with a "drooped shoulder"?

    a. Suprascapular
    b. Axillary
    c. Accessory
    d. Dorsal scapular
    e. Medial pectoral

3. Which of the following describes the medial cord of the brachial plexus?

    a. It is so named because it lies medial to the teres minor muscle.
    b. It supplies fibers to the ulnar, median, and radial nerves.
    c. It gives rise to the lateral and medial pectoral nerves.
    d. It is posterior to the second part of the axillary artery.
    e. It typically contains fibers from spinal cord segments C8 and T1 only.

4. Which of the following muscles is able to compensate in part for paralysis of the supinator muscle?

    a. Brachialis
    b. Brachioradialis
    c. Flexor carpi ulnaris
    d. Biceps brachii
    e. Anconeus

5. Which of the following complications is most likely to result from a fracture of the mid-shaft of the humerus?

    a. Wrist drop
    b. Claw hand
    c. Headwaiter's tip hand
    d. Erb-Duchenne palsy
    e. Klumpke's paralysis

6. All of the following are considered to be "rotator cuff" muscles *except* which of the following?

    a. Teres major
    b. Teres minor
    c. Subscapularis
    d. Supraspinatus
    e. Infraspinatus

7. Your patient has fractured the medial epicondyle of his left humerus. The ulnar nerve has been injured, with some loss of muscle function in his left hand. Which of the following muscles was most likely *not* affected?

    a. Opponens pollicis
    b. Flexor digiti minimi
    c. Fourth lumbrical
    d. First palmar interosseus
    e. First dorsal interosseus

8. Your patient has some loss of sensation over the dorsum of the hand but has normal feeling over all of the little finger. He exhibits no "wrist drop." Which nerve has likely been damaged?

    a. Median
    b. Lateral antebrachial cutaneous
    c. Posterior antebrachial cutaneous
    d. Superficial branch of radial
    e. Deep branch of radial

Questions 9 through 11

    a. Brachial artery
    b. Radial artery
    c. Ulnar artery

For each description select the artery that best matches the description.

9. Gives rise to the common interosseus artery

10. Terminates in the cubital fossa

11. Passes between the heads of the first dorsal interosseus muscle

Chapter 3

Lower Extremity

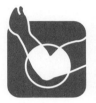

■ **Bones of the Lower Extremity**

● **Pelvic girdle (Fig. 3.1)**

- Through its connection with the axial skeleton, the pelvic girdle transmits the weight of the body to the lower extremity.

- The pelvic girdle contributes to the bony **protective** walls of the pelvic cavity.

- It consists of three separate bones, the **pubis,** the **ilium,** and the **ischium,** which fuse after puberty to form the **coxal,** or **hip bone.**

- Fusion of the three bones is centered at the **acetabulum,** the cup-shaped depression that receives the head of the femur.

- The paired hip bones articulate with each other at the **pubic symphysis** and with the sacrum at the **sacroiliac joint** to form the **bony pelvis.**

— *Pubis*

- Forms the anterior and medial part of the hip bone
- Consists of a **body,** a **superior ramus,** and an **inferior ramus**
- Body

  — **Articulates** with the opposite pubic bone at the **pubic symphysis**

  — On its upper border has a **pubic crest,** which expands laterally into the **pubic tubercle** (for attachment of the inguinal ligament)

- Superior ramus

  — Passes laterally to **articulate** with the **ilium and ischium** at the acetabulum

  — On its upper border has a **pubic pecten** (pectineal line), which passes laterally to become continuous with the **arcuate line** of the ilium

  — On its upper border has an **iliopubic eminence,** which marks the junction of the pubis and ilium

- Inferior ramus

  — Passes laterally, posteriorly, and inferiorly to fuse with the ramus of the ischium

— *Ilium*

- Forms the lateral part of the hip bone
- Consists of a **body** and a **wing** (ala)

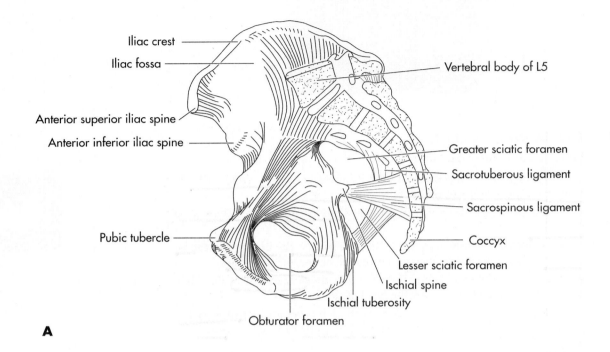

Iliac crest

Iliac fossa

Anterior superior iliac spine

Anterior inferior iliac spine

Pubic tubercle

Vertebral body of L5

Greater sciatic foramen

Sacrotuberous ligament

Sacrospinous ligament

Coccyx

Lesser sciatic foramen

Ischial spine

Ischial tuberosity

Obturator foramen

A

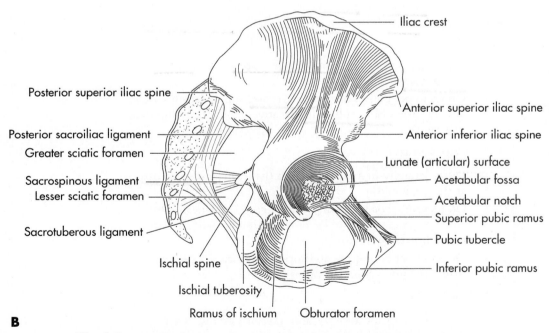

Posterior superior iliac spine

Posterior sacroiliac ligament

Greater sciatic foramen

Sacrospinous ligament

Lesser sciatic foramen

Sacrotuberous ligament

Ischial spine

Ischial tuberosity

Ramus of ischium

Obturator foramen

Iliac crest

Anterior superior iliac spine

Anterior inferior iliac spine

Lunate (articular) surface

Acetabular fossa

Acetabular notch

Superior pubic ramus

Pubic tubercle

Inferior pubic ramus

B

Fig. 3.1 Bony features of the pelvic girdle. **A,** Medial view. **B,** Lateral view.

- Body

  — Contributes to the formation of the acetabulum
  — Has no named features

- Wing

  — Has a thickened upper border, the **iliac crest,** which ends anteriorly as the **anterior superior iliac spine** (to which the inguinal ligament is attached) and posteriorly as the **posterior superior iliac spine**
  — Has a lateral surface presenting the **posterior, anterior, and inferior gluteal lines**, which mark the attachments of the **gluteal muscles**
  — Has a shallow, concave inner surface, the **iliac fossa,** for origin of the iliacus muscle
  — Expands posteriorly to form the medial, ear-shaped, **auricular surface,** which forms the synovial joint with the sacrum
  — Has an **anterior inferior iliac spine** for attachment of the **rectus femoris** muscle and **iliofemoral ligament**
  — Has a **posterior inferior iliac spine** lying at the upper posterior border of the greater sciatic notch

— *Ischium*

  - Forms the posterior and inferior part of the hip bone
  - Consists of a **body and a ramus**
  - Body

    — Contributes to the formation of the acetabulum
    — Has a posteriorly projecting **ischial spine** for attachment of the **sacrospinous ligament**
    — Has an inferiorly projecting **ischial tuberosity** for attachment of the **hamstring muscles**
    — Presents a **lesser sciatic notch** between the ischial spine and the ischial tuberosity
    — Above the ischial spine joins the posterior border of the ilium to form the **greater sciatic notch**

  - **Ramus**

    — Fuses with the inferior ramus of the pubis forming the **ischiopubic ramus**

— *Acetabulum*

  - Is the cup-shaped depression on the outer surface of the hip bone that receives the head of the femur
  - Is formed by the ilium, the ischium, and the pubis
  - Faces downward, forward, and laterally
  - Has a horseshoe-shaped **articular** surface, the **lunate surface,** which is covered with hyaline cartilage
  - Has a depression in the floor, the **acetabular fossa,** which is roughened and **nonarticular**
  - Has an incomplete inferior margin at the **acetabular notch**

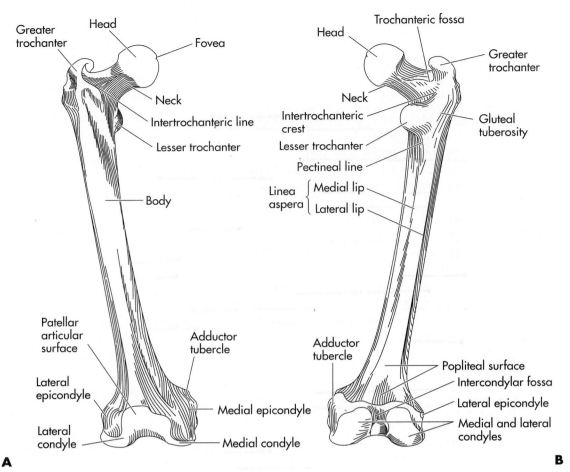

Fig. 3.2 Bony features of the femur. **A,** Anterior view. **B,** Posterior view.

● Femur (Fig. 3.2)

  • **Head**

    — Is ball-like, forming about two thirds of a sphere
    — Is directed upward, medially, and somewhat forward to articulate with the acetabulum of the hip bone
    — Has a small central depression in the articular surface, the **fovea capitis,** for attachment of the **ligament of the head**
    — Is covered by hyaline **cartilage** except at the fovea capitis

  • **Neck**

    — Connects the head to the shaft (body)
    — Is directed downward, laterally, and somewhat posterior
    — Forms an **angle of inclination** of about 125 degrees with the shaft
    — Is a **common site for fractures** of the femur

- Greater trochanter

  — Is a large projection on the upper and lateral surface of the shaft at its junction with the neck
  — Provides attachments for the **gluteus medius, gluteus minimus, and piriformis muscles**
  — On its medial surface has a **trochanteric fossa** for insertion of the **obturator internus tendon**

- Lesser trochanter

  — Is a smaller projection on the posterior and medial surface of the shaft in the angle formed with the neck
  — Provides attachment for the iliopsoas muscle

- Intertrochanteric line

  — Connects the greater and lesser trochanters anteriorly
  — Marks the junction of the neck and the shaft anteriorly
  — Provides attachment for the **iliofemoral ligament**

- Intertrochanteric crest

  — Connects the greater and lesser trochanters posteriorly
  — Marks the junction of the neck and the shaft posteriorly
  — Has a prominent **quadrate tubercle**, which provides attachment for the **quadratus femoris** muscle

- Linea aspera

  — Is a roughened longitudinal line on the **posterior** aspect of the **shaft**, which is otherwise smooth
  — Provides attachment for the **muscles of the thigh and the intermuscular septa**
  — Has a **lateral lip**, which expands proximally near the greater trochanter as the **gluteal tuberosity** (for attachment of the **gluteus maximus**) and is continuous distally with the **lateral supracondylar ridge**
  — Has a **medial lip**, which begins proximally near the lesser trochanter as the **pectineal line** (for attachment of the **pectineus muscle**) and is continuous distally with the **medial supracondylar ridge**

- Medial and lateral femoral condyles

  — Form the distal end of the femur
  — Articulate below with the condyles of the **tibia** and participate in the **knee joint**
  — Are covered on their articular surface by **hyaline cartilage**
  — Blend anteriorly to form the articular surface for the **patella**
  — Are separated posteriorly and inferiorly by the **intercondylar notch**
  — Expand above as the medial and lateral epicondyles

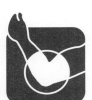

- **Adductor tubercle**

  — Is a prominence on the medial epicondyle

  — Provides attachment for the **adductor magnus muscle**

- **Popliteal surface**

  — Lies between the lips of the linea aspera distally

  — Forms the floor of the **popliteal fossa**

● **Patella**

  - Is the largest bone to develop within the tendon of a muscle (i.e., a **sesamoid bone**)
  - Lies within the tendon of the quadriceps femoris muscle
  - Articulates with the medial and lateral condyles of the femur but not with the tibia
  - Is triangular in shape with a convex upper border and the apex lying inferiorly
  - Is connected to the **tibial tuberosity** by the **patellar ligament,** a continuation of the quadriceps tendon

● **Tibia (Fig. 3.3)**

  - Is the **weight-bearing** bone of the leg
  - Has an expanded upper end for **articulation** with the condyles of the **femur**
  - Has an expanded lower end for **articulation** with the trochlea of the **talus**
  - **Articulates** proximally with the **head** and distally with the **lower end** of the **fibula**
  - **Medial and lateral tibial condyles**

    — Form the expanded proximal end of the tibia

    — Have smooth and slightly concave articular surfaces

    — Are separated from anterior to posterior by the **anterior inter-condylar area,** the **intercondylar eminence** (having medial and lateral intercondylar tubercles), and the **posterior inter-condylar area**

  - **Tibial tuberosity**

    — Is located anteriorly at the junction of the lateral condyle and shaft

    — Provides attachment for the **patellar ligament**

  - **Shaft**

    — Is roughly triangular in cross section; has **medial, lateral, and posterior surfaces** separated by **anterior, medial, and interosseus borders**

    — Is thinnest (and most likely to be fractured) at the junction of the middle and lower thirds

    — Marks the tibial attachment of the soleus muscle

  - **Medial surface**

    — Is broad, subcutaneous, and readily palpable

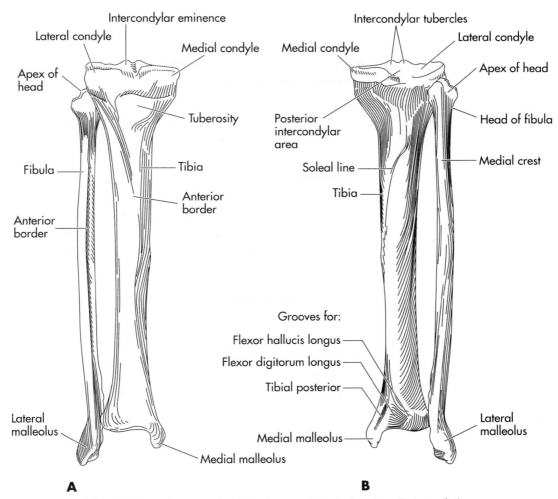

Fig. 3.3 Bony features of the leg bones. **A,** Anterior view. **B,** Lateral view.

- **Lateral and posterior surfaces**

  — Are nonpalpable
  — Provide attachment for muscles of the leg

- **Anterior border**

  — Is subcutaneous and readily palpable
  — Begins laterally at the tibial tuberosity and extends medially and downward to end at the medial malleolus

- **Lateral border**

  — Gives attachment to the interosseus membrane, which joins the tibia and fibula

- **Soleal line**

  — Is located posteriorly on the upper third of the shaft passing obliquely downward from the lateral side
  — Marks the tibial attachment of the soleus muscle

- **Medial malleolus**
  - Is the inferiorly projecting process on the medial side of the expanded lower end of the tibia
  - Is **subcutaneous,** forming the prominent and palpable eminence at the **medial** side of the **ankle**
  - **Articulates** on its lateral surface with the trochlea of the **talus**
  - Is grooved posteriorly by the **tendon** of the **tibialis posterior** muscle (grooves for the flexor hallucis longus and the flexor digitorum longus are on the lower end of the tibia rather than the medial malleolus)

- **Fibular notch**
  - Is the depression on the **lateral side** of the distal end of the tibia for **articulation** with the distal end of the **fibula**

- **Articular facet for the talus**
  - Occupies the distal surface of the tibia and the lateral side of the medial malleolus

- **Fibula (see Fig. 3.3)**
  - Is the **non–weight-bearing** bone of the leg
  - **Articulates** proximally with the lateral condyle of the tibia and distally with the lower end of the tibia and the talus
  - Participates in the ankle joint but **not** in the knee joint
  - **Head**
    - Is the expanded **proximal** end
    - Has a small facet for **articulation** with the lateral condyle of the **tibia**
    - Is connected to the shaft by a slender **neck**
    - Forms a palpable prominence just below the knee on the lateral side

  - **Shaft**
    - Is slender and slightly twisted
    - Is nonpalpable except at its lower end where it becomes subcutaneous and continues as the lateral malleolus
    - Has an **interosseus border** on its medial surface for attachment of the **interosseus membrane**

  - **Lateral malleolus**
    - Is the expanded lower end of the fibula
    - Is **subcutaneous,** forming the prominent, palpable eminence at the **lateral** side of the **ankle**
    - **Articulates** on its medial surface with the trochlea of the **talus**

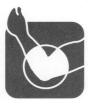

- **Bones of the foot (tarsus) (Fig. 3.4)**
  - Include the **tarsals,** the **metatarsals,** and the **phalanges**
  - *Tarsal bones (see Fig. 3.4)*
    - Are **seven** in number

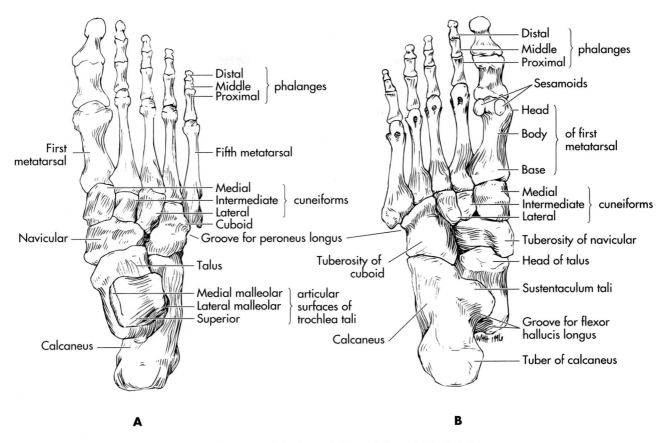

Fig. 3.4 Bones of the foot. **A,** Dorsal view. **B,** Ventral view.

- Are organized with the distal four bones (the cuboid and three cuneiforms) arranged in a row and the proximal three bones arranged irregularly
- Usually **begin ossification** before birth except for the cuneiforms and navicular, which begin at 3 or 4 years of age
- **Talus**

  — Transmits the weight of the body from the tibia to the foot

  — Is the only tarsal bone without muscular or tendinous attachments

  — Begins ossification during the seventh month in utero

  — Has an anterior-projecting **head,** which **articulates** with the **navicular** bone in front and the **calcaneus** and **calcaneonavicular** ligament below

  — Has a **body,** which articulates **above** (as the **trochlea**) with the **tibia and fibula** and **below** with the **calcaneus**

  — Is **grooved** on the posterior body by the **tendon of the flexor hallucis longus** muscle

  — Has **three facets** for articulation with the **calcaneus**

  — Has a deep groove on the inferior body, the **sulcus tali,** which separates the middle and posterior facets for articulation with the calcaneus

- **Calcaneus**

  — Is the **largest** bone of the foot
  — Forms the **heel** of the foot
  — Begins ossification during the sixth month in utero
  — **Articulates** with the **talus** above and the **cuboid** in front
  — Has **three facets** for articulation with the **talus**
  — Has a medial projection, the **sustentaculum tali,** which bears the middle facet for **articulation** with the **talus** and which is **grooved** by the **flexor hallucis longus tendon**
  — Projects posteriorly and inferiorly as the **tuber calcanei,** which supports the weight on the heel
  — Has a deep groove on the upper surface, the **sulcus calcanei,** which separates the middle and posterior facets for articulation with the talus
  — Contributes to formation of the **sinus tarsi,** a space formed by the approximation of **sulcus calcanei** and **sulcus tali** that houses the strong **interosseous talocalcaneal ligament**
  — On its lateral surface has a **peroneal tubercle,** which marks the divergence of the tendons of the **peroneus longus** and the **peroneus brevis**

- **Navicular**

  — Has a concave proximal surface for articulation with the **talus**
  — Has a convex distal surface for articulation with the three **cuneiform** bones
  — Has a prominent, medial **tuberosity** to which most of the **tibialis posterior tendon** is attached

- **Cuboid**

  — **Articulates** proximally with the **calcaneus,** distally with the **lateral two metatarsals,** and medially with the **lateral cuneiform**
  — Is **grooved** on its lateral and plantar surfaces by the **tendon of the peroneus longus muscle**
  — Has a prominent **tuberosity** lying posterior to the lateral end of the groove for the peroneus longus tendon
  — Begins ossification at about the time of birth

- **Medial cuneiform**

  — Is the **largest** of the three cuneiform bones
  — **Articulates** proximally with the **navicular,** distally with the **medial two metatarsals,** and laterally with the **intermediate cuneiform**

- **Intermediate cuneiform**

  — Is the **smallest** of the three cuneiform bones
  — **Articulates** proximally with the **navicular,** distally with

the **second metatarsal,** medially with the **medial cuneiform,** and laterally with the **lateral cuneiform**

- Lateral cuneiform

    — Is **triangular** with the base lying distally
    — **Articulates** proximally with the **navicular,** medially with the **intermediate cuneiform,** laterally with the **cuboid,** and distally mostly with the **second metatarsal** and to a small extent the second and fourth metatarsals

— *Metatarsal bones (see Fig. 3.4)*

- Are the **five** long bones of the **foot**
- Are numbered **1 to 5** from the **great toe to the little toe**
- Have a proximal **base,** a **shaft,** and a distal **head**
- Articulate at their **base** with the distal row of **tarsal bones**
- Articulate at their **head** with the **proximal phalanges**
- Have **facets** at their bases for articulation with the **adjacent metacarpal** (except between the first and second)
- Begin **ossification** at the shaft in the **second to third month** in utero
- First metacarpal

    — Articulates with the **medial cuneiform**
    — Is **shorter and stouter** than the other metatarsals
    — Has a **tuberosity** on the plantar surface of the base for attachment of the peroneus longus tendon

- Second metacarpal

    — Articulates with **all three cuneiform** bones
    — Is the **longest** metacarpal

- Third metacarpal

    — Articulates with the **lateral cuneiform**

- Fourth metatarsal

    — Articulates with the cuboid

- Fifth metatarsal

    — Articulates with the cuboid
    — Has a tuberosity that projects posteriorly from the lateral side of the **fifth metatarsal,** providing attachment for the tendon of the **peroneus brevis**

— *Phalanges (see Fig. 3.4)*

- Are the miniature long bones of the **toes**
- Are **two for the great toe** and **three for the remaining toes**
- Have a proximal **base,** a **shaft,** and a distal **head**
- Begin **ossification** at the shaft in the **third month** in utero

■ Joints of the Lower Extremity

● Sacroiliac joint (see Fig. 3.1)

- Is the only joint between the **pelvic girdle** and the **axial skeleton**

- Is the joint between the **sacrum** and the **auricular surface of the ilium**
- Transfers the **weight** of the upper body to the **lower extremity**
- Is a **synovial joint** with closely applied irregular surfaces allowing for little movement
- Is surrounded by a short, tight fibrous capsule
- Is reinforced by a series of **ligaments** that **stabilize** the joint and further **reduce movement,** including the

    — Short and strong **interosseus ligament,** which connects the **iliac tuberosity** with the **sacral tuberosity**
    — **Dorsal sacroiliac ligament,** which runs downward and medially superficial to and blending with the interosseus ligament
    — **Ventral sacroiliac ligament,** a relatively broad, thin sheet uniting the bones in front of the joint
    — **Iliolumbar ligament,** which joins the transverse process of the fifth lumbar vertebrae to the posterior end of the iliac crest
    — **Sacrospinous ligament,** which connects the side and posterior surface of the **sacrum and coccyx** with the **ischial spine** and **separates the greater and lesser sciatic foramina**
    — **Sacrotuberous ligament** which connects the posterior surface of the **sacrum** with the **ischial tuberosity** thus forming the **medial border of the greater and lesser sciatic foramina**

- **Pubic symphysis**

    - Is the joint in the midline anteriorly between the two hip bones
    - Is a **fibrocartilaginous joint** consisting of a **fibrocartilaginous interpubic disc** connecting the symphyseal surfaces of the bodies of the pubic bones
    - Is reinforced above by the **superior pubic ligament** and below by the **arcuate pubic ligament**
    - Is relatively **immovable** except in the latter stages of **pregnancy,** when hormones cause the ligaments to loosen

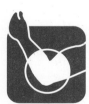

- **Hip joint** (see Figs. 3.1 and 3.2)

    - Is a **synovial ball-and-socket joint** between the **head of the femur** and the **acetabulum** of the hip bone
    - Joins the **lower extremity** to the **pelvic girdle**
    - Is arranged to favor **stability over mobility**
    - Has a fibrocartilage rim, the **labrum acetabulare,** which

        — **Deepens** the acetabular socket and grips the head of the femur
        — Continues across the acetabular notch as the **transverse acetabular ligament**

    - Is surrounded by a **fibrous capsule,** which

        — Is relatively **tight** and restricts **free movement**
        — Encloses the head and most of the neck
        — **Proximally** attaches to the **acetabulum** and the **transverse acetabular ligament**
        — **Distally** attaches laterally to the medial aspect of the **greater**

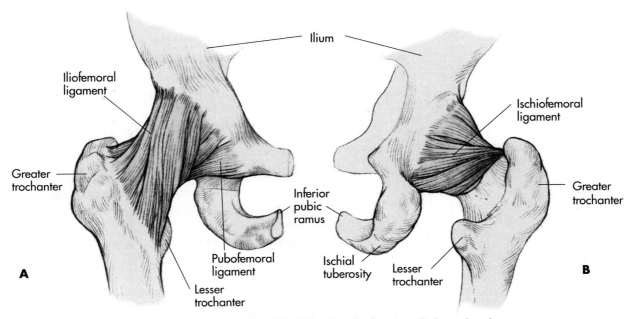

Fig. 3.5 Ligaments of the hip joint. **A,** Anterior view. **B,** Posterior view.

trochanter, anteriorly to the **intertrochanteric line**, and posteriorly to the **base of the neck**

— Is **reinforced** by three strong ligaments extending from the hip bone to the femur, the **iliofemoral, ischiofemoral,** and **pubofemoral** ligaments

• Has a **synovial membrane,** which lines the **fibrous capsule,** covers the fat in the **acetabular fossa,** and excludes the **ligament of the head of the femur** from the joint cavity

• Is most often **dislocated posteriorly** as a result of a severe blow to the knee while the hip is flexed (usually in a head-on automobile accident)

• Has a **wide range of movement,** including flexion and extension, abduction and adduction, and medial and lateral rotation

• Is supplied by the superior and inferior **gluteal,** medial and lateral **femoral circumflex,** and **obturator arteries**

• Is supplied largely by the **femoral and obturator nerves** and to a much lesser extent by the nerve to the quadratus femoris and the superior gluteal nerve

• **Iliofemoral ligament** (Fig. 3.5)

— Is the **strongest** and most important ligament of the hip joint

— Appears as a broad **inverted Y** reinforcing the capsule **anteriorly**

— Attaches proximally to the **anterior inferior iliac spine** and distally along the **intertrochanteric line**

— Strongly **resists hyperextension** and **medial rotation** of the hip joint

— When taut can **balance the trunk on the femoral head** with little activity of the iliopsoas

- **Ischiofemoral ligament** (see Fig. 3.5)

  — Supports the posterior part of the hip joint
  — Is the **thinnest** of the ligaments of the hip joint
  — Arises proximally from the **ischium** near the posterior rim of the acetabulum and spirals forward to attach to the **base of the neck** medial to the greater trochanter
  — **Resists extension** and **medial rotation** of the hip joint

- **Pubofemoral ligament** (see Fig. 3.5)

  — Supports the anterior and inferior part of the hip joint
  — Arises proximally from the **pubis** near the inferior rim of the acetabulum and attaches to the **base of the neck** just above to the lesser trochanter
  — **Resists excessive abduction** of the hip joint

- **Ligament of the head of the femur**

  — Is a flattened band running from the fovea on the head of the femur to the transverse acetabular ligament and the margins of the acetabular notch
  — Probably functions to **resist adduction** of the hip joint in children but not adults
  — Is excluded from the hip joint by the covering synovial membrane
  — Transmits the **artery to the head of the femur** (from the obturator artery), which is an important source of blood to the femoral head in children

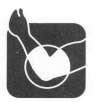

● Knee joint (Fig. 3.6)

  - Is a **synovial hinge joint** of the condylar variety
  - Permits **flexion** and **extension,** with the last part of extension being accompanied by medial **rotation** of the femur on the tibia
    - Consists of

      — An articulation between the **condyles** of the **femur** and the **tibia**
      — An articulation between the **condyles** of the **femur** and the **patella**

  - Is supplied primarily by the **genicular branches** of the **popliteal artery**
  - Is supplied largely by the **femoral, obturator, tibial,** and **peroneal** nerves
  - Is **strengthened medially and laterally** by strong **collateral ligaments**
  - Is **reinforced medially** by the **tendons** of the sartorius, gracilis, semitendinosus, semimembranosus, and medial head of the gastrocnemius muscles
  - Is **reinforced laterally** by the **tendons** of the sartorius, gracilis, semitendinosus, semimembranosus, and medial head of the gastrocnemius muscles

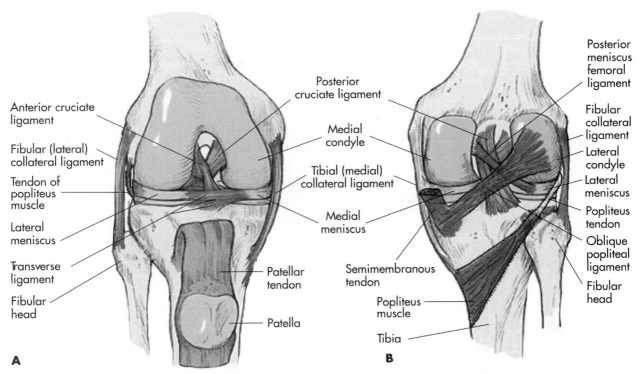

Fig. 3.6 Knee joint opened. **A,** Anterior view. **B,** Posterior view.

- Capsule

  — Is thin, weak, and incomplete

  — Attaches to the margins of the femoral and tibial condyles

  — Is **replaced anteriorly** by the lower part of the **quadriceps tendon,** the **patella,** and the **patellar ligament**

  — Is **deficient** posteriorly and inferiorly, where the **tendon of the popliteus** muscle **penetrates** the **capsule** to pass to its insertion on the tibia; **thickened** portion of the **capsule** above the popliteus tendon is the **arcuate ligament**

  — Is **reinforced** posteriorly by the **oblique popliteal ligament,** an upward and lateral extension of the **semimembranosus tendon;** together they help **resist hyperextension** of the knee

  — Is **reinforced** medially by the **tibial collateral ligament**

  — *Ligaments and menisci (Figs. 3.5 and 3.7)*

    - Tibial collateral ligament

      — Is a broad flat band

      — Extends from the **medial femoral epicondyle** to the **medial tibial condyle**

      — Blends with and **reinforces** the medial part of the **fibrous capsule**

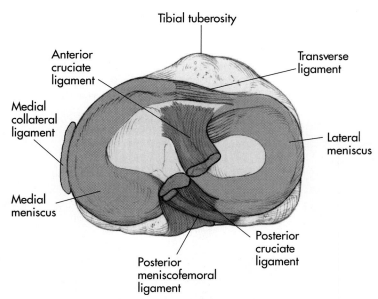

Fig. 3.7 Proximal end of tibia.

— Is firmly **attached to** the **medial meniscus**
— Is a particularly **important stabilizer** of the knee joint because it is taut throughout the range of the joint

• **Fibular collateral ligament**

— Is a rounded cord
— Extends from the **lateral femoral epicondyle** to the **head of the fibula**
— Is distinctly separate from the joint capsule
— Does **not** attach to the **lateral meniscus**
— Is **taut** and stabilizes the joint best when the knee is **fully extended**

• **Anterior cruciate ligament**

— Lies within the fibrous capsule but **outside the synovial cavity**
— Is named for its attachment to the **anterior** intercondylar area of the tibia
— Passes posteriorly, superiorly, and laterally to the medial surface of the lateral femoral condyle
— Limits anterior movement of the tibia on the femur (or posterior movement of the femur on the tibia)
— Is maximally **taut** and stabilizes the joint best when the knee is **fully extended**

• **Posterior cruciate ligament**

— Lies within the fibrous capsule but **outside the synovial cavity**

— Is named for its attachment to the **posterior** intercondylar area of the tibia

— Passes anteriorly, superiorly, and medially to the medial surface of the medial femoral condyle

— Limits posterior movement of the tibia on the femur (or anterior movement of the femur on the tibia)

— Is maximally **taut** and stabilizes the joint best when the knee is **fully extended**

- **Medial meniscus**

— Is a tough **fibrocartilage** wedge in the **shape of a wide C**

— Is **anchored** anteriorly and posteriorly to the **intercondylar area** of the tibia

— Is **anchored** at its periphery to the **fibrous capsule**

— **Increases** the **congruity** between the medial tibial and femoral condyles and may **cushion** compression forces

— Is **more frequently injured** than the lateral meniscus

- **Lateral meniscus**

— Is a tough **fibrocartilage** wedge in the shape of a **closed C**

— Is **anchored** anteriorly and posteriorly to the **intercondylar area** of the tibia

— Is **anchored** at its periphery to the **fibrous capsule** except posteriorly, where it is separated from the capsule by the **popliteus tendon**

— **Increases** the **congruity** between the lateral tibial and femoral condyles and may **cushion** compression forces

— Is **less frequently injured** than the medial meniscus because it is more mobile and lacks the tight peripheral attachment to the capsule and collateral ligament

- **Coronary ligament**

— Is the part of the fibrous capsule between the menisci and the tibial condyles

- **Transverse ligament**

— Variably joins the medial and lateral menisci anteriorly in front of the anterior cruciate ligament

— *Synovial membrane and bursae*

- The synovial cavity is a **horseshoe-shaped cavity** that communicates anterior to the intercondylar area (and thus **excludes the cruciate ligaments**). It commonly communicates with **synovial bursae** around the knee.

- The **suprapatellar bursa** is an upward extension of the synovial cavity lying **between** the lower end of the shaft of the **femur** and the **quadriceps muscle and tendon**. At its proximal extent it receives the insertion of the **articularis genus muscle**.

- The **prepatellar bursa** lies between the superficial surface of the patella and the skin.

- The **infrapatellar bursa** consists of a **subcutaneous infrapa-**

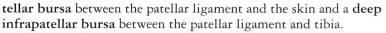

tellar bursa between the patellar ligament and the skin and a **deep infrapatellar bursa** between the patellar ligament and tibia.

    • The **anserine bursa** lies between the **pes anserinus** (the combined tendons of the sartorius, gracilis, and semitendinosus) and the tibial collateral ligament.

    • **Other bursae** around the knee are associated with the **attachments** of the **popliteus, semimembranosus, biceps femoris,** and the medial and lateral heads of the **gastrocnemius** muscle.

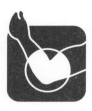

●   Talocrural (ankle) joint (see Figs. 3.3 and 3.4)

    • Is a **synovial hinge joint**

    • Moves on a single plane, allowing **dorsiflexion** (flexion) and **plantar flexion** (extension)

    • Is the joint formed **between** the distal ends of the **tibia** and **fibula** and the trochlea of the **talus**

    • Transmits the weight of the body to the talus

    • Is **most stable in dorsiflexion** because the trochlea tali is wider anteriorly

    • **Capsule**

      — Is thin and loose anteriorly and posteriorly to accommodate movement of the joint

      — Is lined by **synovial membrane**

      — Is **reinforced medially and laterally** by strong collateral ligaments

    • **Medial (deltoid) ligament**

      — Is a strong, triangular ligament with its **apex** attached superiorly to the **medial malleolus**

      — Separates inferiorly into **four parts:** a **tibionavicular part** with attachment to the tuberosity of the navicular bone, a **tibiocalcaneal part** with attachment to the sustentaculum tali, and **anterior** and **posterior tibiotalar parts** with attachment to the medial surface of the talus

      — Resists eversion of the foot

      — May be damaged by extreme eversion of the foot

      — Is so tough that the tip of the corresponding malleolus may fracture without tearing of the ligament

    • **Lateral ligament**

      — Consists of three separate ligaments attached superiorly to the **lateral malleolus:** the **anterior talofibular ligament,** which attaches to the neck of the talus; the **posterior talofibular ligament,** which attaches to the lateral tubercle of the talus; and the **calcaneofibular ligament,** which attaches to the lateral surface of the calcaneus

      — **Resists inversion** of the foot

      — May be damaged by extreme inversion of the foot (particularly the anterior talofibular ligament)

— Is so tough that the tip of the corresponding malleolus may fracture without tearing of the ligament

● **Talocalcaneal (subtalar) joint (see Fig. 3.4)**

- Consists of the **posterior talocalcaneal joint** (posteriorly) and the talocalcaneal part of the **talocalcaneonavicular joint** (anteriorly)
- Is supported by the tough **interosseus talocalcanean ligament,** which fills the **sinus tarsi**
- **Allows** the important movements of **inversion** and **eversion**

● **Talocalcaneonavicular (subtalar) joint**

- Consists of the articulation of the head of the **talus** with the **calcaneus** at the anterior talocalcaneal joint and with the **navicular bone** and the **plantar calcaneonavicular ligament**
- Is defined by a **single joint cavity**
- Is supported by the **plantar calcaneonavicular ligament** (spring ligament), which connects the tuberosity of navicular bone and the sustentaculum tali and on which the **head of the talus** rests

● **Calcaneocuboid joint**

- Consists of the simple articulation between the calcaneus and the cuboid
- Is supported by the

— **Plantar calcaneocuboid** (short plantar) **ligament,** which runs from the calcaneal tuberosity to the plantar surface of the cuboid
— **Long plantar ligament,** which runs from the calcaneal tuberosity to the cuboid and middle three metatarsals
— **Tendon of the peroneus longus** muscle

● **Transverse tarsal joint**

- Is functional rather than an anatomical entity
- Consists of the **calcaneocuboid joint** and the talonavicular part of the **talocalcaneonavicular joint**
- Allows movement between the front and back of the foot
- Is important in **plantar flexion** and **dorsiflexion** and in **eversion** and **inversion**

● **Intertarsal and tarsometatarsal joints**

- Are stable synovial joints
- Are connected by **interosseus, dorsal,** and **plantar ligaments,** the strongest of which are the plantar ligaments, which contribute to the arched shape of the foot
- Allow **limited** sliding movements

● **Metatarsophalangeal and interphalangeal joints**

- Are similar to those of the hand
- Are synovial joints surrounded by articular capsules
- Are reinforced by collateral and plantar ligaments
- Allow mostly flexion and extension

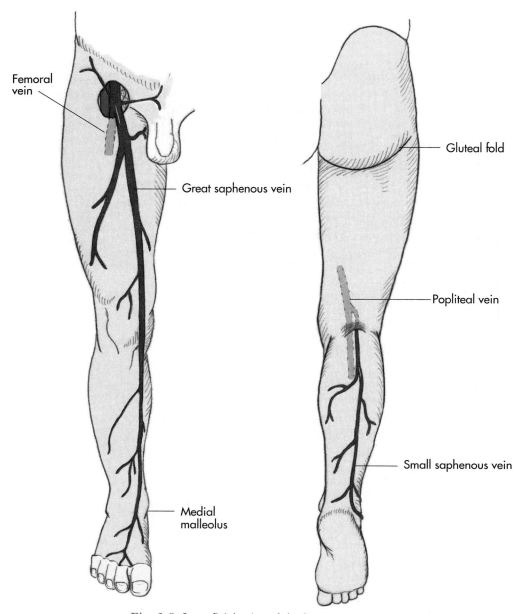

Femoral
vein

Great saphenous vein

Gluteal fold

Popliteal vein

Small saphenous vein

Medial
malleolus

Fig. 3.8 Superficial veins of the lower extremity.

■ Blood Vessels of the Lower Extremity

- ● Superficial veins of the lower extremity (Fig. 3.8)
  - • Dorsal venous arch
    - — Is an irregular venous network on the **dorsum of the foot**
    - — Forms from the **dorsal metatarsal veins** and veins from the sole of the foot via the **medial and lateral marginal veins**
    - — Is drained on the lateral side by the **small saphenous vein** and on the medial side by the **great saphenous vein**

- Small saphenous vein

  — Arises from the **lateral** side of the **dorsal venous arch**
  — Passes **posterior** to the **lateral malleolus**
  — Courses upward on the **posterior side** of the **leg** adjacent to the **sural nerve**
  — At the popliteal fossa pierces the **popliteal fascia** to end in the **popliteal vein**
  — Communicates with deep veins by way of **perforating veins**

- Great saphenous vein

  — Arises from the **medial** side of the **dorsal venous arch**
  — Passes **anterior** to the **medial malleolus**
  — Courses upward on the **medial side** of the leg and thigh
  — In the leg lies adjacent to the **saphenous nerve**
  — Pierces the fascia lata at the **saphenous opening** to end in the **femoral vein**
  — May be harvested for **coronary arterial bypass** surgery or used for **venipuncture** where it lies anterior to the medial malleolus
  — Has numerous **one-way valves** that promote the movement of blood toward the heart
  — Communicates with deep veins by way of **perforating veins**
  — Near its termination receives several tributaries, including the **external pudendal, superficial epigastric, superficial circumflex iliac,** and **accessory saphenous** veins

- Deep veins of the lower extremity
  - Venae comitantes

    — Are deep veins, usually **paired,** that run alongside arteries

  - Femoral vein

    — Is the **main venous structure** draining the **lower extremity**
    — Is formed at the **adductor hiatus** as an upward continuation of the **popliteal vein**
    — **Receives** the **great saphenous vein** and **deep veins** corresponding to the branches of the femoral artery
    — Lies **medial** to the **femoral artery**

- Lymphatics of the lower extremity
  - Lymphatics of the lower extremity can be classified into a **superficial group** and a **deep group.**
  - The **superficial lymph vessels** follow the **superficial veins.**

    — Lymph vessels following the **great saphenous vein** and its tributaries drain to the **superficial inguinal nodes.**
    — Lymph vessels following the **small saphenous vein** and its tributaries drain to the **popliteal nodes.**

  - The **deep lymph vessels** follow the **deep veins** of the lower extremity and drain either to the **popliteal nodes** or to the **deep inguinal nodes.**

- **Efferents** from both the **superficial inguinal nodes** and the deep inguinal nodes drain to **external iliac nodes** and eventually to the aortic nodes.

— *Superficial inguinal nodes*

- The superficial inguinal nodes lie superficial to the fascia lata just below the inguinal ligament.
- Nodes **lying along** the termination of the **great saphenous vein** receive lymph from the **thigh, foot,** and **leg.**
- Nodes that lie parallel to the **inguinal ligament** receive lymph from the **buttock, abdominal wall,** and **perineum.**

— *Deep inguinal nodes*

- Lie deep to the fascia lata just below the inguinal ligament
- Receive lymph from the deep structure of the thigh and leg
- Receive efferents from the popliteal nodes

● **Arteries of the lower extremity**

- The arterial supply to the lower extremity is summarized in Fig. 3.9.

● **Cutaneous innervation of the lower extremity (Fig. 3.10)**

- **Genital branch of the genitofemoral nerve** and the **ilioinguinal nerve** (from the **lumbar plexus**)

— Enter the thigh through the superficial inguinal ring
— Supply the skin **below** the medial part of the **inguinal ligament**

- **Cutaneous branch of the obturator nerve**

— Arises from the anterior branch of the obturator nerve
— Supplies the upper medial thigh

- **Medial and intermediate cutaneous nerves of the thigh** (from the femoral nerve)

— Become cutaneous below the inguinal ligament
— Supply the **anterior and medial thigh** to the knee

- **Lateral femoral cutaneous nerve** (from the **lumbar plexus**)

— Enters the thigh under the inguinal ligament near the anterior superior iliac spine
— Supplies the **anterior and lateral thigh** to the knee

- **Posterior femoral cutaneous nerve of the thigh** (from the sacral plexus)

— Emerges in the posterior thigh from under the inferior border of the gluteus maximus muscle
— Descends in the thigh deep to the fascia lata
— Supplies the skin of the **lower buttock, posterior thigh,** and **upper posterior leg**

- **Saphenous nerve** (from the femoral nerve)

— Descends in the adductor canal to the knee
— Becomes cutaneous at the knee between the tendons of the sartorius and gracilis

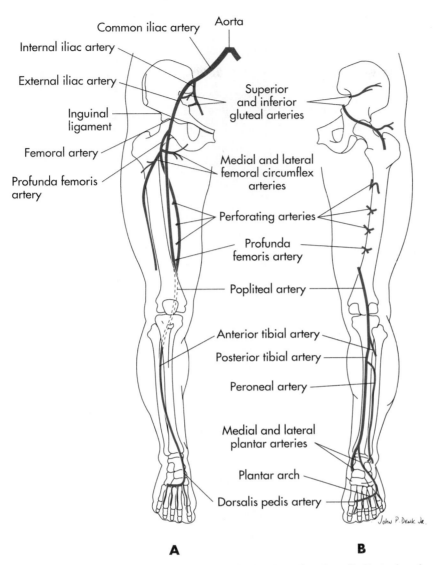

Fig. 3.9 Main arteries of the lower extremity. **A,** Anterior view. **B,** Posterior view.

— Descends on the medial leg with the great saphenous vein
— Supplies skin of the **medial leg and foot**

• **Lateral sural cutaneous nerve** (from the common peroneal)

— Arises in the popliteal fossa
— Supplies the skin on the **posterior and lateral leg**

• **Medial sural cutaneous nerve** (from the tibial nerve)

— Arises in the politeal fossa
— May be joined by the sural communicating branch from the common peroneal to form the **sural nerve**
— Is distributed over the **posterior leg onto the lateral heel and foot**

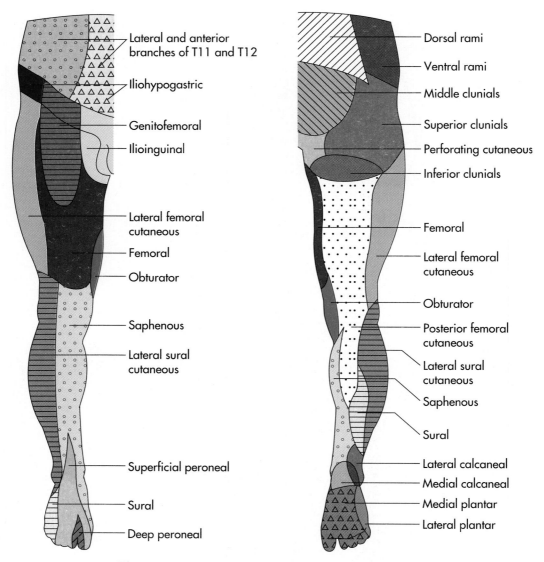

Fig. 3.10 Cutaneous innervation of the lower extremity.

- **Superficial peroneal nerve** (from the common peroneal nerve)

  — Emerges on the lateral leg between the anterior and lateral compartments

  — Descends down the leg and passes onto the foot to divide into **dorsal cutaneous nerves**

  — Supplies the lateral side of the lower leg, the dorsum of the foot, the medial side of the great toe, and adjacent sides of the second, third, and fourth toes

- **Deep peroneal nerve** (from the common peroneal)

  — Becomes cutaneous on the dorsum of the foot

  — Runs with the dorsalis pedis artery

Table 3.1 *Muscles of the Gluteal Region*				
NAME	ORIGIN	INSERTION	ACTION	INNERVATION
Gluteus maximus	Iliac crest, sacrum, coccyx, and sacro- tuberous ligament	Gluteal tuberosity of femur and iliotibial tract	Extends and laterally rotates the thigh	Inferior gluteal nerve
Gluteus medius	Ilium between the an- terior and posterior gluteal lines	Lateral side of greater trochanter of femur	Abducts and medially rotates the thigh	Superior gluteal nerve
Gluteus minimus	Ilium between ante- rior and inferior gluteal lines	Lateral side of greater trochanter of femur	Abducts and medially rotates the thigh	Superior gluteal nerve
Tensor fasciae latae	Anterior iliac crest be- hind the anterior su- perior iliac spine	Iliotibial tract	Flexes, abducts, and medially rotates the thigh	Superior gluteal nerve
Piriformis	Anterior surface of sacrum	Medial side of the upper end of the greater trochanter	Laterally rotates the thigh	Branches of the S1 and S2 root to the lumbosacral plexus
Obturator internus	Medial surface of the obturator membrane and adjacent hip bone	Medial side of the upper end of the greater trochanter	Laterally rotates the thigh	Nerve to the obtura- tor internus
Superior and inferior gemelli	Ischium above and below the lesser sci- atic notch	Obturator internus tendon	Laterally rotates the thigh	Superior: nerve to obturator internus Inferior: nerve to quadratus femoris
Quadratus femoris	Ischial tuberosity	Intertrochanteric crest and quadrate tu- bercle of femur	Laterally rotates the thigh	Nerve to quadratus femoris

— Divides into dorsal digital nerves to the adjacent sides of the first and second toes

Gluteal Region

- **Muscles of the gluteal region**
  - The muscles of the gluteal region are summarized in Table 3.1.

- **Nerves of the gluteal region**
  - *Superior gluteal nerve (L4, L5, S1)*
    - Emerges into the gluteal region through the greater sciatic fora- men **above the piriformis** muscle
    - Runs between the gluteus medius and minimus muscles along with the **superior gluteal artery**
    - Supplies the **gluteus medius** (superior branch) and the **gluteus minimus, tensor fasciae latae,** and **hip joint** (inferior branch)

  - *Inferior gluteal nerve (L5, S1, S2)*
    - Emerges into the gluteal region through the greater sciatic fora- men **below the piriformis** muscle
    - Runs with the **inferior gluteal artery** to supply the **gluteus maximus** muscle
  - *Sciatic nerve (L4, L5, S1, S2, S3)*
    - Is the largest branch of the **lumbosacral plexus** and, as well, is the **largest nerve** in the body

- Is actually two nerves, the **tibial nerve** and the **common peroneal nerve**, bound together by connective tissue
- Emerges into the gluteal region through the greater sciatic foramen **below the piriformis** muscle
- Descends **under** cover of the **gluteus maximus** muscle and **posterior** to the **obturator internus**, the **gemelli**, and the **quadratus femoris** muscles and **between** the **ischial tuberosity** and the **greater trochanter**
- Has **no branches** in the gluteal region **except** articular branches to the **hip joint**
- May be damaged by **posterior dislocations** of the hip or by **intramuscular injection** into the buttock

— *Posterior femoral cutaneous nerve (S1, S2, S3)*

- Emerges from the greater sciatic foramen **inferior** to the piriformis and descends on the posterior surface of the sciatic nerve
- Gives rise to the **inferior cluneal** nerves and a **perineal** branch.
- Descends in the posterior thigh under the **fascia lata;** becomes cutaneous at the popliteal fossa
- Supplies the skin of the **buttocks, posterior thigh, popliteal fossa,** and **external genitalia**

— *Nerve to the obturator internus (L5, S1, S2)*

- Emerges from the greater sciatic foramen inferior to the piriformis muscle
- Descends on the **superior gemellus** muscle to pass below the **ischial spine** and enter the **lesser sciatic foramen**
- Supplies the **superior gemellus** and **obturator internus** muscles

— *Nerve to the quadratus femoris (L4, L5, S1)*

- Enters the gluteal region through the greater sciatic foramen below the piriformis muscle and deep to the sciatic nerve
- Runs deep (anterior) to the **superior and inferior gemellus** and **obturator internus** muscles
- Supplies the **inferior gemellus** and **quadratus femoris** muscles

— *Pudendal nerve (S2, S3, S4)*

- Emerges from the greater sciatic foramen inferior to the piriformis muscle along with the **internal pudendal artery and vein**
- Descends posterior to the **ischial spine** and enters the **lesser sciatic foramen**
- Is distributed to the **perineum** and has **no branches** in the **gluteal region**

● Vessels of the gluteal region

— *Superior gluteal artery*

- Is the largest branch of the internal iliac artery
- Passes between the lumbosacral trunk and the ventral ramus of the first sacral nerve
- Emerges into the gluteal region through the greater sciatic fora-

men **above the piriformis** muscle and divides into **superficial** and **deep** branches

- **Superficial branch**

    — Ramifies to enter and supply the **gluteus maximus** muscle
    — Has no accompanying nerve

- **Deep branch**

    — Runs between the **gluteus minimus** and **medius** muscles
    — Divides into **superior and inferior branches,** which accompany the branches of the **superior gluteal nerve**

— *Inferior gluteal artery*

- Arises from the **internal iliac artery**
- Passes between the ventral rami of the **first** and **second** sacral nerves
- Emerges into the gluteal region through the greater sciatic foramen **below the piriformis** muscle
- Runs on the deep surface of the gluteus maximus muscle with the **inferior gluteal nerve**
- Supplies the **gluteal** and **hamstring** muscles and the **hip joint,** and participates in the **cruciate anastomosis**
- Gives rise to the important **companion artery to the sciatic nerve**

— *Internal pudendal artery*

- Emerges from the greater sciatic foramen inferior to the piriformis muscle along with the **pudendal artery**
- Descends posterior to the **ischial spine** and enters the **lesser sciatic foramen**
- At the ischial spine lies **lateral to the pudendal nerve** and **medial to the nerve to the obturator internus**
- Is distributed to the **perineum** and has **no branches in the gluteal region**

— *Gluteal veins*

- Are usually **double** and accompany the corresponding artery
- Are tributaries of the **internal iliac vein**
- Communicate with tributaries of the **femoral vein** and form an **alternative pathway** for return of blood from the lower extremity

● Important features of the gluteal region

— *Sacrotuberous ligament (see Fig. 3.1)*

- Connects the **posterior iliac spines,** the lower **sacrum,** and the **coccyx** to the ischial tuberosity
- Forms the **medial border of the greater and lesser sciatic foramina**

— *Sacrospinous ligament (see Fig. 3.1)*

- Connects the posterior surface of the **sacrum and coccyx** with the **ischial spine**

Table 3.2   *Muscles of Posterior Thigh*

Name	Origin	Insertion	Action	Innervation
Semitendinosus	Ischial tuberosity	Medial surface of upper tibia	Extends the thigh, flexes the knee, and rotates the leg medially	Tibial division of sciatic nerve
Semimembranosus	Ischial tuberosity	Medial condyle of tibia	Extends the thigh, flexes the knee, and rotates the leg medially	Tibial division of sciatic nerve
Biceps femoris	Long head: ischial tuberosity Short head: lateral lip of linea aspera	Head of fibula	Extends the thigh, flexes the knee, and rotates the leg laterally	Long head: tibial division of sciatic nerve Short head: common peroneal division of sciatic nerve

- • Separates the **greater** and **lesser sciatic foramina**
— *Greater and lesser sciatic foramina (see Fig. 3.1)*
    - • Are bony **notches** on the posterior **hip bone** that are converted to foramina by the **sacrotuberous** and **sacrospinous** ligaments
    - • In life are filled by **muscles, nerves, and vessels** passing from the **pelvis** to the **gluteal region** and **lower extremity**
    - • **Greater sciatic foramen** transmits the
        - — Piriformis muscle
        - — Sciatic nerve
        - — Superior gluteal nerves and vessels
        - — Inferior gluteal nerves and vessels
        - — Pudendal nerve
        - — Internal pudendal artery and vein
        - — Posterior femoral cutaneous nerve
        - — Nerve to the quadratus femoris
        - — Nerve to the obturator internus
    - • **Lesser sciatic foramen** transmits the
        - — Tendon of the obturator internus
        - — Nerve to the obturator internus
        - — Pudendal nerve
        - — Internal pudendal artery and vein

■ **Thigh**
- ● **Muscles of the thigh**
    - • The muscles of the posterior thigh are summarized in Table 3.2.
    - • The muscles of the anterior thigh are summarized in Table 3.3.
    - • The muscles of the medial thigh are summarized in Table 3.4.
- ● **Nerves of the thigh**
    - — *Femoral nerve (L2, L3, L4) (Fig. 3.11)*
        - • Is the largest branch of the **lumbar plexus**
        - • Forms in the substance of the **psoas major** muscle and emerges to lie between the psoas and iliacus muscles

Table 3.3 Muscles of the Anterior Thigh

NAME	ORIGIN	INSERTION	ACTION	INNERVATION
Iliacus	Iliac fossa	Lesser trochanter of femur	Flexes the thigh	Femoral nerve
Psoas major	T12 through L5 vertebrae and intervening intervertebral discs	Lesser trochanter of femur	Flexes the thigh	Ventral rami of L2 and L3
Sartorius	Anterior superior iliac spine	Tibial shaft below the medial condyle	Flexes and laterally rotates the thigh; flexes the knee joint	Femoral nerve
Rectus femoris*	Anterior inferior iliac spine and upper lip of the acetabulum	Patella; by patellar ligament to tibial tuberosity	Flexes the thigh, extends the knee joint	Femoral nerve
Vastus medialis*	Spiral line and the medial lip of the linea aspera of femur; medial intermuscular septum	Patella; by patellar ligament to tibial tuberosity	Extends the knee joint	Femoral nerve
Vastus lateralis*	Intertrochanteric line and lateral lip of the linea aspera; lateral intermuscular septum	Patella; by patellar ligament to tibial tuberosity	Extends the knee joint	Femoral nerve
Vastus intermedius*	Anterior and lateral surfaces of the upper two thirds of femoral shaft	Patella; by patellar ligament to tibial tuberosity	Extends the knee joint	Femoral nerve
Articularis genus	Anterior surface of the lower femoral shaft	Proximal border of the synovial membrane of the knee joint	Retracts the synovial membrane on extension of the knee joint	Femoral nerve

*These four muscles make up the quadriceps femoris.

Table 3.4 Muscles of the Medial Thigh

NAME	ORIGIN	INSERTION	ACTION	INNERVATION
Pectineus	Pectineal line of pubis	Spiral line of femur	Flexes and adducts the thigh	Femoral and obturator nerves
Obturator externus	Lateral surface of the obturator membrane and adjacent hip bone	Trochanteric fossa of femur	Laterally rotates the thigh	Obturator nerve
Gracilis	Body and inferior ramus of pubis	Tibial shaft below the medial condyle	Adducts the thigh; flexes and medially rotates the knee	Obturator nerve
Adductor longus	Body of pubis below the pubic crest	Middle one third of the linea aspera of femur	Adducts and laterally rotates the thigh	Obturator nerve
Adductor brevis	Inferior pubic ramis	Upper part of the linea aspera	Adducts and laterally rotates the thigh	Obturator nerve
Adductor magnus	Ischiopubic ramus	Adductor portion: entire length of the linea aspera; Hamstrings portion: adductor tubercle	Adductor portion: adducts and laterally rotates the thigh; Hamstrings portion: extends the thigh	Adductor portion: obturator nerve; Hamstrings portion: tibial division of the sciatic nerve

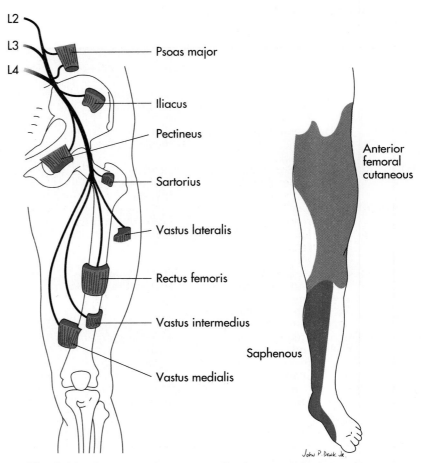

Fig. 3.11 Muscular and cutaneous distribution of the femoral nerve.

- Enters the **femoral triangle** by passing deep to the inguinal ligament
- In the upper femoral triangle branches into terminal **muscular** and **cutaneous** branches
- Gives **articular branches** to both the **hip** and **knee** joints
- **Cutaneous branches** include the

  — Medial cutaneous nerve of the thigh
  — Intermediate cutaneous nerve of the thigh
  — Saphenous nerve

- **Saphenous nerve**

  — Descends through the thigh in the **adductor canal** along with the **femoral artery**
  — Becomes cutaneous at the knee between the sartorius and gracilis tendons
  — Gives an infrapatellar branch and then descends to supply the skin on the medial side of the leg, ankle, and foot

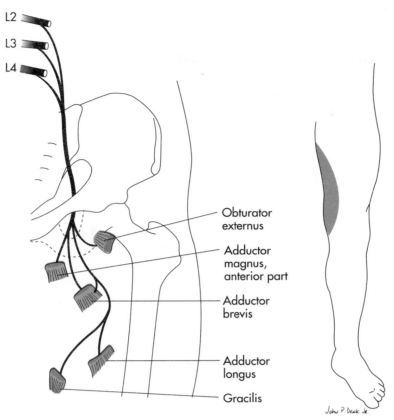

L2

L3

L4

Obturator
externus

Adductor
magnus,
anterior part

Adductor
brevis

Adductor
longus

Gracilis

John P. Denk Jr.

Fig. 3.12 Muscular and cutaneous distribution of the obturator nerve.

— Is the only branch of the femoral nerve to extend below
the knee

• **Muscular branches** innervate the

— Iliacus muscle

— Sartorius muscle

— Pectineus muscle (also receives a branch from the **obturator
nerve**)

— Quadriceps femoris muscles (vastus medialis, vastus intermedius, vastus lateralis, and rectus femoris)

— Articularis genus muscle

• Is particularly **susceptible to injury** because it lies superficially
just below the **inguinal ligament**

— *Obturator nerve (L2, L3, L4) (Fig. 3.12)*

• Forms in the substance of the **psoas major** and emerges on its
medial side to enter the pelvis

• Enters the thigh through the **obturator foramen** along with
the **obturator artery and vein**

- Within the **obturator canal** divides into **anterior** and **posterior branches**
- **Anterior branch**
  - Descends in the adductor compartment **between** the **adductor longus** and **adductor brevis** muscles
  - Provides muscular branches to the **adductor longus, adductor brevis, gracilis,** and **pectineus** muscles (pectineus may also receive a branch from the femoral nerve)
  - Gives a **cutaneous** branch to the **medial thigh**
- **Posterior branch**
  - Descends in the adductor compartment **between** the **adductor brevis** and **adductor magnus** muscles
  - Provides muscular branches to the **obturator externus, adductor brevis,** and **adductor magnus** muscles
- Gives **articular branches** to both the **hip** and **knee** joints

— *Sciatic nerve (L4, L5, S1, S2, S3)*

- Descends in the posterior thigh deep to the long head of the **biceps femoris** muscle
- Separates in the lower third of the thigh into the **tibial nerve** and the **common peroneal nerves**
- **Tibial nerve** (Fig. 3.13)
  - Is the principal nerve to the **posterior thigh, posterior leg,** and **sole of the foot**
  - In the thigh, provides muscular branches to the **semitendinosus, semimembranosus, long head of the biceps femoris,** and lower fibers of the **adductor magnus** (hamstrings portion)
- **Common peroneal nerve**
  - Innervates the **short head of the biceps femoris** muscle

● **Vessels of the thigh region**

— *Femoral artery (see Fig. 3.9)*

- Begins deep to the **inguinal ligament** as a continuation of the **external iliac artery** and ends in the **adductor hiatus** as the **popliteal artery**
  - Is enclosed in the **femoral sheath** along with the **femoral vein**
  - Descends through the femoral triangle **lateral to the femoral vein** and **medial to the femoral nerve**
  - Close to its origin gives rise to the **superficial epigastric artery,** the **superficial circumflex iliac artery,** and the **superficial external pudendal artery**
  - Deep branches include the **deep external pudendal artery,** the **profunda femoris artery,** and the **descending genicular artery**

Superficial epigastric artery

  - Becomes superficial passing through or close to the saphenous hiatus

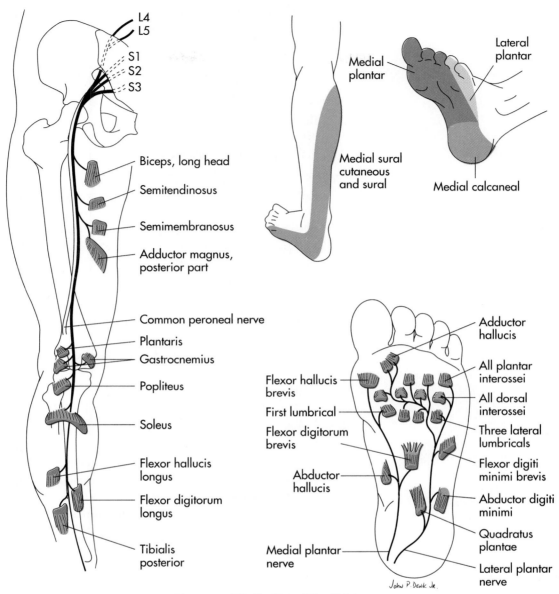

Fig. 3.13 Distribution of the tibial nerve.

- Passes superiorly and medially crossing the inguinal ligament toward the umbilicus
- Supplies the inferior and medial part of the superficial abdominal wall
- Anastomoses with the inferior epigastric artery

Superficial circumflex iliac artery

- Becomes superficial passing through or close to the saphenous hiatus

- Passes superiorly and laterally along the inguinal ligament toward the anterior superior iliac spine
- Supplies the inferior and lateral part of the superficial abdominal wall
- Anastomoses with the deep circumflex iliac artery

Superficial external pudendal artery

- Becomes superficial passing through or close to the saphenous hiatus
- Passes medially toward the external genitalia

Deep external pudendal artery

- Passes medially across the pectineus and adductor longus muscles
- Becomes superficial to supply the external genitalia

Profunda femoris artery (see Fig. 3.9)

- Arises from the deep side of the femoral artery within the **femoral triangle**
- Is the largest branch of the femoral artery
- Leaves the femoral triangle by passing **posterior** to the **adductor longus muscle**
- Usually gives rise to the **medial** and **lateral femoral circumflex** arteries
- Gives rise to the **perforating arteries** to the posterior thigh
- Typically **ends** as the **fourth perforating artery**

Medial femoral circumflex artery (see Fig. 3.9)

- Often arises as a branch of the proximal **profunda femoris artery** but can arise directly from the **femoral artery**
- Passes medially and posteriorly to leave the femoral triangle **between** the **iliopsoas** and **pectineus** muscles
- Winds around the femur to enter the gluteal region between the quadratus femoris muscle and the upper border of the adductor magnus
- Gives an **ascending branch,** which **anastomoses** with the **inferior gluteal artery**
- Gives a **transverse branch,** which **anastomoses** with the corresponding branch of the **lateral femoral circumflex artery**
- Supplies the **hip joint** and the muscles of the upper **thigh** and **gluteal region**
- Participates in the **cruciate anastomosis**

Lateral femoral circumflex artery (see Fig. 3.9)

- Usually arises as a branch of the **femoral artery** but can arise directly from the proximal **profunda femoris artery**
- Passes laterally deep to the rectus femoris and sartorius muscles
- Gives an **ascending branch,** which passes deep to the tensor fascia latae muscle to supply the hip joint and **anastomose** with the **superior gluteal artery**

- Gives a **transverse branch,** which **anastomoses** with the corresponding branch of the **medial femoral circumflex artery**
- Gives a **descending branch,** which descends behind the **rectus femoris** muscle to reach the knee and **anastomose** with the **genicular arteries**
- Supplies the **hip joint** and the muscles of the upper **thigh** and **gluteal region**
- Participates in the **cruciate anastomosis**

Perforating arteries (see Fig. 3.9)

- Are posterior **branches** (usually four in number) of the **profunda femoris** artery
- Pierce the **adductor magnus** muscle to supply the posterior compartment of the thigh
- Are the major supply to the **posterior thigh**
- Participate in the **cruciate anastomosis via the first perforating artery**

Descending genicular artery

- Arises from the **femoral artery** in the adductor canal just before it passes through the **adductor hiatus**
- Gives a **musculoarticular branch,** which descends on the femur to participate in the **genicular anastomosis**
- Gives a **saphenous branch,** which runs superficially with the **saphenous nerve**

Cruciate anastomosis

- Provides an important potential **collateral pathway** to bypass an **obstruction** of the **external iliac** or **femoral artery**
- Joins the **internal iliac** artery to the **femoral** artery
- Includes the **medial femoral circumflex** artery, the **lateral femoral circumflex** artery, the **inferior gluteal artery,** and the **first perforating** artery
- Forms by an anastomoses between the inferior gluteal branch of the internal iliac artery and the femoral circumflex branches of the **femoral artery,** which in turn anastomoses with the first perforating branch of the **profunda femoris** artery
- May also participate in an expanded anastomosis between the internal iliac and the popliteal arteries if anastomoses are present between the perforating arteries and branches of the popliteal artery

— **Obturator artery**

- Arises from the **internal iliac artery** in the pelvis
- Enters the thigh through the **obturator canal** with the anterior and posterior branches of the **obturator nerve**
- Gives rise to **anterior** and **posterior** branches, which encircle the obturator foramen and obturator externus muscle
- Gives rise to an **acetabular artery,** which provides the small but important artery that reaches the head of the femur in the **ligament of the head of the femur**

- Generally does **not** accompany the **obturator nerve** distally into the thigh

● **Important features of the thigh region**

— *Fascia lata*

- Is the deep **investing fascia** of the thigh
- Ensheaths the muscles of the thigh like a **tight stocking**
- Gives rise to the **medial and lateral intermuscular septa,** which pass deep to attach to the **linea aspera** of the femur
- Is attached **superiorly** to the margins of the **hip bone,** the **sacrum and coccyx,** and the **inguinal ligament**
- Inferiorly attaches to the **tibial condyles** and **patella** and extends over the **popliteal fossa**

— *Iliotibial tract*

- Is a **bandlike thickening** of the fascia lata on the **lateral** side of the thigh
- Arises from the tubercle of the **iliac crest** and passes distally to the **lateral condyle of the tibia**
- Receives insertions from the **tensor fasciae latae** and **gluteus maximus** muscles
- Is functionally important in **maintaining posture** and in **locomotion**

— *Saphenous opening (fossa ovalis)*

- Is a large, oval gap in the **fascia lata** just below the inguinal ligament
- Transmits the **great saphenous vein** as it passes to the femoral vein
- Also transmits the small **superficial branches** of the **femoral artery**
- Is covered by the **cribriform fascia,** which is perforated by numerous small **lymphatic vessels**

— *Femoral sheath*

- Is a downward extension of the **transversalis fascia** and **iliacus fascia** from the abdomen into the thigh
- Passes deep to the inguinal ligament
- From **lateral to medial,** invests the **femoral artery,** the **femoral vein,** and the **femoral canal**

— *Femoral canal*

- Is the most **medial compartment** of the femoral sheath
- Lies on the **pectineus muscle**
- Contains fat, loose connective tissue, and lymphatics
- Is a **potential weak area** in the abdominal wall; may allow a **femoral hernia**

— *Femoral ring*

- Is the proximal end of the **femoral canal**
- Is normally closed by extraperitoneal connective tissue (called the **femoral septum**) and a single lymph node

- **Important relationships** are

    — Medially: lacunar ligament
    — Laterally: femoral vein
    — Anteriorly: inguinal ligament
    — Posteriorly: superior ramus of pubis and pectineal ligament

— *Femoral triangle*

- Lies at the junction of the trunk and the lower extremity

- Contains the **femoral nerve** and the **femoral artery, vein, and canal** (within the femoral sheath) as they lie **anterior to the hip joint**

- Is covered only by skin and fascia, leaving its contents **vulnerable to injury**

- **Relationships** are

    — Base: inguinal ligament
    — Lateral border: medial margin of the sartorius muscle
    — Medial border: lateral border of the adductor longus
    — Apex: junction of the medial and lateral borders
    — Floor: iliopsoas and pectineus

— *Adductor canal*

- Extends from the **apex** of the femoral triangle to the **adductor hiatus**

- Lies between the **vastus medialis** and the **adductor brevis and magnus**

- Is covered by the **sartorius muscle** and thus is also called the **subsartorial canal**

- Contains the **femoral artery and vein**, the **saphenous nerve**, and the **nerve to the vastus medialis**

■ Leg and Popliteal Region

● Muscles of the leg

- The muscles of the posterior leg are summarized in Table 3.5.
- The muscles of the anterior and lateral leg are summarized in Table 3.6.

● Popliteal fossa

- Is the diamond-shaped area behind the knee that contains the important nerves and vessels passing from the thigh to the leg
- **Relationships** are

    — Superiorly and medially: semimembranosus and semitendinosus
    — Superiorly and laterally: biceps femoris
    — Inferiorly and medially: medial head of the gastrocnemius
    — Inferiorly and laterally: lateral head of the gastrocnemius
    — Floor (anteriorly): popliteal surface of distal femur
    — Roof (posteriorly): deep (popliteal) fascia

Table 3.5 *Muscles of the Posterior Compartment of the Leg*

Name	Origin	Insertion	Action	Innervation
Superficial Group				
Gastrocnemius* (medial and lateral heads)	Posterior surface of femur above the medial and lateral condyles	Posterior calcaneus by way of the tendo calcaneus (Achilles tendon)	Plantar flexes the foot at the ankle joint; weakly flexes the knee joint	Tibial nerve
Soleus*	Upper shaft and head of fibula, soleal line of tibia	Posterior calcaneus by way of the tendo calcaneus (Achilles tendon)	Plantar flexes the foot at the ankle joint	Tibial nerve
Plantaris	Lateral condyle of femur	Posterior surface of the calcaneus	Insignificant plantar flexor at the ankle	Tibial nerve
Deep Group				
Popliteus	Posterior tibia above the soleal line	Lateral condyle of femur	Laterally rotates the femur on the tibia at the initiation of flexion from full extension	Tibial nerve
Tibialis posterior	Posterior tibia, fibula, and interosseus membrane	Tubercle of the navicular bone with secondary slips to all tarsals, except the talus, and all metatarsals, except the first	Plantar flexes at the ankle joint and inverts the foot	Tibial nerve
Flexor hallucis longus	Lower two thirds of posterior fibula, the interosseus membrane, and the intermuscular septum	Base of the distal phalanx of the great toe	Flexes the big toe and plantar flexes the foot at the ankle joint	Tibial nerve
Flexor digitorum longus	Posterior surface of the tibia distal to the soleal line	Base of the distal phalanx of the lateral four toes	Flexes the toes and plantar flexes the foot at the ankle	Tibial nerve

*These muscles make up the so-called triceps surae.

- **Contents** are

    — In the middle from **superficial to deep**, the **tibial nerve**, the **popliteal vein**, and the **popliteal artery**

    — Laterally along the medial border of the biceps femoris, the **common peroneal nerve**

- **Nerves of the leg**

    — *Tibial nerve (L4, L5, S1, S2, S3) (see Fig. 3.13)*

        - **Supplies** all of the muscles of the **posterior compartment** of the leg

        - Gives **articular branches** to both the **knee** and **ankle** joints

        - Separates from the **sciatic nerve** in the posterior thigh

        - Descends behind the knee joint in the **popliteal fossa** lying **superficial and lateral** to the **popliteal vessels**

        - Enters the posterior compartment of the leg passing **deep** to the **gastrocnemius** and **soleus** muscles

Table 3.6 *Muscles of the Anterior and Lateral Compartments of the Leg*

NAME	ORIGIN	INSERTION	ACTION	INNERVATION
Anterior Group				
Tibialis anterior	Lateral condyle, lateral surface of tibia, and adjacent interosseus membrane	Medial cuneiform and first metatarsal bones	Dorsiflexes the ankle joint and inverts the foot	Deep peroneal nerve
Extensor digitorum longus	Lateral condyle of tibia, anterior surface of fibula, and adjacent interosseus membrane	Middle and distal phalanges of lateral four toes	Extends the toes and dorsiflexes the foot	Deep peroneal nerve
Extensor hallucis longus	Anterior fibula and adjacent interosseus membrane	Distal phalanx of the great toe	Extends the great toe and dorsiflexes the foot	Deep peroneal nerve
Peroneus tertius	Anterior surface of the distal fibula	Dorsum of the base of the fifth metatarsal	Dorsiflexes and everts the foot	Deep peroneal nerve
Lateral Group				
Peroneus longus	Lateral condyle of tibia and lateral surface of the upper fibula	Plantar surface of the medial cuneiform and first metatarsal bones	Everts the foot	Superficial peroneal nerve
Peroneus brevis	Lateral surface of the lower fibula	Tuberosity at the base of the fifth metatarsal	Everts the foot	Superficial peroneal nerve

- Passes with the **posterior tibial artery** posterior to the medial malleolus and lies **between** the **flexor hallucis longus** and the **flexor digitorum longus**
- Ends **deep** to the **flexor retinaculum** by dividing into **medial and lateral plantar nerves**
- Gives rise to the **medial sural cutaneous nerve** and to the **medial calcaneal nerve**

— *Common peroneal nerve (L4, L5, S1, S2) (Fig. 3.14)*

- Arises from the **sciatic nerve** midway down the posterior thigh
- Enters the **popliteal fossa** at its apex
- Courses along the medial margin of the **biceps femoris muscle** to leave the popliteal fossa
- Passes superficially around the **neck of the fibula** and divides into the **superficial and deep peroneal nerves**
- Can be readily **palpated** as a firm cord at the **neck of the fibula,** where it is particularly **vulnerable to injury**
- Gives rise to the **lateral sural cutaneous nerve,** the **sural communicating nerve,** and the **recurrent articular branch**

— *Deep peroneal nerve (L4, L5, S1) (see Fig. 3.14)*

- Arises from the **common peroneal nerve** in the **lateral compartment** of the leg
- Enters the **anterior compartment** by passing through or deep to the extensor digitorum longus
- Descends in the leg with the **anterior tibial artery**

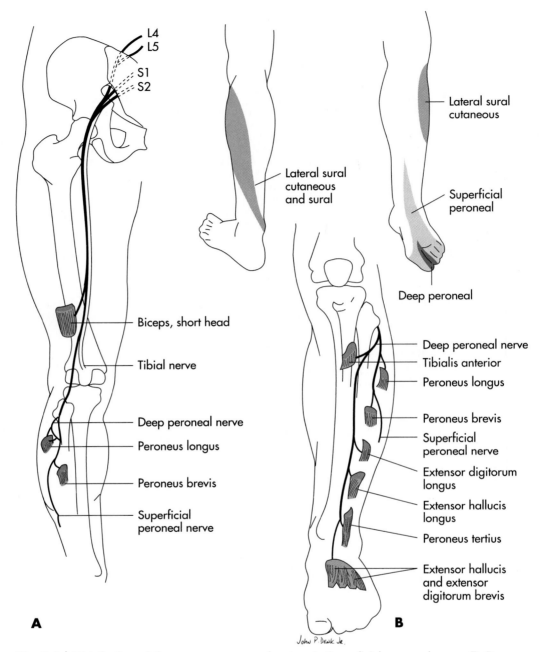

Fig. 3.14 Distribution of the common peroneal nerve. **A,** Superficial peroneal nerve. **B,** Deep peroneal nerve.

- Lies at first between the **tibialis anterior** and the **extensor digitorum longus** and then between the **tibialis anterior** and the **extensor hallucis longus**
- At the ankle lies deep to the **extensor retinaculum** and between the **extensor digitorum longus** and **extensor hallucis longus**

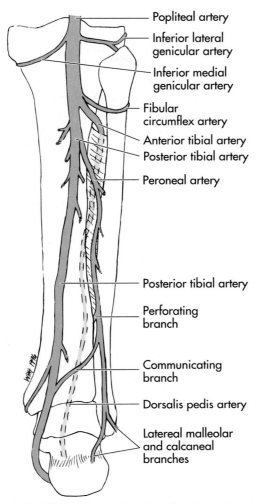

Fig. 3.15 The main arteries of the leg. Posterior view.

- **Supplies** all muscles of the **anterior compartment** of the leg
- Becomes **cutaneous** over the **dorsum of the foot**

— *Superficial peroneal nerve (L5, S1, S2) (see Fig. 3.14)*

- Arises from the **common peroneal nerve** in the **lateral compartment** within the **peroneus longus** muscle
- Descends **between the peroneus longus** and **peroneus brevis** muscles
- Becomes **superficial** in the lower leg to supply the skin of the **lateral leg and foot**

● Arteries of the leg and popliteal region

— *Popliteal artery (Fig. 3.15)*

- Is a continuation of the **femoral artery** beginning at the adductor hiatus

- Ends at the lower border of the popliteus muscle by dividing into the anterior and posterior tibial arteries
- Is the most **anterior** structure in the **popliteal fossa** lying against the popliteal surface of the **femur,** the capsule of the **knee joint,** and the **popliteus** muscle
- Is **vulnerable** to injury in **fractures** of the lower end of the femur and in **dislocation** of the **knee joint**
- Includes the medial and lateral **superior genicular arteries,** the **middle genicular artery,** the medial and lateral **inferior genicular arteries,** and the **sural artery**
  - **Medial superior genicular artery**
    — Passes over the **medial epicondyle** deep to the **semimembranosus** and **semitendinosus** muscles to end in the vastus medialis

  - **Lateral superior genicular artery**
    — Passes over the **lateral epicondyle** deep to the **biceps femoris** muscle

  - **Medial inferior genicular artery**
    — Passes around the **medial tibial condyle** deep to the **medial head** of the **gastrocnemius** muscle

  - **Lateral inferior genicular artery**
    — Passes around the **lateral tibial condyle** deep to the **lateral head** of the **gastrocnemius** muscle

  - **Middle genicular artery**
    — Pierces the **oblique popliteal ligament** and **joint capsule** to be distributed within the joint

  - **Sural arteries**
    — Are the largest branches of the popliteal artery other than the terminal branches
    — Supply the gastrocnemius and soleus muscles

— *Genicular anastomosis (Fig. 3.16)*
  - Receives contributions from
    — Genicular branches of the **popliteal artery**
    — Descending branches of the **femoral** and **profunda femoris arteries**
    — Ascending branches of the **anterior and posterior tibial arteries**

  - Allows blood to flow to the leg and foot when the popliteal artery is blocked (as when the knee is fully flexed)

— *Posterior tibial artery (see Fig. 3.15)*
  - Is a **terminal branch** of the popliteal artery
  - Arises in the popliteal fossa at the lower border of the **popliteus muscle**

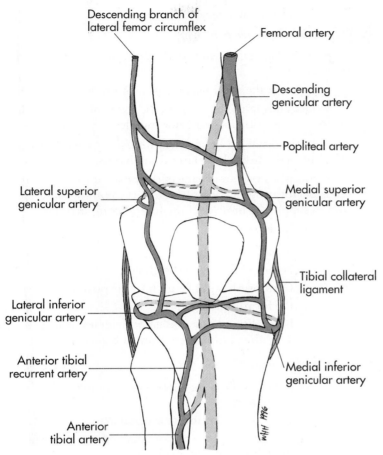

Fig. 3.16 Collateral circulation around the knee. Anterior view.

- Supplies the **posterior compartment** of the leg
- Descends with the **tibial nerve** on the posterior surface of the **tibialis posterior** muscle
- Terminates deep to the **flexor retinaculum** and posterior to the **medial malleolus** by dividing into the **medial and lateral plantar arteries**
- Is frequently **palpable behind** the **medial malleolus**
- Gives rise to the

    — **Nutrient artery** to the tibia
    — **Circumflex fibular artery,** which passes around the neck of the fibula to supply the peroneus muscles and contribute to the genicular anastomosis
    — **Medial posterior malleolar branches,** which pass over the lower end of the tibia
    — **Medial calcaneal branches,** which supply the medial side of the heel

— Peroneal artery

— *Peroneal artery (see Fig. 3.15)*

- Is the largest branch and often of equal size with the posterior tibial artery
- Arises at the proximal end of the posterior tibial artery
- Descends in the leg close to the fibula between the **flexor hallucis longus** and **tibialis posterior** muscles
- In the distal leg lies on the **interosseus membrane** giving terminal branches behind the **lateral malleolus**
- **Supplies** the lateral side of the **posterior compartment** and sends **perforating branches** through the posterior intermuscular septum to supply the muscles of the **lateral compartment**
- Gives rise to the

    — **Muscular branches**
    — **Nutrient artery** to the fibula
    — **Communicating branch** to the **posterior tibial** artery
    — **Perforating branch**
    — **Lateral posterior malleolar arteries,** which are **terminal branches** ending as **calcaneal** branches

- **Perforating branch**

    — Passes through the **interosseus membrane** to the anterior compartment
    — **Reinforces** the **anterior tibial artery**
    — **May give rise** to the **dorsalis pedis artery** when the anterior tibial artery is small
    — **May continue** into the foot as the **plantar arteries** when the posterior tibial artery is deficient

— *Anterior tibial artery (see Fig. 3.15)*

- Arises on the posterior surface of the **popliteus muscle** as a terminal branch of the **popliteal artery**
- Passes below the muscle and above the **interosseus membrane** to reach the **anterior compartment** of the leg
- Descends on the anterior surface of the **interosseus membrane** accompanied by the **deep peroneal nerve**
- Is changed in name to the **dorsalis pedis** as it crosses the ankle joint
- May be **deficient** in the lower leg, in which case the **dorsalis pedis** artery will arise **from the perforating branch of the peroneal artery**
- On the dorsum of the foot lies **between** the tendons of the **extensor hallucis longus** and the **extensor digitorum longus**
- Gives rise to the

    — **Muscular branches**
    — **Posterior tibial recurrent artery,** an **inconstant** branch arising near its origin and ascending in front of the popliteus muscle

Table 3.7 *Muscles of the Dorsum of the Foot*

NAME	ORIGIN	INSERTION	ACTION	INNERVATION
Extensor digitorum brevis	Dorsal surface of the calcaneus	Joins the tendons of the extensor digitorum longus to the second, third, and fourth toes	Extends the toes	Deep peroneal nerve
Extensor hallucis brevis	Dorsal surface of the calcaneus	Joins the extensor tendon to the great toe	Extends the great toe	Deep peroneal nerve

— **Anterior tibial recurrent artery,** which arises at the **interosseus membrane** to enter the **tibialis anterior** muscle before continuing to participate in the **genicular anastomosis**

— **Medial and lateral anterior malleolar** branches

— **Dorsalis pedis artery**

■ **Foot**

● Muscles of the foot

- The intrinsic muscles of the dorsum of the foot are summarized in Table 3.7.
- The intrinsic muscles of the sole of the foot are summarized in Table 3.8.

● Nerves of the foot

— *Deep peroneal nerve (see Fig. 3.14)*

- Passes onto the **dorsum** of the foot **between** the tendons of the **extensor digitorum longus** and the **extensor hallucis longus**
- Supplies the **extensor digitorum brevis** and the **extensor hallucis brevis** muscles
- Branches into cutaneous **digital nerves** to supply **adjacent sides of the first and second toes**

— *Medial plantar nerve (L4, L5) (see Fig. 3.13)*

- Is a terminal branch of the **tibial nerve** arising deep to the **flexor retinaculum**
- Passes **deep** to the **abductor hallucis** and then forward **between** the **abductor hallucis** and the **flexor digitorum brevis** muscles
- Supplies the **abductor hallucis**, the **flexor hallucis brevis**, the **flexor digitorum brevis**, and the **first lumbrical** muscles
- Supplies the **skin** over the **medial two thirds** of the **sole**
- Gives rise to **common plantar digital nerves,** which branch as **proper plantar digital nerves;** digital nerves supply the **medial 3½ digits,** including the dorsum of the distal phalanges and the nail beds

— *Lateral plantar nerve (S1, S2) (see Fig. 3.14)*

- Is a terminal branch of the **tibial nerve** arising deep to the **flexor retinaculum**

Table 3.8 *Muscles of the Plantar Surface of the Foot*

NAME	ORIGIN	INSERTION	ACTION	INNERVATION
First Layer				
Abductor hallucis	Medial side of the tubercle of the calcaneus	Medial side of base of the proximal phalanx of the great toe	Abducts the great toe	Medial plantar nerve
Flexor digitorum brevis	Tubercle of the calcaneus	Middle phalanges of the lateral four toes	Flexes the lateral four toes at the proximal interphalangeal joint	Medial plantar nerve
Abductor digiti minimi	Tubercle of the calcaneus	Lateral side of the proximal phalanx of the little toe	Abducts the little toe	Lateral plantar nerve
Second Layer				
Quadratus plantae	Medial and lateral sides of the plantar surface of the calcaneus	Tendon of the flexor digitorum longus	Flexes the toes when the foot is plantar flexed; corrects the angle of pull for the long flexor tendons	Lateral plantar nerve
Lumbrical (4)	Tendons of the flexor digitorum longus	Medial side of the dorsal digital expansion of the lateral four toes	Flex the metatarsophalangeal and extend the interphalangeal joints	Lumbrical 1: medial plantar nerve Lumbrical 2-4: lateral plantar nerve
Third Layer				
Flexor hallucis brevis	Plantar surface of the cuboid and lateral cuneiform bones	Proximal phalanx of great toe	Flexes the metatarsophalangeal joint of the great toe	Medial plantar nerve
Adductor hallucis	Oblique head: bases of second to fourth metatarsal and the long plantar ligament Transverse head: capsules of medial four metatarsophalangeal joints	Lateral side of base of the proximal phalanx of the great toe	Adducts the great toe	Lateral plantar nerve
Flexor digiti minimi brevis	Plantar surface of the base of the fifth metatarsal and the long plantar ligament	Plantar surface of the base of the proximal phalanx of the little toe	Flexes the metatarsophalangeal joint of the little toe	Lateral plantar nerve
Fourth Layer				
Plantar interossei (3)	Medial sides of third to fifth metatarsals	Medial side of the base of the corresponding proximal phalanx	Adduct the toes; flex the metatarsophalangeal joint and extend the interphalangeal joints	Lateral plantar nerve
Dorsal interossei (4)	Sides of adjacent metatarsals	Medial and lateral sides of the base of proximal phalanx of the second toe; lateral side of base of proximal phalanx of the third and fourth toes	Abduct the toes; flex the metatarsophalangeal joint and extend the interphalangeal joints	Lateral plantar nerve

- Passes **laterally** across the foot **between** the **flexor digitorum brevis** (first layer) and the **quadratus plantae** (second layer)
- Supplies the **quadratus plantae** and the **abductor digiti minimi**
- On reaching the fifth metatarsal, divides into a **superficial** and **deep** branch
- Superficial branch

    — Gives rise to **common plantar digital nerves,** which branch as **proper plantar digital nerves**
    — Supplies the **lateral 1½ digits,** including the dorsum of the distal phalanges and the nail beds
    — Supplies the **skin** over the **lateral one third of the sole**
    — Supplies the **flexor digiti minimi brevis** and the **plantar and dorsal interossei** of the fourth interspace

- Deep branch

    — Passes medially along the interosseus muscles with the **plantar arterial arch**
    — Supplies the remaining **interossei,** the **lateral three lumbricals,** and the **adductor hallucis**

- **Arteries of the foot (Fig. 3.17)**

    — *Medial plantar artery (see Fig. 3.17)*

        - Is a terminal branch of the **posterior tibial artery** arising deep to the flexor retinaculum
        - Courses in the foot with the **medial plantar nerve**
        - Gives rise to

            — The **plantar digital artery** to the **medial side of the great toe**
            — **Anastomotic branches** to the plantar metatarsal arteries

    — *Lateral plantar artery (see Fig. 3.17)*

        - Is a terminal branch of the **posterior tibial artery** arising deep to the flexor retinaculum
        - Courses in the foot with the **lateral plantar nerve**
        - Is called the **plantar arch** as it passes on the inferior surfaces of the interossei muscles
        - **Plantar arch**

            — Gives rise to **plantar metatarsal arteries,** which branch to **plantar digital arteries** to the **lateral 4½ toes**
            — Is completed medially by anastomosis with the **deep plantar artery** from the **dorsalis pedis**

    — *Dorsalis pedis artery (see Fig. 3.17)*

        - Is the distal continuation of the **anterior tibial artery** as it crosses the ankle joint
        - May arise from the **perforating branch of the peroneal artery** if the anterior tibial is deficient distally
        - Gives rise to the

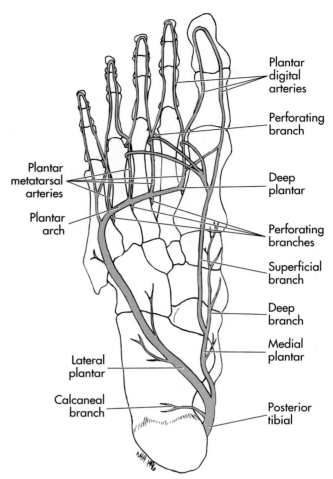

Fig. 3.17 Arteries of the foot. Plantar view.

— **Medial and lateral tarsal arteries**
— **First dorsal metatarsal artery**

- Terminates by dividing into the

    — **Arcuate artery,** which gives rise to **dorsal metatarsal arteries**
    — **Deep plantar artery**

- **Deep plantar artery**

    — Passes between the two heads of the **first dorsal interosseus** muscle into the plantar surface of the foot
    — Anastomoses with the **plantar arch**

- **Dorsal metatarsal arteries**

    — End as **dorsal digital arteries**
    — Anastomose with the **plantar metatarsal arteries**

● **Important features of the leg and foot**

— *Crural fascia*

- The crural fascia is the deep **investing fascia** of the leg.
- It attaches proximally to the margins of the **tibial condyles** except posteriorly, where it is continuous with the **fascia lata** over the popliteal region.
- It **closely binds** the muscles of the **anterior and lateral compartments**, where it provides attachment for some muscles.
- It gives rise to sheetlike inward extensions, the **anterior, posterior,** and **transverse intermuscular septa.**

   — The **anterior intermuscular septum** attaches to the anterior fibula and separates the **anterior** and **lateral** compartments of the leg.
   — The **posterior intermuscular septum** attaches to the posterior fibula and separates the **posterior** and **lateral** compartments of the leg.
   — The **transverse intermuscular septum** is an extension of the **posterior septum** to the **medial crural fascia** separating the **superficial** and **deep** muscles of the posterior leg.

— *Flexor retinaculum*

- Is a localized thickening of **crural fascia** at the **medial** side of the **ankle and foot**
- Extends posteriorly from the medial malleolus to the calcaneus and plantar fascia
- Binds down the tendons and synovial sheaths of the **flexor hallucis longus, flexor digitorum longus,** and **tibialis posterior** muscles
- Also covers the **tibial nerve** and the **posterior tibial artery**

— *Extensor retinacula*

- Are localized thickenings of the **anterior crural fascia** at the ankle arranged as **superior** and **inferior** bands
- Binds down the tendons and synovial sheaths of the **tibialis anterior, extensor hallucis longus, extensor digitorum longus,** and **peroneus tertius** muscles
- Covers the **deep peroneal nerve** and the **anterior tibial artery**

Superior extensor retinaculum

- Extends from the anterior border of the tibia to the anterior border of the fibula

Inferior extensor retinaculum

- Is a **Y**-shaped band lying in front of the ankle joint
- Has a stem, which attaches laterally to the calcaneus
- Has a superior limb, which attaches to the medial malleolus
- Has an inferior limb, which attaches medially to the plantar fascia

— *Peroneal retinacula*

- Are localized thickenings of the **deep fascia** as it extends onto the **lateral foot**

- Bind down the tendons and synovial sheaths of the **peroneus longus** and **peroneus brevis**
- Are arranged as **superior** and **inferior** bands
  - The **superior peroneal retinaculum** passes from the **lateral malleolus** to the **calcaneus**.
  - The **inferior peroneal retinaculum** extends from the **upper lateral** to the **lower lateral calcaneus**.

— *Plantar aponeurosis*

- Is a central thickening of the **deep fascia** on the sole of the foot
- Attaches proximally to the **calcaneal tuberosity** and extends distally to end in **slips** to the **five** digital **tendon sheaths**
- Is a thick, tough layer that **protects** the important underlying **plantar nerves and vessels**

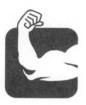

Movements of the Lower Extremity

Movements of the hip joint

- Flexion: iliopsoas but also pectineus, rectus femoris, and sartorius
- Extension: gluteus maximus but also the hamstrings muscles
- Abduction: gluteus medius, gluteus minimus, tensor fasciae latae
- Adduction: adductor magnus, longus, and brevis, pectineus, gracilis
- Medial rotation: tensor fasciae latae, anterior fibers of gluteus medius and minimus
- Lateral rotation: obturator internus, obturator externus, piriformis, quadratus femoris, superior and inferior gemelli, gluteus maximus

Movements of the knee joint

- Flexion: hamstrings but also sartorius, gracilis, and gastrocnemius
- Extension: quadriceps femoris
- Medial rotation: popliteus, semitendinosus, semimembranosus
- Lateral rotation: biceps femoris

Movements of the ankle (talocrural) joint

- Dorsiflexion: tibialis anterior, extensor digitorum longus, extensor hallucis longus, peroneus tertius
- Plantar flexion: gastrocnemius, soleus, tibialis posterior, flexor digitorum longus, flexor hallucis longus, peroneus longus

Movements of the subtalar joint

- Inversion: tibialis anterior, tibialis posterior
- Eversion: peroneus longus, peroneus brevis

Movements of the metatarsophalangeal joints (of the second to fifth toes)

- Flexion: lumbricals, interossei
- Extension: extensor digitorum longus and brevis
- Abduction: dorsal interossei
- Adduction: plantar interossei

Movements of the interphalangeal joints (of the second to fifth toes)

- Flexion: flexor digitorum longus, flexor digitorum brevis

- Extension: extensor digitorum longus and brevis, lumbricals, interossei

- **Movements of the great toe**
  - Flexion: flexor hallucis longus, flexor hallucis brevis
  - Extension: extensor hallucis longus and brevis
  - Abduction: abductor hallucis
  - Adduction: adductor hallucis

Summary of the Innervation of the Lower Extremity

- **Summary of motor innervation by nerve**

  - **Femoral nerve** (see Fig. 3.11)

    — Anterior (extensor) compartment of the thigh: all muscles, including pectineus

  - **Obturator nerve** (see Fig. 3.12)

    — Medial (adductor) compartment of the thigh: all muscles except hamstrings part of adductor magnus (tibial nerve), but including the pectineus

  - **Tibial nerve** (see Fig. 3.13)

    — Posterior (flexor) compartment of the thigh: all muscles except the short head of the biceps femoris
    — Medial (adductor) compartment of the thigh: hamstrings part of adductor magnus
    — Posterior (flexor) compartment of leg: all muscles
    — Plantar foot: all intrinsic muscles

  - **Common peroneal nerve** (see Fig. 3.14)

    — Posterior (flexor) compartment of the thigh: short head of the biceps femoris

  - **Deep peroneal nerve** (see Fig. 3.14)

    — Anterior (extensor) compartment of the leg: all muscles

  - **Superficial peroneal nerve** (see Fig. 3.14)

    — Lateral compartment of the leg: all muscles
    — Dorsum of foot: extensor digitorum brevis, extensor hallucis brevis

  - **Medial plantar nerve** (see Fig. 3.13)

    — Plantar foot: abductor hallucis, flexor hallucis brevis, flexor digitorum brevis, first lumbrical

  - **Lateral plantar nerve** (see Fig. 3.13)

    — Plantar foot: quadratus plantae, abductor digiti minimi, flexor digiti minimi brevis, adductor hallucis, all interossei, lateral three lumbricals

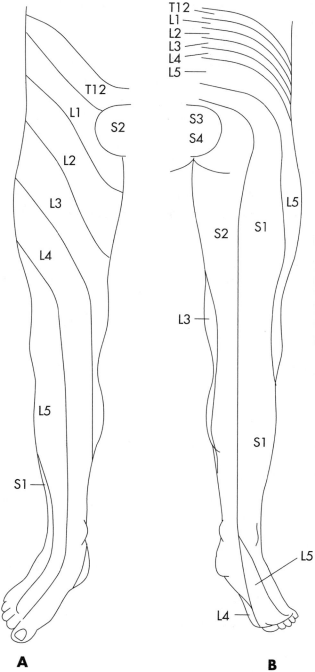

A   **B**

Fig. 3.18 Dermatomes of the lower extremity. **A,** Anterior view. **B,** Posterior view.

● **Dermatomes of the lower extremity (Fig. 3.18)**

■ **Nerve Injuries of the Lower Extremity**

- Nerve injuries are much **less common in the lower extremity** than in the upper extremity.
- Direct injuries to the brachial plexus are common, but the **lumbosacral plexus** is rarely damaged directly.

● Injuries of individual nerves

— *Injury to the femoral nerve (see Fig. 3.11)*

- Is seldom completely cut in the thigh because it terminates just below the inguinal ligament
- May be sectioned by a penetrating wound into the lower abdomen above the inguinal ligament
- May occur during catherization of the femoral artery
- Produces a variable **loss of extension at the knee** by the quadriceps femoris muscle
- May also produce some **weakness of hip flexion**
- Results in a **loss of sensation** over the **anterior thigh** and the **medial leg and foot**

— *Injury to the obturator nerve (see Fig. 3.12)*

- Is uncommon
- May occur in obstetric procedures and in pelvic disease
- Will affect adduction of the thigh
- Does not greatly affect walking but is noticeable when attempting to cross the legs while sitting
- May result in reduced sensation over the upper medial thigh

— *Injury to the sciatic nerve (see Figs. 3.13 and 3.14)*

- Is most often caused by misplaced **intramuscular injection** into the gluteal region
- May be damaged in **posterior dislocation** of the **hip**
- Results in an **inability** to **extend the hip, flex the knee,** and **dorsiflex** or **plantar flex the foot**
- Will result in an obvious **footdrop**
- Will also result in a loss of cutaneous sensation **over the leg and foot** except on the medial side (because of saphenous nerve distribution)

— *Injury to the common peroneal nerve (see Fig. 3.14)*

- Often results from direct **trauma** to the nerve as it passes **superficially** around the **neck of the fibula**
- May result from **compression** by the upper end of a plaster **leg cast**
- Results in the characteristic **footdrop** caused by **paralysis of extensors** of the foot and toes
- Produces a **variable degree of paralysis** of the extensor muscles of the leg depending on the extent to which the nerve is injured
- May result in little or no **sensory loss** because of sensory overlap

— *Injury to the tibial nerve (see Fig. 3.13)*

- Is uncommon
- May occur by compression behind the knee or by a puncture wound because the tibial nerve lies superficially in the **popliteal fossa**
- Results in a **loss of plantar flexion** of the foot
- Can be tested by **standing on the tiptoes**

MULTIPLE CHOICE
REVIEW QUESTIONS

1. Injury to the tibial nerve would likely result in which of the following?

    a. A complete loss of sensation on the dorsum of the foot
    b. An inability to abduct and adduct the toes
    c. An impaired ability to dorsiflex the foot
    d. An impaired ability to evert the foot
    e. An inability to extend the knee

2. The femoral sheath is a continuation of which of the following?

    a. Scarpa's fascia
    b. External oblique aponeurosis
    c. Superficial perineal fascia
    d. Transversalis fascia
    e. Peritoneum

3. Which of the following is *not* found in the adductor canal?

    a. Saphenous nerve
    b. Great saphenous vein
    c. Femoral vein
    d. Femoral artery
    e. Nerve to the vastus medialis

4. Which of the following muscles can both flex the knee and plantar flex at the ankle?

    a. Tibialis posterior
    b. Flexor digitorum longus
    c. Peroneus longus
    d. Soleus
    e. Gastrocnemius

5. The plantar arterial arch is formed by the lateral plantar artery and which of the following?

    a. Anterior tibial artery
    b. Posterior tibial artery
    c. Medial plantar artery
    d. Peroneal artery
    e. Deep plantar artery

6. Which of the following structures typically exits the pelvis via the greater sciatic foramen superior to the piriformis muscle?

    a. Internal pudendal artery
    b. Superior gluteal nerve
    c. Sciatic nerve
    d. Obturator artery
    e. Obturator internus muscle

7. The important ligament that resists hyperextension and medial rotation of the hip joint is which of the following?

    a. Iliofemoral ligament
    b. Ischiofemoral ligament
    c. Pubofemoral ligament
    d. Ligament of the head of the femur
    e. Transverse acetabular ligament

8. The nerve most likely to be injured by a fracture of the neck of the fibula is which of the following?

    a. Saphenous nerve
    b. Tibial nerve
    c. Common peroneal nerve
    d. Deep peroneal nerve
    e. Femoral nerve

9. Lateral rotation of the hip joint is a powerful movement, but medial rotation is relatively weak. Which of the following is *not* a lateral rotator of the hip?

    a. Gluteus medius
    b. Gluteus maximus
    c. Obturator internus
    d. Obturator externus
    e. Quadratus femoris

10. An examination of your patient's injured knee reveals excessive anterior movement of the tibia on the femur. This is most likely a result of damage to which of the following?

    a. Medial meniscus
    b. Anterior cruciate ligament
    c. Posterior cruciate ligament
    d. Coronary ligament
    e. Fibular collateral ligament

Chapter 4

Thorax

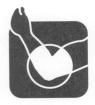

■ The Thoracic Wall

● Thoracic skeleton

— *Ribs*

- There are 12 pairs of ribs; they are attached posteriorly to the thoracic vertebrae.
- The first seven ribs are connected to the sternum by their costal cartilages and are called **true ribs.**
- The lower five are called **false ribs** because their costal cartilages do not reach the sternum.

    — The cartilages of the eighth, ninth, and tenth ribs join the cartilage immediately above.

    — The eleventh and twelfth ribs lie free and are called **floating ribs.**

Typical ribs (Fig. 4.1)

- Ribs 3 through 9 have similar characteristics and are called **typical ribs.**
- Each has a **head, neck, tubercle,** and **body.**
- The **head** has two facets for articulation with the body of its numerically equivalent vertebra and with the one above.
- The **tubercle** has a facet for articulation with the transverse process of the corresponding vertebra.
- The **body** is twisted about its long axis, turns sharply forward at the **angle,** and has an inferior **costal groove,** which contains the intercostal vessels and nerves.

Atypical ribs (see Fig. 4.1)

- **First rib**

    — Is short and flattened
    — Has a single facet on its head for articulation with the first thoracic vertebra
    — On its upper surface has a **scalene tubercle,** which marks the attachment of the anterior scalene muscle and separates shallow **grooves for the subclavian artery and vein**

- **Second rib**

    — Is strongly curved but is not twisted about its long axis
    — Has **two facets on its anterior tip** for articulation with the manubrium and with the body of the sternum

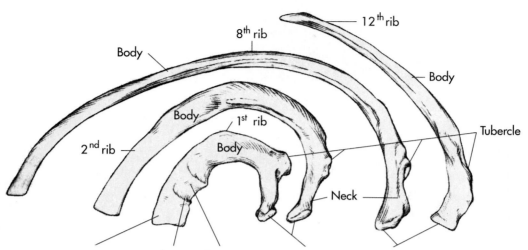

Fig. 4.1 A comparison of four ribs.

  — Is distinguished by the **tuberosity of the serratus anterior muscle**

- **Tenth rib**

  — Has a single facet on its head for articulation with the tenth thoracic vertebra

- **Eleventh and twelfth ribs**

  — Have a single facet on the head for articulation with the corresponding vertebra

  — Have no tubercle or facet for articulation with the transverse process

Cervical rib

- A cervical rib occurs in 0.5% to 1% of persons.

- It arises from the transverse process of the seventh cervical vertebra.

- It may be unattached anteriorly or may be attached to the first rib, first costal cartilage, or the manubrium by a fibrous band, cartilage, or bone.

- It may **compress the subclavian artery and the lower trunk of the brachial plexus** as they pass over it between the anterior and middle scalene muscles, particularly when the limb is hanging to the side. The symptoms are referred to as **thoracic outlet syndrome.**

— *Sternum (Fig. 4.2)*

- The sternum is elongated and flat.

- It has a marrow cavity, which, because of its accessibility, may be used for bone marrow biopsy.

- Until puberty it consists of a series of **six sternebrae** joined by hyaline cartilage. All but the first and last fuse to form the **body.** The

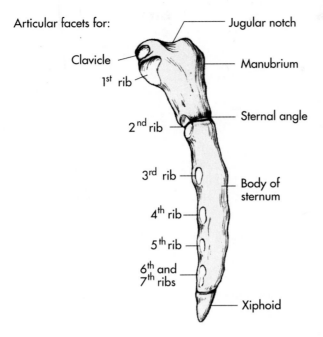

Articular facets for: Jugular notch
Clavicle   Manubrium
1st rib
Sternal angle
2nd rib
3rd rib   Body of sternum
4th rib
5th rib
6th and 7th ribs
Xiphoid

Fig. 4.2 The sternum.

first and the last sternebrae become the **manubrium sterni** and the **xiphoid process,** respectively.

Manubrium

- Is the widest and thickest of the three parts
- On its upper border has an easily palpable **jugular (suprasternal) notch,** which lies in the midline at the root of the neck
- Articulates with the clavicle, the first costal cartilage, the upper part of the second costal cartilage, and the body of the sternum

Body

- Articulates with the manubrium at the fibrocartilaginous **manubriosternal joint**
- Is notched on the sides for articulation with the second through seventh costal cartilages

Xiphoid process

- Is a thin plate of hyaline cartilage at birth
- Is frequently bifid or perforated
- Ossification begins in childhood in the central core, increases with age, and may eventually fuse with the body
- Can be palpated in the infrasternal angle

Sternal angle (of Louis)

- Is the **manubriosternal joint**
- Can be palpated as a **transverse ridge,** which reflects the slight angle of the union of the manubrium and sternum
- Marks the level of the second costal cartilage and is a convenient starting place for counting the ribs

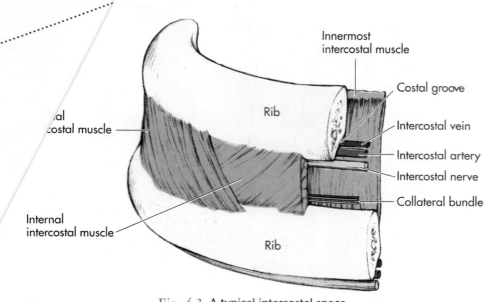

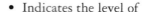

Fig. 4.3 A typical intercostal space.

- Indicates the level of

  — The boundary between the superior mediastinum and the inferior mediastinum
  — The beginning and ending of the arch of the aorta
  — The bifurcation of the trachea
  — The lower border of the fourth thoracic vertebra

— ***Muscles of the thoracic wall (Fig. 4.3, Table 4.1)***
Intercostal muscles

- Fill the intercostal spaces
- Are innervated by their associated intercostal nerve
- Function to move the ribs, although their specific action is not well defined; are classically described as elevators or depressors of the ribs
- Alternatively may function as a group to relay upward or downward pull to the adjacent rib and to resist the inward and outward forces associated with changes in intrathoracic pressure

  - **External intercostal muscles**

    — Pass **obliquely downward and forward** between adjacent ribs
    — Are said to assist inspiration by **elevating** the ribs
    — Are deficient anterior to the costochondral junction being replaced by the **external intercostal membrane**

  - **Internal intercostal muscles**

    — Pass **obliquely downward and backward** between adjacent ribs
    — Are said to assist **expiration** by **depressing** the ribs

Table 4.1	*Muscles of the Thoracic Wall*			
NAME	ORIGIN	INSERTION	ACTION	INNERVATION
External intercostals	Inferior border of rib	Superior border of rib below	Assist in inspiration and expiration by elevating and depressing the ribs*	Intercostal nerve
Internal intercostals	Inferior border of rib	Superior border of rib below	Assist in inspiration and expiration by elevating and depressing the ribs*	Intercostal nerve
Innermost intercostals	Inferior border of rib	Superior border of rib below	Assist in inspiration and expiration by elevating and depressing the ribs*	Intercostal nerve
Subcostals	Inferior border of rib	Superior border of second or third rib below	Assist in inspiration and expiration by elevating and depressing the ribs*	Intercostal nerve
Transversus thoracis	Posterior surface of sternum and xiphoid	Inner surface of lower costal cartilages	Assist in inspiration and expiration by elevating and depressing the ribs*	Intercostal nerve
Levator costarum	Transverse processes of seventh cervical through the eleventh thoracic vertebrae	Between the tubercle and angle of the rib below	Elevates the rib	Dorsal rami of C8-T11 spinal nerves
Serratus posterior superior	Ligamentum nuchae and the upper thoracic spinous processes	Upper borders of ribs 2-5	Assists in inspiration by elevating the ribs	T1-T4 intercostal nerves
Serratus posterior inferior	Spinous processes of the lower two thoracic and the first two lumbar vertebrae	Lower borders of the last three or four ribs	Assists in expiration by depressing the ribs	Lower four intercostal nerves

*It is likely that these muscles can act as either elevators or depressors of the ribs depending on whether the proximal or distal attachment is fixed; consequently, they may function in both inspiration and expiration.

    — Are deficient posterior to the angle of the rib being replaced by the **internal intercostal membrane**

- **Innermost intercostal muscles**

  — May be considered to be part of the internal intercostals from which they are separated by the intercostal vessels and nerve

  — Are best developed in the middle of the intercostal space

- **Subcostal muscles**

  — Are considered to be innermost intercostal muscles that bridge two or three intercostal spaces

  — Are variable but are best developed on the lower posterior thoracic wall

- **Transversus thoracis muscles**

    — Are continuous below the attachment of the diaphragm with the transversus abdominis muscles

    — Connect the inner surface of the lower sternum with adjacent costal cartilages

    — Lie deep to the internal thoracic vessels as they descend over the inner surface of the costal cartilages

Serratus posterior muscles

- **Serratus posterior superior**

    — Arises from the ligamentum nuchae and the upper thoracic spinous processes

    — Runs downward to insert into the upper borders of ribs 2 through 5

    — Assists in inspiration by elevating the ribs

    — Receives innervation from the upper four intercostal nerves

- **Serratus posterior inferior**

    — Arises from the spinous processes of the lower two thoracic and the first two lumbar vertebrae

    — Runs upward to insert into the lower borders of the last three or four ribs

    — Assists in expiration by depressing the ribs

    — Receives innervation from the lower four intercostal nerves

— *Intercostal space (see Fig. 4.3)*

- The intercostal space contains the intercostal muscles.
- It is covered on its deep surface by endothoracic fascia.
- It contains a neurovascular bundle in the plane between the internal and innermost intercostals.
- The **vein, artery,** and **nerve** lie, in that order from above downward, immediately inferior to the rib. The pneumonic **VAN** is helpful in remembering this relationship.
- A collateral bundle runs forward along the lower border of the space.
- A needle to be placed into the pleural cavity should be inserted midway between the ribs to avoid the neurovascular bundle and its collateral bundle.

— *Intercostal nerves*

- The intercostal nerves are the ventral rami of the first eleven spinal nerves.
- They lie in the intercostal space between the internal and innermost intercostal muscles.
- Branches arising in the intercostal space include the following:

    — A **collateral branch** passes forward in the lower part of the intercostal space immediately above the rib below.

    — A **lateral cutaneous branch** pierces the external intercostal muscle along the midaxillary line and divides into anterior

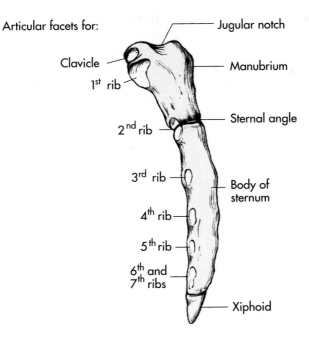

Articular facets for:

Clavicle

1st rib

2nd rib

3rd rib

4th rib

5th rib

6th and
7th ribs

Jugular notch

Manubrium

Sternal angle

Body of
sternum

Xiphoid

Fig. 4.2 The sternum.

first and the last sternebrae become the **manubrium sterni** and the **xiphoid process,** respectively.

Manubrium

- Is the widest and thickest of the three parts
- On its upper border has an easily palpable **jugular (suprasternal) notch,** which lies in the midline at the root of the neck
- Articulates with the clavicle, the first costal cartilage, the upper part of the second costal cartilage, and the body of the sternum

Body

- Articulates with the manubrium at the fibrocartilaginous **manubriosternal joint**
- Is notched on the sides for articulation with the second through seventh costal cartilages

Xiphoid process

- Is a thin plate of hyaline cartilage at birth
- Is frequently bifid or perforated
- Ossification begins in childhood in the central core, increases with age, and may eventually fuse with the body
- Can be palpated in the infrasternal angle

Sternal angle (of Louis)

- Is the **manubriosternal joint**
- Can be palpated as a **transverse ridge,** which reflects the slight angle of the union of the manubrium and sternum
- Marks the level of the second costal cartilage and is a convenient starting place for counting the ribs

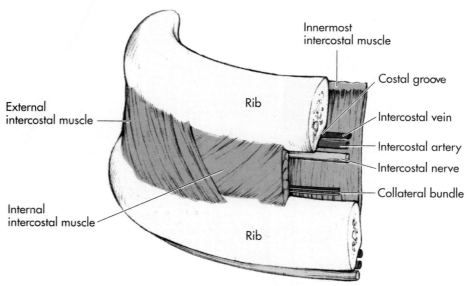

Innermost
intercostal muscle

Costal groove

Intercostal vein

Intercostal artery

Intercostal nerve

Collateral bundle

Rib

External
intercostal muscle

Internal
intercostal muscle

Rib

Fig. 4.3 A typical intercostal space.

- Indicates the level of

  — The boundary between the superior mediastinum and the inferior mediastinum
  — The beginning and ending of the arch of the aorta
  — The bifurcation of the trachea
  — The lower border of the fourth thoracic vertebra

— ***Muscles of the thoracic wall (Fig. 4.3, Table 4.1)***
Intercostal muscles

  - Fill the intercostal spaces
  - Are innervated by their associated intercostal nerve
  - Function to move the ribs, although their specific action is not well defined; are classically described as elevators or depressors of the ribs
  - Alternatively may function as a group to relay upward or downward pull to the adjacent rib and to resist the inward and outward forces associated with changes in intrathoracic pressure
  - **External intercostal muscles**

    — Pass **obliquely downward and forward** between adjacent ribs
    — Are said to assist inspiration by **elevating** the ribs
    — Are deficient anterior to the costochondral junction being replaced by the **external intercostal membrane**

  - **Internal intercostal muscles**

    — Pass **obliquely downward and backward** between adjacent ribs
    — Are said to assist **expiration** by **depressing** the ribs

and posterior branches to supply the skin of the lateral thoracic wall.

— An **anterior cutaneous branch** arises as a continuation of the intercostal nerve at the lateral border of the sternum and supplies the skin of the anterior thoracic wall.

• Only a small part of the ventral ramus of the first thoracic spinal nerve continues in the intercostal space as the first intercostal nerve. The major portion joins the ventral ramus of the eighth cervical spinal nerve to form the **lower trunk of the brachial plexus.**

• The lateral cutaneous branch of the second intercostal nerve is called the **intercostobrachial nerve** and joins the medial brachial cutaneous nerve to supply the medial side of the arm.

• The **seventh to eleventh intercostal nerves** are often called **thoracoabdominal nerves** because they leave the intercostal space anteriorly to supply the skin and muscles of the anterolateral abdominal wall.

• The ventral ramus of the twelfth thoracic spinal nerve lies immediately below the twelfth rib and is called the **subcostal nerve.**

Mediastinum and Pleura

Mediastinum The mediastinum is the space that lies between the paired pleural sacs. It contains all of the thoracic organs except the lungs. For descriptive purposes and to assist in clinical localization, the mediastinum is divided into a superior and an inferior mediastinum. The inferior mediastinum is further divided into an anterior, middle, and posterior mediastinum (Fig. 4.4).

— *Superior mediastinum*

• Is bounded superiorly by the superior thoracic aperture
• Is bounded inferiorly by a line joining the manubriosternal joint to the lower border of the fourth thoracic vertebra
• From anterior to posterior, the contents of the superior mediastinum are (Fig. 4.5)

— Remains of the thymus
— Right and left brachiocephalic veins uniting to form the superior vena cava
— Arch of the aorta and its branches
— Phrenic and vagus nerves
— Trachea
— Esophagus
— Thoracic duct

— *Inferior mediastinum*
Anterior mediastinum

• Lies between the body of the sternum and the pericardium
• In the adult contains only lymph nodes and remnants of the thymus
• In children may contain much of the thymus

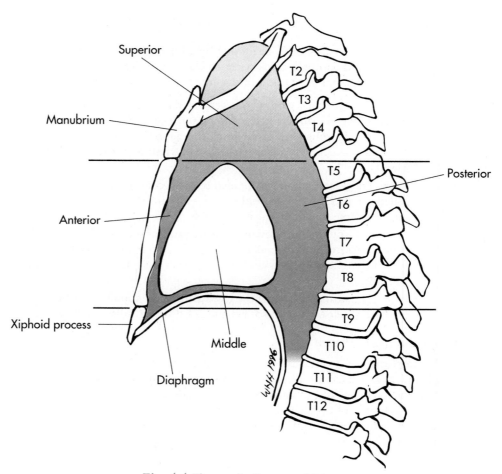

Fig. 4.4 **The mediastinum and its parts.**

Middle mediastinum

- Is largely filled by the pericardium, heart, and roots of the great vessels
- Also contains the

  — Phrenic nerves
  — Tracheal bifurcation and primary bronchi
  — Arch of the azygous vein

Posterior mediastinum

- Lies anterior to the bodies of the fifth to twelfth thoracic vertebrae
- Lies posterior to the pericardium and sloping diaphragm
- Main contents are the

  — Descending thoracic aorta
  — Esophagus and esophageal plexus
  — Thoracic duct
  — Azygous and hemiazygous veins

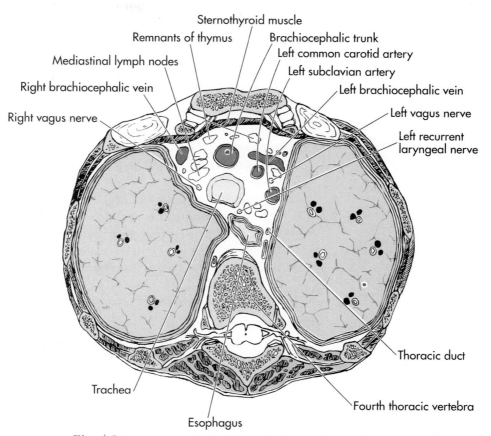

Fig. 4.5 A transverse section through the superior mediastinum.

● **Pleura** Each lung is invaginated into a **pleural sac** composed of a thin serous membrane. The **pleural cavity** is a closed space, containing a small amount of serous fluid, which separates the inner layer of the sac, the **visceral pleura,** from the outer layer of the sac, the **parietal pleura.**

— *Parietal pleura*

- Is a continuous sheet given different names in different locations
- Is highly sensitive to pain
- **Costal pleura**

  — Lines the thoracic wall
  — Is supplied by intercostal nerves

- **Diaphragmatic pleura**

  — Covers the upper surface of the diaphragm forming the floor of the pleural cavity
  — Is supplied by the phrenic nerve

- **Mediastinal pleura**

  — Forms the lateral boundary of the mediastinum
  — Is reflected around the root of the lung and pulmonary ligament to become continuous with the visceral pleura

— Is continuous anteriorly and posteriorly with the costal pleura and inferiorly with the diaphragmatic pleura

— Is supplied by the phrenic nerve

- **Cervical pleura**

  — Is also known as the **cupula of the pleura**

  — Rises above the level of the first rib to lie in the neck

  — Is continuous with the costal and mediastinal pleura

— *Visceral pleura*

- Covers the surface of the lung and extends into the fissures between the lobes
- Is reflected around the root of the lung and pulmonary ligament to become continuous with the mediastinal pleura
- Receives its blood supply from bronchial arteries but is drained by pulmonary veins
- Receives visceral afferent innervation through the pulmonary plexus
- Is sensitive to stretching but is insensitive to pain

— *Endothoracic fascia*

- A thin layer of connective tissue that binds the parietal pleura to the inner surface of the thoracic wall

— *Suprapleural membrane*

- A thickening of the endothoracic fascia above the first rib that reinforces the cervical pleura

— *Pleural recesses*

- Are parts of the pleural cavity that do not contain lung during quiet respiration
- Become almost filled with lung during very deep inspiration
- Normally have parietal pleura in contact with parietal pleura
- **Costodiaphragmatic recess**

  — Occurs between the lowest margin of the lung and the attachment of the diaphragm to the ribs

  — Has diaphragmatic pleura in contact with costal pleura

  — Is the lowest part of the pleural cavity and may accumulate abnormal pleural fluid

- **Costomediastinal recess**

  — Is the narrow anterior and medial extension of the pleural cavity to the midline

  — Has costal pleura in contact with mediastinal pleura

■ The Trachea, Bronchi, and Lungs

● Trachea

- Begins in the neck at the lower border of the cricoid cartilage (at the level of the sixth cervical vertebra) as a continuation of the larynx
- Is a fibromuscular tube reinforced by a series of 16 to 20 horseshoe-shaped hyaline cartilages that prevent collapse of its wall during inspiration
- Is 10 to 12 cm long and 2.5 cm in diameter in the male and slightly smaller in the female

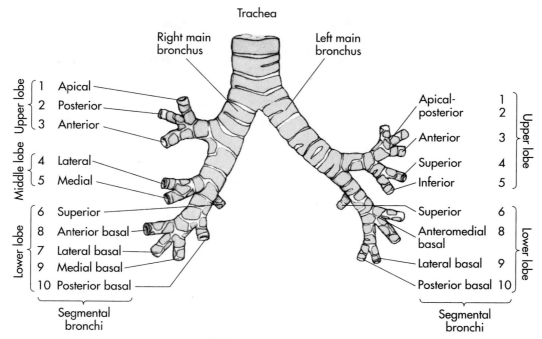

Fig. 4.6 The trachea and bronchi.

- Is midline in the neck and deviates slightly to the right in the thorax
- Ends by dividing into the two main bronchi at the level of the sternal angle
- **Important relationships** of the trachea in the superior mediastinum (see Fig. 4.5)

— **Anteriorly**—arch of the aorta, origins of the brachiocephalic trunk and the left common carotid artery, and the deep cardiac plexus

— **Right side**—right vagus nerve and pleura

— **Left side**—left vagus nerve, arch of the aorta, the left common carotid artery, and the left subclavian artery

— **Posteriorly**—esophagus and left recurrent laryngeal nerve

● **Bronchi**

— *Right main bronchus (Fig. 4.6)*

- Is shorter, wider, and more vertical than the left main bronchus.
- Is more likely to contain inhaled objects because it more closely continues the course of the trachea
- Gives rise to the right upper lobe bronchus (the **epiarterial bronchus**) outside the hilum
- Ends within the hilum by dividing into middle and lower lobe bronchi
- Is crossed superiorly by the azygous vein as it passes to the superior vena cava

— *Left main bronchus (see Fig. 4.6)*

- Is longer, narrower, and more horizontal than the right main bronchus
- Passes below the arch of the aorta and anterior to the esophagus

- Ends within the hilum by dividing into superior and inferior lobe bronchi

— *Epiarterial bronchus*

- Is another name for the right upper lobe bronchus
- Is so named because it arises above the point where the right pulmonary artery crosses the right main bronchus
- Is the most superior of the lobar bronchi; the others are called *hyparterial*

● **Lungs (Fig. 4.7)**

- The lungs are situated on each side of the mediastinum, each within its own half of the thoracic cavity.
- They are covered by a visceral layer of pleura.
- Each has a main bronchus, one pulmonary artery, and two pulmonary veins, which divide within the substance of the lung.
- The lungs are connected by their roots to the mediastinum.
- The **root** of the lung consists of the structures passing between the lung and the mediastinum.
- The **hilum** is the region on the mediastinal surface of the lung where structures enter or leave the lung.
- The pleura covering the root extends inferiorly as a loose sleeve to form the **pulmonary ligament.**

— *Surfaces and borders*

- The **diaphragmatic surface** of each lung is concave inferiorly to fit the diaphragm.
- The **costal surface** is convex to fit against the thoracic wall.
- The **mediastinal surface** is concave to fit against the pericardium and other mediastinal structures.
- The **posterior border** where the costal and mediastinal surfaces meet posteriorly is thick and rounded.
- The **inferior border** is sharp and separates the diaphragmatic surface from the costal and mediastinal surfaces.
- The thin **anterior border** is where the costal and mediastinal surfaces meet anteriorly.
- The **base** is the diaphragmatic surface of the lung.
- The **apex** is the rounded superior projection of the lung into the root of the neck.

— *Right lung (see Fig. 4.7)*

- The right lung is shorter than the left because of the higher right dome of the diaphragm.
- It is divided into **upper, middle, and lower lobes** by the oblique and horizontal fissures.
- The upper and middle lobes together correspond to the upper lobe of the left lung.
- The right lung has three lobar and ten segmental bronchi.
- Important relationships at the hilum:

  — The pulmonary veins lie anteriorly and inferiorly.

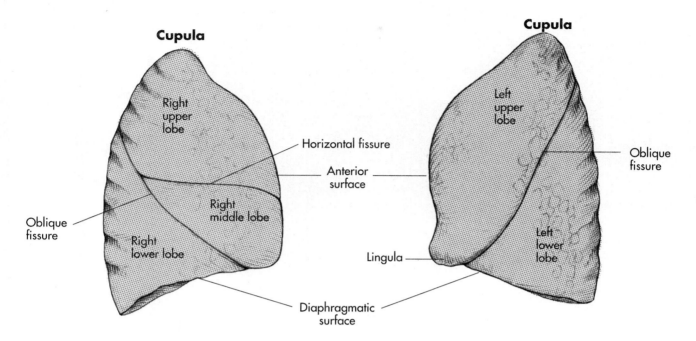

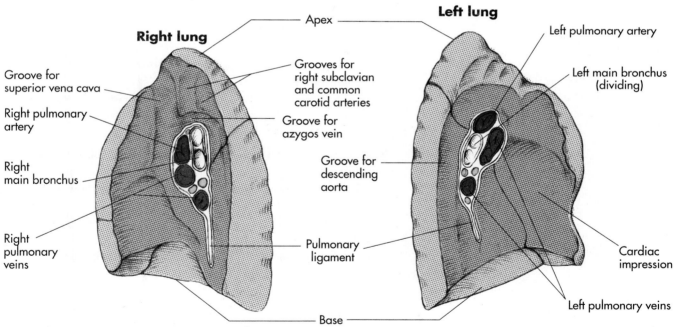

Fig. 4.7 Medial and lateral views of the lungs.

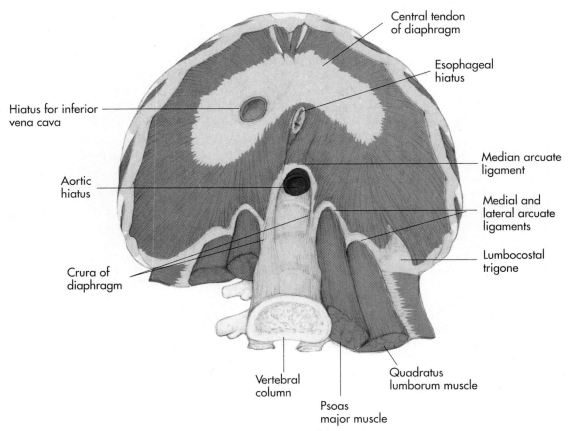

Fig. 4.8 Inferior view of the respiratory diaphragm.

— The main bronchus and epiarterial bronchus lie posteriorly and superiorly.

— The pulmonary artery lies superiorly between the vein and bronchus.

— *Left lung (see Fig. 4.7)*

- The left lung is divided into **upper and lower lobes** by the oblique fissure.
- It has an anterior deficiency, the **cardiac notch,** where it overlies the heart and pericardium.
- The lowest part of the upper lobe forms a thin tongue, the **lingula.**
- The left lung has two lobar and eight segmental bronchi.
- Important relationships at the hilum:

   — The pulmonary veins lie anteriorly and inferiorly.
   — The main bronchus lies posteriorly.
   — The pulmonary artery lies superiorly.

— *Bronchopulmonary segment (Fig. 4.8)*

- The bronchopulmonary segment is the portion of a lung lobe supplied by a segmental (tertiary) bronchus and its accompanying branch of the pulmonary artery.

- It is pyramidal in shape with its apex directed toward the hilum.
- There are ten bronchopulmonary segments on the right side and eight on the left.
- The bronchopulmonary segments are important because disease processes often follow a segmental pattern.
- Bronchopulmonary segments can be surgically removed without compromising the function of surrounding segments because segmental bronchi and arteries do not communicate to adjoining segments.
- Veins draining adjacent segments communicate freely and are said to be intersegmental.

— ***Blood vessels of the lungs***

Pulmonary arteries

- Carry deoxygenated blood to the alveolar capillary plexuses
- Arise within the pericardial sac
- **Left pulmonary artery**

    — Is attached to the aortic arch by the ligamentum arteriosum, the remnant of the ductus arteriosus
    — Crosses above the left main bronchus to reach the hilum

- **Right pulmonary artery**

    — Is longer than the left
    — Crosses under the arch of the aorta and anterior to the right main bronchus to reach the hilum

Pulmonary veins

- Carry oxygenated blood from the lung to the left atrium
- Are intersegmental and do not conform to the pattern of the bronchopulmonary segments
- Are five in number because one major vein drains each lobe
- At the root are two on each side because the upper and middle lobe veins on the right side unite in the hilum

Bronchial arteries

- Bronchial arteries supply oxygenated blood to the bronchial tree and visceral pleura.
- On the left there are two bronchial arteries; they arise from the descending thoracic aorta.
- On the right there is usually only one artery; it arises from the third right posterior intercostal artery.
- Considerable anastomoses occur between the capillaries of the bronchial and pulmonary systems.

Bronchial veins

- Drain deoxygenated blood from the bronchial tree and visceral pleura
- Usually number two on each side
- On the right empty into the azygous vein and on the left into the hemiazygous vein

— *Lymphatic drainage of the lungs*

- A **superficial lymphatic plexus** lies just beneath the visceral pleura and drains toward the hilus.
- A **deep lymphatic plexus** follows along the bronchial tree to the hilus.
- Vessels in the deep plexus begin around the bronchioles because there are no lymphatic vessels in the alveolar walls.
- Many small **peribronchial (pulmonary) nodes** occur within the substance of the lung along the course of the deep plexus.
- The two plexuses end in the **bronchopulmonary nodes** at the root of the lung.
- Lymph leaves the root of the lung to join the **tracheobronchial nodes** and eventually empties into the left and right subclavian veins through the **bronchomediastinal lymph trunks.**

— *Nerve supply of the lungs*

- The lungs receive sympathetic, parasympathetic, and visceral afferent innervation through the pulmonary plexuses.
- **Parasympathetic fibers** are derived from the vagus nerves. On stimulation, they produce **bronchial constriction and mucus secretion.**
- **Sympathetic fibers** are derived from the upper five thoracic sympathetic ganglia. On stimulation, they produce **relaxation** of bronchial smooth muscle.
- **Visceral afferent fibers** from the vagus nerves are sensitive to stretch and participate in the reflex control of respiration. They end in the bronchial mucosa and participate in the cough reflex.

■ **Respiration**

- In the physiologic sense, respiration refers to the exchange of oxygen and carbon dioxide that occurs in the lungs.
- In the anatomic sense, respiration refers to the rhythmic increase and decrease of the thoracic volume that results in the regular exchange of air within the lungs (**inspiration** and **expiration**).
- Fluid adhesion between the visceral and parietal pleura allows the size of the lungs to vary with movement of the diaphragm and thoracic wall.
- During inspiration, enlargement in the volume of the thoracic cavity and lungs creates a negative pressure drawing air into the lungs.

- Efficient respiration requires intimate contact between the parietal and visceral pleura. The presence of air or gas in the pleural cavity (**pneumothorax**) separates these surfaces, resulting in a collapse of the lung.
- Fluid can collect in the pleural cavity and preclude proper inflation of the lung. Fluid may be removed by **thoracentesis,** a surgical procedure in which the thoracic wall is punctured in the intercostal space posterior to the midaxillary line.

● Quiet inspiration

- Almost all of the movement in quiet inspiration is **diaphragmatic.**
- Contraction of the diaphragm pulls the central tendon downward, increasing the **vertical diameter** of the thoracic cavity.
- Quiet inspiration results mainly in ventilation of the lower lobes.

- **Forced inspiration**

  - The need for increased ventilation may occur in exercise or disease.
  - Additional excursion of the diaphragm further increases the vertical diameter of the thoracic cavity.
  - Contraction of the **intercostal muscles** elevates the ribs, carrying the sternum upward and forward. This action is analogous to raising the handle of a bucket and increases the **anteroposterior and lateral diameters** of the thoracic cavity.
  - Further increasing the depth of inspiration (or difficulty in inspiration) will recruit **accessory muscles of respiration** to assist in elevating the ribs.

- **Quiet expiration**

  - Is a passive process largely caused by the elastic recoil of the lungs and relaxation of the diaphragm
  - Requires no direct muscle action

- **Forced expiration**

  - Forced expiration is an active process that reinforces normally passive quiet expiration.
  - Contraction of the muscles of the anterior abdominal wall actively depresses the ribs and increases the intraabdominal pressure, forcing the relaxed diaphragm up into the thorax.

- **Muscles of respiration**

  - Include the respiratory diaphram and those muscles whose only action is to move the rib cage during respiration

    — The external, internal, and innermost intercostal muscles, the subcostal muscles, and the transversus thoracis muscles
    — To a lesser degree, the serratus posterior superior and inferior and the levatores costarum

- **Accessory muscles of respiration**

  - Include muscles of the head, neck, and upper limb that have attachment to the rib cage, manubrium, or sternum
  - Can be called on to assist in respiration if the opposite ends are appropriately fixed
  - Include the

    — Sternocleidomastoid
    — Scalenus anterior and medius
    — Serratus anterior
    — Pectoralis major and minor

- **Respiratory diaphragm (see Fig. 4.8)**

  - The respiratory diaphragm separates the thoracic and abdominal cavities.
  - It is the most important muscle of respiration and is mostly responsible for quiet inspiration.
  - It receives its motor innervation entirely from the phrenic nerve.
  - It receives its sensory innervation from the phrenic nerve except for a narrow peripheral rim supplied by intercostal nerves.

- The **central tendon** is derived embryologically from the **septum transversum** and the **muscular diaphragm** from **myoblasts of the third, fourth, and fifth cervical myotomes** that invaded the septum transversum in its caudal migration.

— *Muscular diaphragm*

- The muscular portion is divided into three parts, each of which inserts into the **central tendon**:

   — The **sternal part** arises from the posterior surface of the **xiphoid process**.
   — The **costal part** arises from the costal cartilages and adjacent parts of the **lower six ribs** and forms the domes.
   — The **lumbar part** arises from the **medial and lateral arcuate ligaments** and from the lumbar vertebrae as the **right and left crura**.

- The **medial arcuate ligament** is a thickening of the fascia over the upper part of the psoas major muscle extending from the body to the transverse process of the first lumbar vertebra.
- The **lateral arcuate ligament** is a thickening of the fascia over the upper part of the quadratus lumborum muscle extending from the twelfth rib to the transverse process of the first lumbar vertebra.
- The **right crus** is longer and larger than the left and takes origin from the bodies of the upper three lumbar vertebrae.
- The **left crus** takes origin from the bodies of the upper two lumbar vertebrae.
- The crura are joined across the midline in front of the aorta by the **median arcuate ligament**.

— *Openings in the diaphragm*

- **Esophageal hiatus**

   — Lies at the level of the tenth thoracic vertebra
   — Lies within the right crus
   — Transmits the esophagus, the vagus nerves, and the esophageal branches of the left gastric vessels

- **Aortic hiatus**

   — Lies at the level of the twelfth thoracic vertebra
   — Lies between the crura and behind the median arcuate ligament
   — Transmits the aorta, the thoracic duct, and sometimes the azygous vein

- **Vena caval hiatus**

   — Lies at the level of the eighth thoracic vertebra
   — Lies within the central tendon to the right of midline
   — Transmits the inferior vena cava and branches of the right phrenic nerve

◼ Pericardium and Heart

● **Pericardium** The pericardium is a sac that encloses the heart, the proximal segments of the great vessels, and the terminal segment of the inferior vena cava. The sac consists of two layers, an outer fibrous layer and an inner serous layer.

— *Fibrous pericardium*

- Is a tough fibrous sac surrounding the heart
- Fuses firmly with the adventitia of the ascending aorta and pulmonary trunk and to a lesser degree with the six veins that pierce it
- Rests inferiorly on and fuses with the central tendon of the diaphragm

— *Serous pericardium*

- The serous layer of pericardium is a single sheet that covers the heart as the **visceral layer** and the inner surface of the fibrous pericardium as the **parietal layer.**
- The two layers become continuous at the roots of the great vessels forming the closed **pericardial cavity.**
- The cavity is a potential space that is normally empty except for a small amount of lubricating fluid, which allows the heart to move freely as it beats.
- Rapid accumulation of blood or other fluids within the pericardial cavity (**cardiac tamponade**) may compromise the normal function of the heart because the fibrous pericardium resists sudden distention.

— *Pericardial sinuses*

- The points at which the visceral layer of serous pericardium reflects from the heart onto the fibrous pericardium as the parietal layer of serous pericardium are the **pericardial reflections.** These reflections occur at the roots of the great vessels entering and leaving the heart.
- One line of reflection surrounds the pulmonary veins and vena cava, thus forming a ∪-shaped blind pocket dorsal to the left atrium, the **oblique pericardial sinus.**
- A second line of reflection surrounds the aorta and pulmonary trunk. A finger passed from the right side of the pericardial cavity to the left side between these two lines of reflection traverses the **transverse pericardial sinus.** The finger lies anterior to the superior vena cava, posterior to the ascending aorta and pulmonary trunk, and superior to the pulmonary veins and left atrium.

● **Heart**

— *Structure of the heart*

- The **epicardium** covers the outside of the heart and is composed of the visceral layer of serous pericardium and a thin subserous layer of connective tissue.
- The **myocardium** consists of cardiac muscle fibers arranged as spiraling and looping bundles of fibers.

- The **endocardium** lines the interior of the heart and consists of endothelial cells continuous with the endothelial lining of the great vessels.

- The **skeleton of the heart** consists of four firmly connected, fibrous connective tissue rings, the annuli fibrosi, and is continuous with the membranous portion of the interventricular septum. It provides a relatively rigid attachment for the myocardial fiber bundles and the pulmonary, aortic, and atrioventricular valves.

— *External form, surfaces, and borders*

- The **base** is the posterior aspect of the heart and is formed largely by the left atrium but also by a narrow portion of the right atrium.

- The heart projects downward, forward, and to the left from the base to terminate as the blunt **apex.** The apex is located at the level of the fifth intercostal space medial to the nipple and is formed by the left ventricle.

- The **diaphragmatic surface** rests on the diaphragm and is formed largely by the left ventricle but also by a narrow portion of the right ventricle.

- The **sternocostal surface** faces anteriorly and is composed largely of the right atrium and right ventricle but also a narrow portion of the left ventricle.

- The **obtuse margin** is the rounded left side of the heart formed entirely by the left ventricle.

- The **acute margin** is the narrowed inferior border where the sternocostal and diaphragmatic surfaces meet. It is formed largely by the right ventricle.

- The **right margin** is formed on radiographs by the superior vena cava and right atrium.

- The **left margin** is formed on radiographs mainly by the left ventricle and to a small extent by the left atrium.

— *Chambers and valves*

Right atrium

- The right atrium receives blood from the superior and inferior venae cavae, the coronary sinus, and the anterior cardiac veins.

- It is larger and thinner walled than the left atrium.

- It communicates with the right ventricle through the **right atrioventricular orifice,** which is guarded by the **tricuspid valve.**

- The posteriorly situated main cavity, the **sinus venarum cavarum,** is smooth walled. It is derived from incorporation of the right sinus horn into the developing right atrium.

- The anterior portion, including the ear-shaped appendage, the **auricle,** is rough walled because of the presence of pectinate muscles. This portion corresponds to the primitive atrium of the embryonic heart.

- The two parts are separated internally by a longitudinal ridge, the **crista terminalis,** and externally by the **sulcus terminalis.** Their superior end marks the location of the **sinoatrial node,** the "pacemaker" of the heart.

- **Pectinate muscles** are ridgelike thickenings of the atrial musculature found in the anterior half of the right atrium and in both auricles.

- The **coronary sinus** opens between the atrioventricular orifice and the inferior vena cava.

- The **valve of the coronary sinus** and the **valve of the inferior vena cava** are rudimentary endothelial folds. They and the crista terminalis are derived from the right sinus valve of the embryonic heart. In the embryonic heart the valve of the inferior vena cava helps direct blood from the inferior vena cava into the left atrium through the patent foramen ovale.

- The **fossa ovalis** is an oval-shaped depression in the interatrial septum and marks the site of the **foramen ovale** of the embryonic heart through which blood passes from the right atrium to the left atrium before birth. The upper margin of the fossa is formed by the **limbus fossa ovale.**

- The **interatrial septum** forms part of the posterior wall.

Triscuspid valve

- Guards the **right atrioventricular orifice**
- Has **anterior, posterior,** and **septal cusps**
- Allows the flow of blood from the right atrium to the right ventricle during ventricular relaxation (diastole)
- Closes during ventricular contraction (systole)
- Is prevented from being everted into the right ventricle by the papillary muscles and chordae tendinae attached to their margins

Right ventricle

- The right ventricle is considerably thicker walled than the right atrium.

- It forms much of the sternocostal (anterior) surface of the heart and a small part of the diaphragmatic surface.

- It lies anterior to most of the left ventricle.

- The superior portion is the funnel-shaped outflow tract, the **conus arteriosus** or **infundibulum,** which leads to the pulmonary trunk. It is smooth walled and is separated from the ventricle proper by the **supraventricular crest.**

- The ventricle proper is rough walled because of the presence of prominent, irregular muscular projections, the **trabeculae carnae.**

- **Papillary muscles** are projecting cones of ventricular musculature that give rise at their apex to the **chordae tendinae.** The right ventricle typically has three papillary muscles named according to the location of their bases (**anterior, posterior,** and **septal**).

- **Chordae tendinae** are fibrous strands that extend from the apices of the papillary muscles to the free margin of the atrioventricular valve cusps. Chordae tendinae from a single papillary muscle typically connect to more than one cusp.

- The **septomarginal trabecula** or **moderator band** is a relatively constant trabeculae carnae in the form of a free band that passes as a bridge between the interventricular septum and the anterior wall of the ventricle. It conveys the right branch of the atrioventricular bundle.

Pulmonary valve

- The pulmonary valve has **three semilunar cusps,** which are named according to their fetal position.
- In the adult heart, the **right** cusp lies posteriorly and the **anterior** and **left** cusps lie anteriorly.
- The pulmonary valve is forced closed by pressure in the pulmonary trunk during relaxation of the right ventricle.
- It has associated **pulmonary sinuses,** which are dilations of the pulmonary trunk adjacent to each cusp.

Left atrium

- The left atrium receives blood from the four pulmonary veins.
- It is smaller and thicker walled than the right atrium.
- It communicates with the left ventricle through the **left atrioventricular orifice,** which is guarded by the **mitral valve.**
- The posterior portion is smooth walled and receives the four pulmonary veins. It is derived from the incorporation of the proximal portions of the embryonic pulmonary veins.
- The anterior portion, including the ear-shaped appendage, the **auricle,** is rough walled because of the presence of pectinate muscles. This portion is derived from the embryonic atrium.
- The **interatrial septum** forms part of the anterior wall.

Mitral valve

- Guards the **left atrioventricular orifice**
- Has anterior and posterior cusps

Left ventricle

- Forms much of the diaphragmatic surface of the heart and a small part of the sternocostal surface
- Lies largely behind the right ventricle
- Has a wall two to three times as thick as that of the right ventricle because it works harder pumping against the systemic resistance
- Has **trabeculae carnae** that are less coarse than those of the right ventricle
- Has no **moderator band**
- Has two large **papillary muscles, anterior** and **posterior,** each of which sends chordae tendinae to both mitral cusps

Aortic valve

- The aortic valve resembles the pulmonary valve except that it is somewhat more robust to accommodate the higher systemic pressure.
- It has **three semilunar cusps** and **sinuses** named according to their fetal position.
- In the adult heart, the **right** cusp lies anteriorly and the **posterior** and **left** cusps lie posteriorly.

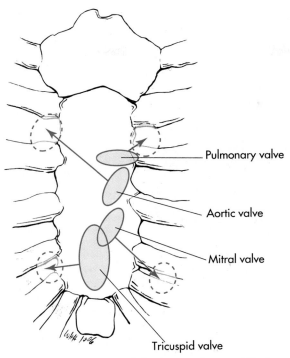

Fig. 4.9 Surface projection of the heart valves and their sounds.

- The **left and right coronary arteries** open from the **left and right sinuses,** respectively.

— *Heart sounds* Normal function of the heart produces two sounds: *lub* and *dup.* The first sound coincides with the closure of the atrioventricular valves at the start of systole. The second sound is produced by the closure of the aortic and pulmonary valves at the end of systole. Significantly, the position at which the sound of each heart valve is best heard **does not** correspond to the surface projection of the valve (Fig. 4.9). The positions at which the sounds of individual valves are best heard are as follows:

- Tricuspid valve—lower end of sternum opposite fourth to sixth intercostal spaces
- Mitral valve—at apex in the left fifth intercostal space in the midclavicular line
- Pulmonary valve—medial end of left second intercostal space
- Aortic valve—medial end of right second intercostal space

— *Conducting system (Fig. 4.10)* The conducting system is necessary for the orderly synchronous rhythm of atrial and ventricular contraction and to establish a common rate at which these chambers will contract. It is composed of modified, specialized cardiac muscle cells lying immediately beneath the endocardial layer.

Sinoatrial node

- The sinoatrial node is also known as the **pacemaker** of the heart because it initiates the stimulus that causes contraction of the heart.

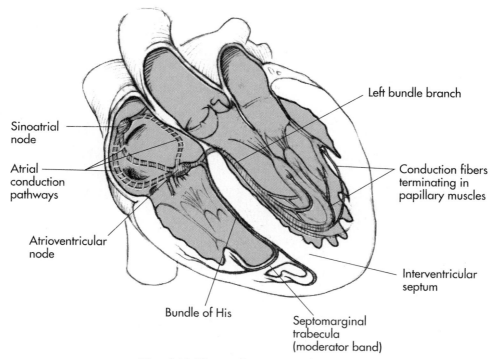

Sinoatrial
node

Atrial
conduction
pathways

Atrioventricular
node

Bundle of His

Septomarginal
trabecula
(moderator band)

Left bundle branch

Conduction fibers
terminating in
papillary muscles

Interventricular
septum

Fig. 4.10 The conducting system of the heart.

• Its location in the atrial wall is marked by the superior end of the sulcus terminalis near the opening of the superior vena cava.

• The wave of contraction it generates spreads over both atria but does not reach the ventricles directly because the atrial and ventricular musculature are nowhere continuous.

• Although the sinoatrial node possesses an **inherent rhythmicity**, direct stimulation by the **sympathetic cardiac nerves increases** the rate of contraction, and direct stimulation by the **parasympathetic cardiac nerves decreases** the rate of contraction.

• The **sinoatrial artery** (artery to the sinoatrial node) usually arises from the right coronary artery but may be a branch of the left coronary artery.

Atrioventricular node

• The atrioventricular node is a collection of specialized cardiac muscle cells in the interatrial septum posterior to the attachment of the septal cusp of the tricuspid valve and above the opening of the coronary sinus.

• It receives the impulse generated in the sinoatrial node and passes it to the **atrioventricular bundle.**

• The **artery to the atrioventricular node** arises from the right coronary artery as it turns from the coronary sulcus into the posterior interventricular sulcus.

Atrioventricular bundle

• Begins as a continuation of the atrioventricular node and ends as the plexus of subendocardial **Purkinje fibers** in the ventricular wall.

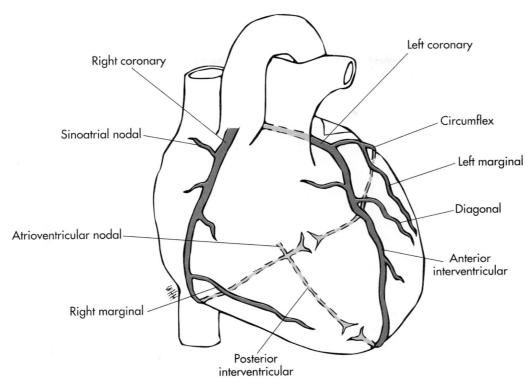

Fig. 4.11 The coronary arteries.

• The bundle descends through a channel in the fibrous skeleton to reach the **membranous interventricular septum.** This is the only connection between the myocardium of the atria and the ventricles.

• In the muscular interventricular septum, the bundle divides into branches to each ventricle, the **right and left crus.** Clinicians refer to these as **bundle branches.**

• The **right crus** passes through the **septomarginal trabecula.**

• The atrioventricular bundle ensures that ventricular contraction begins in the region of the apex.

— *Blood supply of the heart*

• The heart is supplied entirely by the right and left coronary arteries, which are the only branches of the ascending aorta.

• The flow of blood through the coronary arteries is greatest during filling of the heart (diastole) while the myocardium is relaxed and the aortic valve is closed.

• The coronary arteries are essentially end arteries. Anastomoses between these vessels are inadequate to maintain the heart muscle in the event of a sudden major reduction of flow through either vessel or its branches. The resulting damage to the heart muscle is referred to as a **myocardial infarction.**

Right coronary artery (Fig. 4.11)

• Arises from the **right aortic sinus** and passes between the pulmonary trunk and right auricle to reach the **coronary sulcus**

- Follows the coronary sulcus to the diaphragmatic surface where it terminates by anastomosing with branches of the left coronary artery

- Mainly supplies the right atrium, the right ventricle, and the posterior half of the interventricular septum

  - **Important named branches** of the right coronary artery

    — **Artery to the sinoatrial node,** which also supplies adjacent parts of the right atrium

    — **Artery to the atrioventricular node,** which arises as the right coronary descends into the posterior interventricular sulcus

    — **Right marginal artery,** which runs along the acute margin of the right ventricle to the apex.

    — **Posterior interventricular artery,** which passes in the posterior interventricular sulcus to the apex (clinicians frequently refer to this vessel as the **posterior descending artery [PDA]**)

Left coronary artery

- Arises from the **left aortic sinus** and passes to the left between the pulmonary trunk and left auricle to reach the **coronary sulcus**

  - Is typically larger than the right coronary artery

- Terminates in the coronary sulcus by dividing into two branches of comparable size, the **circumflex branch** and the **anterior interventricular branch**

- Mainly supplies the left atrium, the left ventricle, and the anterior half of the interventricular septum

  - **Important named branches**

    — **Anterior interventricular artery,** which descends to the apex in the anterior interventricular sulcus to anastomose with the posterior interventricular artery (clinicians frequently refer to this vessel as the **left anterior descending [LAD] artery**)

    — **Circumflex artery,** which passes posteriorly in the coronary sulcus to anastomose with terminal branches of the right coronary artery

    — **Left marginal artery,** a branch of the circumflex artery, which runs along the obtuse margin of the left ventricle

    — **Diagonal arteries** (one or more), which arise from the anterior interventricular artery to supply the left ventricle

    — **Posterior ventricular arteries** (one or more), which arise from the circumflex artery to supply the left ventricle

Variations in arterial supply The usual arrangement with the posterior interventricular artery arising from the right coronary artery is said to be **right dominant** even though the right and left coronary arteries have about equal distribution. When the circumflex branch of the left coronary terminates as the posterior interventricular artery, the pattern is referred to as **left dominant.**

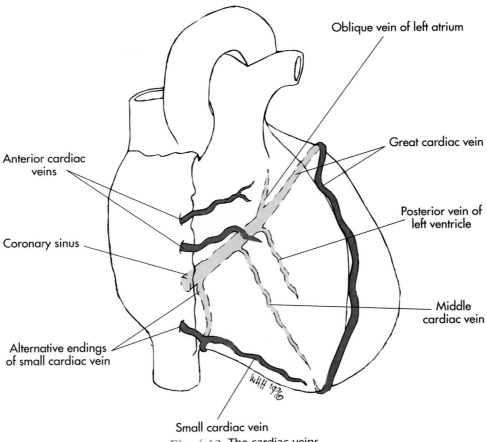

Fig. 4.12 The cardiac veins.

— *Venous drainage of the heart (Fig. 4.12)*

   • Blood from the coronary circulation returns to the right atrium through **cardiac veins,** the largest of which is the coronary sinus.

   • The **coronary sinus** lies in the posterior part of the coronary sulcus and opens into the right atrium between the tricuspid valve and the orifice of the inferior vena cava. It may be considered to be a direct continuation of the **great cardiac vein.**

   • The **tributaries of the coronary sinus** include the following:

   — The **great cardiac vein** begins at the apex and ascends in the anterior interventricular sulcus to reach the coronary sulcus and drain into the left end of the coronary sinus. In its course it lies alongside the **anterior interventricular artery.**

   — The **middle cardiac vein** begins at the apex and ascends in the posterior interventricular sulcus to reach the coronary sulcus and empty along the midpoint of the coronary sinus. In its course it lies alongside the **posterior interventricular artery.**

   — The **small cardiac vein** runs along the acute margin of the right ventricle to terminate in the right end of the coronary sinus. In its course it accompanies the **right marginal artery.**

— The **oblique vein of the left atrium** runs downward on the left atrium to end in the coronary sinus. It is of interest because it represents a remnant of the embryonic left common cardinal vein.

— The **posterior vein of the left ventricle** drains the diaphragmatic surface of the left ventricle and enters the first part of the coronary sinus.

• Cardiac veins that **do not end in the coronary sinus** include the following:

— Two or three small **anterior cardiac veins** drain the sternocostal surface of the right ventricle and empty directly into the right atrium.

— Numerous **smallest cardiac veins** (venae cordis minimae) arise in the walls of the heart and open directly into the chambers. They are most numerous in the right atrium.

— *Nerve supply of the heart*

• The heart is innervated by **sympathetic and parasympathetic fibers** of the autonomic nervous system and by their accompanying **visceral afferent fibers** through the cardic plexuses.

• The cervical origin of the heart innervation attests to the original location of the **cardiogenic area** in the splanchnic mesoderm at the cranial end of the embryonic germ disk.

Sympathetic innervation to the heart

• Is distributed primarily to the conducting system and the coronary arteries

• When stimulated causes increased heart rate, increased force of ventricular contraction, and dilation of coronary arteries

• Is derived mostly from cardiac branches of the superior, middle, and inferior cervical sympathetic ganglia

• Includes **preganglionic neurons** in the **intermediolateral cell column** (IMLCC) of the upper thoracic spinal cord segments and **postganglionic neurons** in the **cervical sympathetic ganglia**

Parasympathetic innervation to the heart

• Is distributed primarily to the conducting system

• When stimulated causes decreased heart rate and decreased force of ventricular contraction

• Is derived from cardiac branches of the cervical and thoracic **vagus nerves**

• Includes **preganglionic neurons** in the **dorsal motor nucleus** in the brain stem and **postganglionic neurons** in **terminal ganglia** scattered in the cardiac plexuses

Visceral afferent fibers traveling with sympathetic fibers

• Originate in the **dorsal root ganglia** of the upper thoracic segments of the spinal cord

• Provide sensory input for important **cardiac reflexes** and are the sole conductors of **pain** from the heart

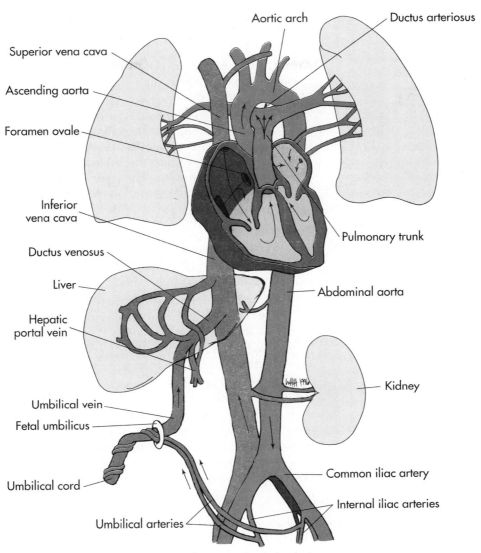

Superior vena cava
Aortic arch
Ductus arteriosus
Ascending aorta
Foramen ovale
Inferior vena cava
Pulmonary trunk
Ductus venosus
Liver
Abdominal aorta
Hepatic portal vein
Kidney
Umbilical vein
Fetal umbilicus
Common iliac artery
Internal iliac arteries
Umbilical cord
Umbilical arteries

Fig. 4.13 The fetal circulation.

- Account for referred heart pain (**angina pectoris**) to the up-per thoracic wall and the ulnar border of the left upper ex-tremity

Visceral afferent fibers *traveling with* ***parasympathetic fibers***

- Originate in the **inferior vagal ganglion** located at the base of the skull
- Provide sensory input for important **cardiac reflexes**

- **Fetal circulation and changes at birth (Fig. 4.13)**
  - *Fetal circulation*
    - **Oxygenated blood** from the placenta enters the fetus through the **umbilical vein** and passes to the **liver.**
    - This blood is largely shunted through the **liver to the inferior vena cava** via the **ductus venosus.**

• Blood from the **inferior vena cava** reaches the **right atrium** where it is directed by the valve of the inferior vena cava toward the **foramen ovale.**

• It passes from the right atrium to the **left atrium** through the foramen ovale. In this way most oxygenated blood bypasses the lungs and directly enters the left side of the heart to be distributed to the systemic circulation.

• The blood pumped by the **right ventricle** into the **pulmonary trunk** is largely **deoxygenated** and is derived mostly from the superior vena cava. Most of this blood bypasses the lungs via the **ductus arteriosus,** a shunt that joins the aortic arch.

• **Deoxygenated blood** returns to the **placenta** through the **umbilical arteries.**

— *Changes at birth*

• The fetal circulation functions until shortly after the newborn infant takes its first breath. Within minutes the adult pattern of circulation is established.

• Contraction of the **umbilical arteries** stops the flow of blood to the placenta. The remnants of these vessels form the **medial umbilical ligaments.**

• Blood flow from the placenta stops. The **umbilical vein** closes and obliterates to form the **ligamentum teres hepatis.**

• The **ductus venosus** closes and obliterates to form the **ligamentum venosum,** establishing normal circulation to the liver.

• With expansion of the lungs and the rise in the left atrial pressure, the **foramen ovale** closes and its flaplike valve eventually fuses with the interatrial septum giving rise to the **fossa ovalis.**

• The **ductus arteriosus** closes and eventually obliterates giving rise to the **ligamentum arteriosum.**

▪ Blood Vessels of the Thorax

● **Aorta and its branches** For descriptive purposes, the aorta may be divided into four parts, three of which are in the thorax (Fig. 4.14).

— *Ascending aorta*

• The ascending aorta begins within the pericardial sac at the aortic valve and ascends behind the sternum to end at the level of the **sternal angle.**

• The wall has three **aortic sinuses** located immediately above the cusps of the aortic valve.

• The **only branches** of the ascending aorta are the **right and left coronary arteries,** which begin at the right and left aortic sinuses.

— *Arch of the aorta*

• The arch of the aorta lies within the **superior mediastinum.**

• It begins as a continuation of the ascending aorta lying behind the manubrium and in front of the trachea.

• It arches posteriorly and slightly to the left over the right pulmonary artery and the left main bronchus.

• The **apex** of the arch reaches the **middle of the manubrium**

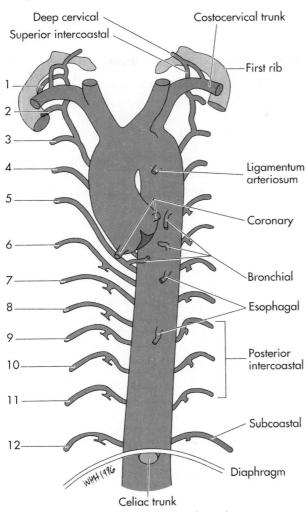

Fig. 4.14 Branches of the thoracic aorta.

where it gives rise to its **three main branches,** which ascend to the superior thoracic aperture in relationship to the trachea:

— **Brachiocephalic artery** (ends by dividing into the **right subclavian** and **right common carotid** arteries)
— **Left common carotid artery**
— **Left subclavian artery**

• A much smaller inconstant branch, **the thyroid ima artery,** may arise from the apex of the arch between the brachiocephalic and left common carotid arteries to supply the thyroid gland.

• **Important relationships** of the arch include the following:

— **Anteriorly**—left phrenic nerve, left vagus nerves, superficial cardiac plexus, mediastinal pleura
— **Inferiorly**—left recurrent laryngeal nerve, ligamentum arteriosum, pulmonary trunk, left main bronchus
— **Posteriorly**—trachea, left recurrent laryngeal nerve

— *Descending thoracic aorta*

- Lies within the **posterior mediastinum**
- Begins at the level of the **sternal angle** (the lower border of the body of the fourth thoracic vertebra)
- Ends over the front of the twelfth thoracic vertebral body
- Is continuous with the abdominal aorta through the aortic hiatus in the respiratory diaphragm
- Important named branches

    — Paired **posterior intercostal arteries** supplying the lower nine intercostal spaces
    — Paired **subcostal arteries** running beneath the twelfth rib
    — Two or more **bronchial arteries** (commonly, the right bronchial artery arises from the third right posterior intercostal artery rather than the aorta)
    — Two to five **esophageal arteries,** one of which may arise in common with the right bronchial artery.

- **Other arteries of the thorax** Apart from the brachiocephalic artery, the large branches of the aortic arch normally give no branches in their thoracic course. The subclavian arteries, however, give rise to vessels that reenter the superior thoracic aperture to supply thoracic structures.

    - The **supreme intercostal artery** arises from the costocervical trunk of the subclavian artery to supply the **first two intercostal spaces.**
    - The **internal thoracic artery** arises in the root of the neck and descends vertically just lateral to the sternum.
    - Important named **branches of the internal thoracic artery** include the following:

        — **Anterior intercostal arteries** supply the first five or six intercostal spaces.
        — **Musculophrenic artery,** a terminal branch, supplies the diaphragm and the seventh to ninth intercostal spaces.
        — **Superior epigastric artery,** a terminal branch, descends in the rectus sheath to supply the abdominal wall and anastomose with the inferior epigastric artery.
        — **Pericardiacophrenic artery** accompanies the phrenic nerve and supplies the pericardium, mediastinal pleura, and diaphragm.
        — **Perforating branches** accompany the anterior cutaneous branches of the intercostal nerves. They are largest in the second to fourth intercostal spaces of the female where they supply the breast.

- **Great systemic veins of the thorax** The right atrium receives blood from the superior vena cava and inferior vena cava. The superior vena cava returns blood from the head, neck, upper extremities, and thorax; the inferior vena cava returns blood from the abdomen, pelvis, and lower extremity (Fig. 4.15).

    — *Right brachiocephalic vein*

        - Begins with the union of the **right internal jugular** and **right subclavian veins**

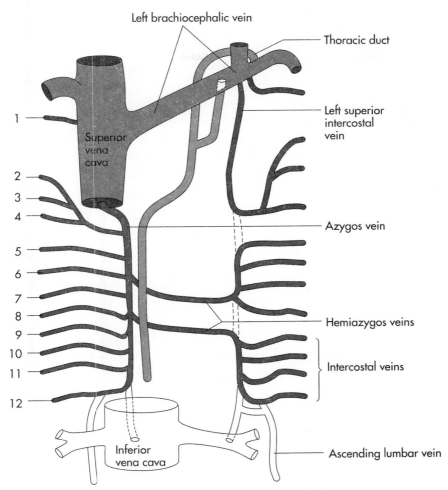

Fig. 4.15 The azygous system of veins.

- Forms in the root of the neck behind the medial end of the right clavicle
- In its course lies close to the right border of the manubrium
- Receives the **right internal thoracic vein** as its only thoracic tributary

— *Left brachiocephalic vein*

- Begins with the union of the **left internal jugular** and **left subclavian veins**
- Forms in the root of the neck behind the medial end of the left clavicle
- In its course passes obliquely down and to the right behind the manubrium
- Receives three tributaries, the **left internal thoracic vein,** the **left superior intercostal vein,** and the **inferior thyroid veins**

— *Superior vena cava*

- Begins with the union of the **right and left brachiocephalic veins**

- Forms behind the right first costal cartilage
- Enters the right atrium behind the right third costal cartilage
- Lower half lies within the pericardial sac
- Receives one major tributary, the **azygous vein,** just before it enters the pericardial sac

— *Inferior vena cava*

- Is formed in the abdomen
- Passes through an opening in the central tendon of the diaphragm at the level of the eighth thoracic vertebra
- Pierces the pericardial sac to end in the right atrium

● **Azygous system of veins (see Fig. 4.15)**

- Drains most of the blood from the thoracic wall
- Is composed of longitudinal veins lying on the sides of the thoracic vertebral bodies
- Is prone to largely insignificant variation from the basic pattern
- Forms an important potential anastomosis between the superior and inferior vena caval systems

— *Azygous vein*

- Forms in the abdomen by union of the **right subcostal** and **right ascending lumbar veins**
- Enters the thorax through the aortic hiatus
- Drains all of the **right posterior intercostal veins** except the first
- Receives the second through fourth right posterior intercostal veins through the **right superior intercostal vein**
- At the level of the fourth thoracic vertebra arches over the root of the right lung to join the **superior vena cava**
- Important tributaries include **bronchial, esophageal, hemiazygous,** and **accessory hemiazygous veins**

— *Hemiazygous vein*

- Forms in the abdomen by union of the **left subcostal** and **left ascending lumbar veins**
- Enters the thorax through the aortic hiatus
- Receives the **lower four left posterior intercostal veins**
- Crosses to the right at the level of the **eighth thoracic vertebra** to end in the **azygous vein**

— *Accessory hemiazygous vein*

- Drains the **fourth to the seventh or eighth intercostal spaces**
- Crosses to the right at the level of the **seventh thoracic vertebra** to end in the **azygous vein**
- Often joins the hemiazygous vein before draining to the azygous vein

— *Intercostal veins not joining the azygous system of veins*

- The **first intercostal space** on both sides is drained by the **supreme intercostal vein,** which empties into the corresponding **brachiocephalic vein.**

• The **left superior intercostal vein** drains the **left second and third intercostal spaces** and crosses the arch of the aorta to end in the left brachiocephalic vein.

■ Nerves of the Thorax

● **Phrenic nerves**

• Phrenic nerves arise in the neck from the ventral rami of the third, fourth, and fifth cervical spinal nerves. The major contribution is from C4.

• They are the sole motor innervation to the respiratory diaphragm.

• They provide sensory fibers to the pericardium, mediastinal pleura, and the pleural and peritoneal coverings of the central part of the diaphragm.

• Pain from the areas supplied by the phrenic nerves is usually referred to the base of the neck and to the tip of the shoulder.

• The C5 contribution may arise from the nerve to the subclavius and is designated an **accessory phrenic nerve.**

• **Important relationships** of the phrenic nerves include the following:

— Both nerves descend through the **middle mediastinum** between the fibrous pericardium and the mediastinal pleura.

— In the **superior mediastinum** the **right nerve** lies at the right side of the superior vena cava.

— In the **superior mediastinum** the **left nerve** descends between the left subclavian and left common carotid arteries and crosses the aortic arch laterally.

— Both are accompanied in their course by the **pericardiacophrenic** branches of the internal thoracic vessels.

● **Vagus nerves**

• After arising from the brain stem, the vagi exit the skull and descend through the neck to enter the superior thoracic aperture.

• They supply **parasympathetic** and **general visceral afferent** innervation to the thoracic viscera.

• **Parasympathetic preganglionic** cell bodies are located in **dorsal motor nucleus** in the brain stem.

• **Parasympathetic postganglionic** cell bodies are located in **terminal ganglia** located in the autonomic plexuses or in the wall of the organ supplied.

• **Visceral afferent fibers** in the vagus nerves are from cell bodies in the **inferior vagal (nodose) ganglia.**

• **Important relationships** of the **right vagus** nerve include the following:

— It crosses anterior to the first part of the right subclavian artery.

— It descends in the superior mediastinum on the right side of the trachea.

— It passes posterior to the root of the right lung and onto the posterior esophagus contributing to the esophageal plexus.

• **Important relationships** of the **left vagus** nerve include the following:

— It enters the thorax between the left common carotid and left subclavian arteries.

— It crosses the left side of the aortic arch.

— It passes posterior to the root of the left lung and onto the anterior esophagus contributing to the esophageal plexus.

• **Important branches** of the **vagus** nerves in the thorax include the following:

— **Cardiac branches** of the vagi and the left recurrent laryngeal nerve to the cardiac plexuses.

— **Pulmonary branches** contribute to autonomic plexuses to the lungs.

— **Esophageal branches** contribute to the esophageal plexuses.

— The **left recurrent laryngeal nerve** arises from the left vagus at the aortic arch, hooks below the arch to the left of the **ligamentum arteriosum,** and ascends between the trachea and esophagus.

— The **right recurrent laryngeal nerve** arises in the neck, not in the thorax, and loops around the first part of the subclavian artery.

 Autonomic plexuses of the thorax

• The viscera of the thorax are innervated by **sympathetic and parasympathetic (GVE) fibers** of the autonomic nervous system and by their accompanying **general visceral afferent (GVA) fibers** through the thoracic **autonomic plexuses.**

• **Sympathetic and parasympathetic fibers** are motor to cardiac muscle, smooth muscle, and glands of the thoracic viscera and generally function below the level of consciousness.

• **General visceral afferent fibers** function as the sensory limb of the **autonomic reflex arc.**

• The **visceral nerves** of the thorax are of great importance because they control the function of the heart and lungs.

— *Superficial cardiac plexus*

• Lies just below the arch of the aorta
• Receives contributions from

— Superior cervical cardiac branch of the left sympathetic trunk
— Inferior cervical cardiac branch of the left vagus nerve
— Communicates with the deep cardiac plexus

— *Deep cardiac plexus*

• Lies between the arch of the aorta and the bifurcation of the trachea
• Receives contributions from

— All cervical and thoracic cardiac branches of the **right sympathetic trunk** and **right vagus nerves**
— All cervical and thoracic cardiac branches of the **left sympathetic trunk** and **left vagus nerves** not going to the superficial plexus

— *Coronary plexuses*

- Are extensions of the cardiac plexuses along the coronary arteries to supply the heart

— *Pulmonary plexus*

- Constitutes the nerve supply to the lungs
- Is divided into an **anterior** and **posterior pulmonary plexus** lying anterior and posterior to the pulmonary artery at the root of the lung
  - Receives contributions from

    — Vagus nerves
    — Branches of the upper five thoracic sympathetic ganglia
    — Deep cardiac plexus

— *Esophageal plexus*

- The esophageal plexus is formed by strands of the vagus nerves leaving the posterior pulmonary plexuses.
- The right and left vagus nerves lose their identity in this plexus.
- The esophageal plexus receives contributions from the upper five thoracic sympathetic ganglia.
- It reunites at the lower end of the esophagus into anterior and posterior vagal trunks.

● **Thoracic sympathetic trunk**

- The thoracic sympathetic trunk descends anterior to the heads of the ribs and the intercostal vessels and nerves.
- It leaves the thorax by passing behind the medial arcuate ligament.
- It has 11 or 12 segmentally arranged ganglia corresponding to the spinal nerves.
- The inferior cervical and the first thoracic ganglia often fuse to form the **cervicothoracic, or stellate, ganglion.**
- Sympathetic ganglia contain the cell bodies of sympathetic postganglionic neurons.

● **Thoracic sympathetic nerves**

- Contain preganglionic sympathetic fibers from cell bodies located in the IMLCC of the thoracic spinal cord segments
- Contain postganglionic sympathetic fibers from cell bodies located in the thoracic sympathetic chain ganglia
- Contain visceral afferent fibers from cell bodies located in the dorsal root ganglia of thoracic spinal nerves
- **Gray ramus communicans**

  — Connects each ganglion to a corresponding thoracic spinal nerve
  — Contains postganglionic sympathetic fibers that end on sweat glands, vascular smooth muscle, and arrector pili muscles

- **White ramus communicans**

  — Connects each ganglion from T1 to L2 to a corresponding thoracic spinal nerve

— Is found only between T1 and L2 because this represents the craniocaudal extent of the IMLCC
— Contains preganglionic sympathetic fibers and visceral afferent fibers
— Carries preganglionic sympathetic fibers for the entire body including the head

- **Visceral branches** from the upper five thoracic ganglia

  — Are distributed through the aortic, pulmonary, and esophageal plexuses
  — Contain postganglionic sympathetic fibers and visceral afferent fibers

- **Thoracic splanchnic nerves**

  — Are visceral branches of the fifth through twelfth thoracic ganglia
  — Supply abdominal organs rather than thoracic organs
  — Contain mostly preganglionic sympathetic fibers that synapse in abdominal prevertebral ganglia and visceral afferent fibers
  — **Greater splanchnic** nerve (arises from the fifth to ninth ganglia)
  — **Lesser splanchnic** nerve (arises from the tenth and eleventh ganglia)
  — **Least splanchnic** nerve (arises from the twelfth ganglion)

■ Lymphatic Drainage of the Thorax

- Lymph nodes of the thoracic wall

  — *Parasternal nodes*

    - Lie behind the sternum along the course of the internal thoracic artery
    - Receive lymph from the thoracic wall, the upper anterior abdominal wall, and the diaphragm
    - Are clinically important because they also receive a significant amount of lymph from the mammary gland
    - Efferent channel is the **parasternal lymph trunk**

  — *Posterior intercostal nodes*

    - Lie in the posterior intercostal space near the heads of the ribs
    - Receive lymph from the thoracic wall and the paravertebral region
    - Efferent vessels from the left and lower right nodes drain to the **thoracic duct**
    - Efferent vessels from the upper right nodes drain to the **right lymphatic duct**

  — *Diaphragmatic nodes*

    - Lie on the upper surface of the diaphragm
    - Receive lymph from the diaphragm, pericardium, and upper surface of the liver
    - Efferent vessels drain to the parasternal and posterior mediastinal nodes

- Lymph nodes of the thoracic cavity
  — *Posterior mediastinal nodes*
    - Lie along the esophagus and the descending thoracic aorta
    - Receive lymph from the pericardium and esophagus
    - Also receive afferents from the diaphragmatic nodes
    - Efferents drain to the bronchomediastinal nodes
  — *Brachiocephalic nodes*
    - Lie in the superior mediastinum along the brachiocephalic veins
    - Receive afferents from the heart, pericardium, thymus, and thyroid
    - Efferents drain to the bronchomediastinal lymph trunk
  — *Tracheobronchial nodes*
    - Lie around the bifurcation of the trachea and the main bronchi
    - Are some of the largest lymph nodes in the body
    - Receive the lymphatic drainage of the lung through the bronchopulmonary nodes
    - Efferents drain to the bronchomediastinal lymph trunk
  — *Bronchomediastinal lymph trunks*
    - Are formed in the superior mediastinum by a joining of efferent vessels from
      — Posterior mediastinal nodes
      — Brachiocephalic nodes
      — Tracheobronchial nodes
      — Parasternal nodes
    - End on the right side in **right lymphatic duct**
    - On the left side join the **thoracic duct** near its termination
- **Thoracic duct**
  - Begins in the abdomen behind the right crus of the diaphragm
  - Receives the majority of lymph from the body below the respiratory diaphragm into its dilated lower end, the **cysterna chyli**
  - In the thorax drains the left and lower right posterior intercostal nodes
  - Passes through the aortic hiatus to lie between the descending thoracic aorta and the azygous vein in the posterior mediastinum
  - In the superior mediastinum ascends to the left of the esophagus to reach the root of the neck
  - Terminates by opening near the union of the left **internal jugular and left subclavian veins**
  - Near its termination **receives lymph from**
    — Left side of the head and neck through the **left internal jugular lymph trunk**
    — Left upper extremity through the **left subclavian lymph trunk**
    — Left side of the thoracic cavity through the **left bronchomediastinal lymph trunk**

■ **Esophagus and Thymus**

● **Esophagus**

- Is a muscular tube that begins in the neck as a continuation of the pharynx and ends in the abdomen where it joins the stomach

- Is about 25 cm (10 in.) in length

- Consists of

    — Skeletal muscle in its proximal one third continuous with the muscle of the pharynx

    — Smooth muscle in its distal one third continuous with the muscle of the gut tube

    — A mixture of skeletal and smooth muscle in its middle one third

- Passes through the diaphragm at the level of the tenth thoracic vertebra

- Has obvious constrictions that can be demonstrated on barium swallow

    — At its beginning at the level of the sixth cervical vertebra

    — Where it is crossed by the left main bronchus

    — Where it lies behind the left atrium when the left atrium is enlarged

    — Where it passes through the diaphragm

    — *Relationships of the esophagus*

        - Important relationships in the **superior mediastinum**

            — Anteriorly—the trachea to its bifurcation

            — Posteriorly—the bodies of the upper four thoracic vertebrae

            — To the left—the arch of the aorta, the thoracic duct, and the left recurrent laryngeal nerve

            — To the right—mediastinal pleura

        - Important relationships in the **posterior mediastinum**

            — Anteriorly—the left main bronchus, the pericardium and left atrium (in the middle mediastinum), and the sloping posterior diaphragm

            — Posteriorly—in its upper part, the bodies of the thoracic vertebrae, and in its lower part, the descending thoracic aorta

            — To the left—in its upper part, the descending thoracic aorta, and in its lower part, mediastinal pleura

            — To the right—mediastinal pleura and the arch of the azygous vein

    — *Blood vessels of the esophagus*

        - The esophagus receives its blood supply from the inferior thyroid artery to its upper third, esophageal branches of the descending thoracic aorta to its middle third, and left gastric and inferior phrenic arteries to its lower third.

        - Venous drainage is to the inferior thyroid veins in the upper third, azygous veins in the middle third, and left gastric vein in the lower third.

  • An important **portocaval anastomosis** occurs in the lower esophagus between left gastric veins of the **hepatic portal system** and the esophageal tributaries of the **azygous system.**

— *Nerve supply of the esophagus*

  • The esophagus receives sympathetic, parasympathetic, and visceral afferent innervation from the esophageal plexuses.
  • **Sympathetic fibers** are primarily **vasomotor,** producing vasoconstriction when stimulated.
  • Vagal **parasympathetic fibers** primarily affect **peristalsis** and act through the enteric nervous system.
  • Vagal visceral afferent fibers are concerned with **reflex activity** of the esophagus.
  • **Pain** sensation is carried by visceral afferent fibers traveling with the sympathetic nerves.

● Thymus

  • Is a bilobed lymphoid organ lying behind the sternum in the superior mediastinum
  • Is an important source of T-lymphocytes and is crucial to the establishment of immune competence after birth
  • Relative to body size is largest at birth
  • At birth may extend from the superior mediastinum upward into the root of the neck and downward into the anterior mediastinum
  • Continues to grow until puberty but becomes increasingly smaller relative to body size
  • Begins involution after puberty
  • Is supplied by branches of the internal thoracic and inferior thyroid arteries
  • Drains largely to the left brachiocephalic vein

Multiple Choice Review Questions

1. The sound of which of the heart valves is transmitted to the region of the apex beat?

    a. Valve of the inferior vena cava
    b. Left atrioventricular valve
    c. Right atrioventricular valve
    d. Aortic semilunar valve
    e. Pulmonary semilunar valve

2. The posterior interventricular sulcus contains which of the following?

    a. Small cardiac vein
    b. Middle cardiac vein
    c. Great cardiac vein
    d. Coronary sinus
    e. Oblique vein of the left atrium

3. The superior mediastinum is mostly situated posterior to which of the following?

    a. Arch of the aorta
    b. Heart
    c. Manubrium
    d. First rib
    e. Body of the sternum

4. Afferent fibers, which conduct the sensation of pain from the heart, are from cell bodies located in which of the following?

    a. Inferior vagal ganglion
    b. IMLCC at T1-T4
    c. Dorsal root ganglia at T1-T4
    d. Superior, middle, and inferior cervical ganglia
    e. Paravertebral ganglia at T1-T4

5. A cardiothoracic surgeon places his finger into the transverse pericardial sinus from the right side and, with his thumb, clamps the vessel lying just in front of his finger. Which vessel has he occluded?

    a. Superior vena cava
    b. Ascending aorta
    c. Arch of the aorta
    d. Pulmonary trunk
    e. Right pulmonary artery

6. The superficial and deep lymphatic drainage of the lungs unites at the hilus, where they end in which group of nodes?

    a. Thoracic duct nodes
    b. Tracheobronchial nodes
    c. Bronchomediastinal nodes
    d. Parasternal nodes
    e. Bronchopulmonary nodes

7. A tumor limited to the posterior mediastinum would most likely involve which of the following?

    a. Recurrent laryngeal nerves
    b. Trachea
    c. Thoracic duct
    d. Phrenic nerve
    e. Left atrium

8. Which of the following is *true* of the sinoatrial node?

    a. It gives rise to the atrioventricular bundle.
    b. It is located in the interatrial septum.
    c. It lies outside the pericardium.
    d. It is supplied by the right coronary artery.
    e. It receives no innervation from the vagus nerves.

9. Damaged heart muscle resulting from occlusion of the circumflex branch of the left coronary artery would most likely be found in which of the following?

    a. Left atrium and left ventricle
    b. Right atrium and right ventricle
    c. Apex of the heart
    d. Right and left ventricles
    e. Left ventricle and posterior interventricular septum

10. The posterior intercostal artery in the right second intercostal space typically arises from which of the following?

    a. Ascending thoracic aorta
    b. Descending thoracic aorta
    c. Right bronchial artery
    d. Internal thoracic artery
    e. Supreme intercostal artery

Chapter 5

Abdomen

■ **Anterior Abdominal Wall**

● Fasciae of the anterior abdominal wall

— *Superficial layer of superficial fascia*

- Is known as **Camper's fascia**
- Is continuous with the superficial fascia superiorly over the thorax and inferiorly over the thigh
- Is the **fatty layer** and is of variable thickness

— *Deep layer of superficial fascia*

- Is known as **Scarpa's fascia**
- Is the membranous layer
- Is most apparent on the **lower abdominal wall**
- In the lower midline forms the **suspensory** (fundiform) **ligament** of the penis
- Continues into the perineum as the **superficial perineal fascia** (Colles' fascia)
- Fuses with the fascia lata of the thigh below the inguinal ligament

— *Deep fascia*

- Is a thin layer covering the external surface of the abdominal muscles

● Muscles of the anterior abdominal wall (Table 5.1)

- Take the form of three large, flat sheets (the **external and internal abdominal oblique** and the **transversus abdominis** muscles) connecting the **rib cage** above to the **hip bone** below
- Are **muscular** posteriorly and laterally and **aponeurotic** anteriorly and medially
- Are innervated by the lower **intercostal, subcostal,** and **first lumbar** spinal nerves

● Important features of the anterior abdominal wall

— *Linea alba*

- Is a **median raphe** extending from the xiphoid process above to the pubic symphysis below
- Lies between the rectus abdominis muscles
- Represents a fusion of the **aponeuroses** of the **transversus abdominis, internal abdominal oblique,** and **external abdominal oblique** muscles from both sides

Table 5.1 *Muscles of the Anterior Abdominal Wall*

NAME	ORIGIN	INSERTION	ACTION	INNERVATION
External abdominal oblique	External surface of the lower eight ribs	Anterior half of the iliac crest, pubic crest and tubercle, linea alba, and xiphoid process	Flexes and rotates the trunk, compresses the abdominal contents, depresses the ribs in forced expiration	T7-T11 intercostal nerves, subcostal nerve (T12), and iliohypogastric and ilioinguinal nerve (L1)
Internal abdominal oblique	Lateral two-thirds of inguinal ligament, anterior two-thirds of the iliac crest, thoracolumbar fascia	Lowest four ribs, linea alba via the rectus sheath, pubic crest and pectineal line via the conjoint tendon	Flexes and rotates the trunk, compresses the abdominal contents, depresses the ribs in forced expiration	T7-T11 intercostal nerves, subcostal nerve (T12), and iliohypogastric and ilioinguinal nerve (L1)
Transversus abdominis	Lower six costal cartilages, thoracolumbar fascia, iliac crest, lateral one-third of inguinal ligament	Xiphoid process, linea alba via the rectus sheath, pubic crest and pectineal line via the conjoint tendon	Compresses the abdominal contents, depresses the ribs in forced expiration	T7-T11 intercostal nerves, subcostal nerve (T12), and iliohypogastric and ilioinguinal nerve (L1)
Rectus abdominis	Pubic crest and symphysis	Xiphoid process, costal cartilages 5 through 7	Flexes the trunk, depresses the ribs in forced expiration	T7-T11 intercostal nerves, subcostal nerve (T12)
Pyramidalis (sometimes absent)	Body of the pubis	Linea alba	Tenses the linea alba	Subcostal nerve (T12)

— *Linea semilunaris*

  • Is the shallow groove along the curved lateral margin of the **rectus abdominis muscle**

  • Crosses the **costal margin** near the tip of the **ninth costal cartilage**

— *Arcuate line*

  • Is the lower free edge of the **posterior lamina** of the **rectus sheath**

  • Lies midway between the umbilicus and pubis

— *Inguinal ligament*

  • Is the thickened **lower border** of the **external oblique aponeurosis**

  • Extends from the **anterior superior iliac spine** to the **pubic tubercle**

  • Is **curved inward** to form a shallow trough that contains the structures in the **inguinal canal**

  • Fuses inferiorly with the **fascia lata** of the thigh

— *Lacunar ligament*

  • Is the medial extension of the **inguinal ligament** posteriorly and laterally along the **pectineal line** on the superior ramus of the pubis

- Is **continuous** along the pectineal line with the strong fibrous **pectineal ligament** (Cooper's ligament)
  - Forms the medial border of the **femoral ring**
— *Conjoint tendon*
  - Is formed by the **fusion** of the lower parts of the **transversus abdominis aponeurosis** and the **internal oblique aponeurosis**
    - Inserts into the **pubic crest** and the **pectineal line**
    - Lies behind the **spermatic cord** or **round ligament** at the superficial inguinal ring
    - Strengthens the **abdominal wall** behind the **superficial inguinal ring**
— *Reflected inguinal ligament*
  - Arises from the **deep surface** of the **medial end** of the **inguinal ligament**
  - Passes upward over the conjoint tendon to end at the **linea alba**
  - Lies in the **posterior wall** of the **superficial inguinal ring**
— *Rectus sheath*
  - Is a long fibrous **envelope** enclosing the **rectus abdominis** muscle and **pyramidalis** muscle (if present)
  - Contains the **superior and inferior epigastric arteries** and the distal portions of the **thoracoabdominal, subcostal, and iliohypogastric** nerves
  - Is formed by **fusion** of the **aponeuroses** of the **transversus abdominis, internal abdominal oblique, and external abdominal oblique muscles**
  - Has **anterior** and **posterior** layers
  - Is firmly attached to the **tendinous intersections** of the rectus abdominis on the deep surface of the **anterior layer**

Composition of the rectus sheath
  - The aponeurosis of the **external abdominal oblique** muscle contributes to the **anterior layer.**
  - The aponeurosis of the **internal abdominal oblique** muscle **splits** around the rectus abdominis muscle **contributing to** both the **anterior layer** and the **posterior layer.**
  - The aponeurosis of the **transversus abdominis** muscle contributes to the **posterior layer.**

Arcuate line
  - Is the lower free edge of the **posterior lamina** of the **rectus sheath**
  - Marks the point where **all aponeuroses pass anterior** to the **rectus abdominis** muscle and the rectus abdominis rests directly on the **transversalis fascia**
  - Lies midway between the **umbilicus** and **pubis**

● **Topography of the anterior abdominal wall (Fig. 5.1)**
  - The anterior abdominal wall is divided into **nine regions** by **two vertical planes** and **two horizontal planes.**

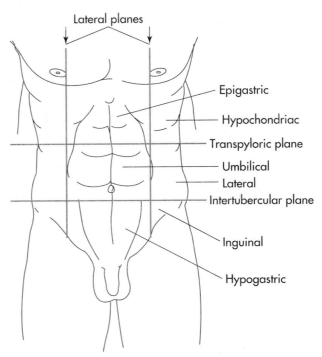

Fig. 5.1 Planes and regions of the anterior abdominal wall.

• The **vertical planes** are the **right and left lateral planes,** which approximate the **midclavicular lines** of the thorax and extend caudally to the midpoint of the **inguinal ligament.**

• The **horizontal planes** are the **transpyloric plane** and the **intertubercular plane.**

• The **transpyloric plane lies midway between the jugular notch** and the **pubic symphysis** (or between the xiphoid and umbilicus). It passes through the lower body of the **first lumbar vertebra,** normally passes through the **pylorus** of the stomach, and intersects the lateral plane at the tip of the **ninth costal cartilage.**

• The **intertubercular plane** passes through the **tubercles of the iliac crest.** It lies at the highest level of the iliac crest, passes through the body of the fifth lumbar vertebra (or the spine of the fourth), and is an important landmark in performing a spinal tap.

• The **lateral regions** are the **right hypochondriac** region, containing the liver; the **left hypochondriac** region, containing the fundus of the stomach and the spleen; the **right lateral** (lumbar) region, containing the ascending colon; the **left lateral** (lumbar) region, containing the descending colon; the **right inguinal** (iliac) region, containing the iliocecal junction and appendix; and the **left inguinal** (iliac) region, containing the sigmoid colon.

• The **midline regions** are the **epigastric** region, containing the liver, stomach, and pancreas; the **umbilical** region, containing the small intestine, transverse colon, and greater omentum; and the **hypogastric** (pubic) region, containing the small intestine, full urinary bladder, or pregnant uterus.

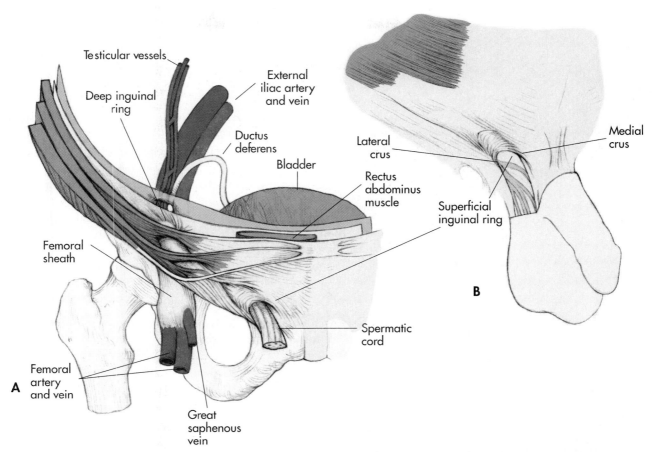

Fig. 5.2 **A,** The relationship of the inguinal canal and spermatic cord to the layers of the anterior abdominal wall. **B,** The external oblique aponeurosis and the superficial inguinal ring.

● Inguinal region (Fig. 5.2)

— *Superficial inguinal ring*

- Is a triangular defect in the **aponeurosis** of the **external abdominal oblique** muscle
- Is the superficial opening of the **inguinal canal**
- Lies above and lateral to the **pubic tubercle**
- Is larger in the **male**, transmitting the **spermatic cord**
- In the **female** transmits the **round ligament of the uterus**
- At its margins is continuous with the **external spermatic fascia**

— *Deep inguinal ring*

- Is the **mouth** of the tubular evagination of the **transversalis fascia**, which becomes the **internal spermatic fascia**
- Lies just **above** the **inguinal ligament** midway between the **anterior superior iliac spine** and the **pubic tubercle**
- Lies just **below** the lower free border of the **transversus abdominis** muscle

- Lies just **lateral** to the **inferior epigastric artery** as it passes upward to enter the rectus sheath

— *Inguinal canal (see Fig. 5.2)*

- Is an oblique passage through the lower abdominal wall
- Is the site of a **potential weakness** in the lower abdominal wall
- Transmits the **spermatic cord** in the **male** and the **round ligament of the uterus** in the **female**
- Extends from the deep inguinal ring to the superficial inguinal ring
- Lies above and parallel to the medial half of the inguinal ligament
- Passes through the **inferior** margin of the **internal abdominal oblique** muscle where some fibers invest the spermatic cord as the **cremasteric muscle and fascia**
- Is said to have a **roof**, a **floor**, an **anterior wall**, and a **posterior wall**

  - Roof

    — Arching fibers of the **transversus abdominis** and **internal abdominal oblique** muscles

  - Floor

    — Medial half of the **inguinal ligament** and the **lacunar ligament**

  - Anterior wall

    — Medially, the **external oblique aponeurosis**
    — Laterally, fibers of the **internal abdominal oblique** muscle arising from the inguinal ligament

  - Posterior wall

    — Medially, the **conjoint tendon**
    — Laterally, the **transversalis fascia**

— *Inguinal triangle (Hesselbach's triangle)*

- Is the triangular interval between the

  — **Rectus abdominis muscle,** medially
  — **Inferior epigastric vessels,** laterally
  — **Inguinal ligament,** inferiorly

- Lies in the abdominal wall **behind** the **superficial inguinal ring**
- Has a posterior wall formed by **transversalis fascia** and the **conjoint tendon** with its strength depending on the adequacy of the conjoint tendon
- Is the site of a potential weakness, which may allow a **direct inguinal hernia**

— *Direct inguinal hernia*

- Occurs in older men (rarely in women)

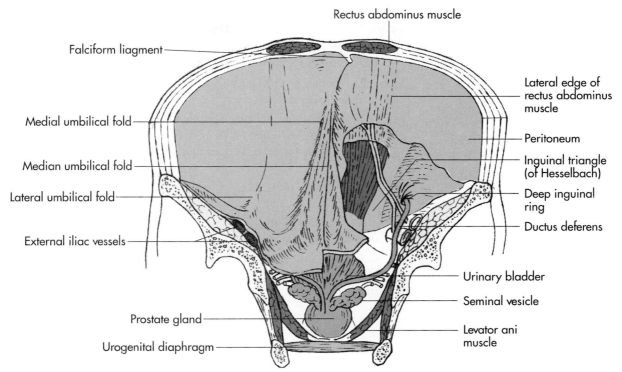

Fig. 5.3 Internal surface of the anterior abdominal wall.

- Results from a **weakness** in the **abdominal wall** behind or just lateral to the superficial inguinal ring
- Passes **directly** through the abdominal wall to reach the superficial inguinal ring
- Does not lie within the coverings of the spermatic cord and does not descend into the scrotum
- Lies **medial** to the **inferior epigastric vessels**
- Has a **sac** formed by the **peritoneum**

— *Indirect inguinal hernia*

- Traverses the **deep inguinal ring,** the **inguinal canal,** and the **superficial inguinal ring**
- Lies **alongside** the **spermatic cord** and **within** the **coverings** of the cord
- May descend into the **scrotum**
- Passes **lateral** to the **inferior epigastric vessels**
- Is said to be **congenital** if it is associated with a persisting **processus vaginalis**
- Is more common than a direct inguinal hernia
- Is more common in boys and young men

● Inner aspect of the lower anterior abdominal wall (Fig. 5.3)

— *Median umbilical fold*

- Is a **midline** peritoneal fold on the inner abdominal wall above the bladder

- Contains the **median umbilical ligament**, a remnant of the embryonic **urachus**
- Extends from the apex of the **bladder** to the **umbilicus**

— *Medial umbilical folds*

- Are paired peritoneal folds lying on each **side** of the **median umbilical fold**
- Contain the **medial umbilical ligament**, a fibrous remnant of the obliterated distal end of the **umbilical artery**
- Extend from the lateral margin of the **bladder** to the **umbilicus**

— *Lateral umbilical folds*

- Are paired peritoneal folds lying on the **lateral** sides of the **medial umbilical folds**
- Contain the **inferior epigastric vessels**
- Extend from medial to the **deep inguinal ring** to the **arcuate line** of the rectus sheath

— *Median inguinal fossa*

- Is the depression in the peritoneal lining of the lower abdominal wall between the **medial** and **lateral** umbilical folds
- Represents the peritoneal covering of the **inguinal triangle (of Hesselbach)**
- Is the area through which **direct inguinal hernias** occur

— *Lateral inguinal fossa*

- Is the depression in the peritoneal lining of the lower abdominal wall **lateral** to the **lateral umbilical fold**

— *Supravesical fossa*

- Is the depression in the peritoneal lining of the lower abdominal wall above the bladder and on each side of the **median umbilical fold**

● **Spermatic cord, scrotum, and testis**

— *Spermatic cord (Fig. 5.4)*

- Is the collection of structures that traverse the inguinal canal passing to or from the testis
- Contains the

  — Ductus deferens
  — Artery of the ductus deferens
  — Testicular artery
  — Testicular veins (pampiniform plexus)
  — Testicular lymph vessels
  — Cremasteric artery
  — Genital branch of the genitofemoral nerve
  — Periarterial autonomic plexus

- Is covered by **three concentric layers** derived from the anterior abdominal wall

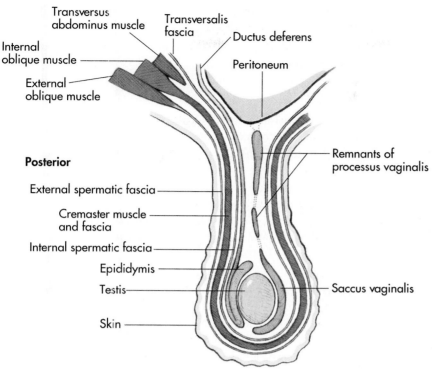

Fig. 5.4 Coverings of the spermatic cord and testis.

— **Internal spermatic fascia** from the **transversalis fascia**
— **Cremasteric muscle and fascia** from the **internal abdominal oblique muscle**
— **External spermatic fascia** from the **external oblique aponeurosis**

Pampiniform plexus of veins

- Consists of 10 to 12 veins that emerge from the back of the **testis**
- Ascends in the **spermatic cord** in an anastomosing network around the **testicular artery**
- Merges in the inguinal canal to form a single **testicular vein** at the **deep inguinal ring**

Cremasteric artery

- Arises from the **inferior epigastric artery** to enter the **deep inguinal ring**
- Supplies the cremaster muscle

Artery of the ductus deferens

- Arises from the **superior vesical artery** to enter the **deep inguinal ring**
- Supplies the **ductus deferens** and **epididymis**
- Anastomoses with the **testicular artery** within the spermatic cord

Testicular artery

- Arises from the **abdominal aorta**
- Descends behind the peritoneum on the posterior body wall to enter the **deep inguinal ring**
- Supplies the testis

Processus vaginalis

- Is an **evagination** of the **parietal peritoneum** into the **inguinal canal** and **scrotum** in the fetus
- Is applied to the back side of the **testis** as the **tunica vaginalis testis**
- **Normally** closes off from the peritoneal cavity with **no remnant** except the tunica vaginalis testis
- When persistent, forms a direct **tubular connection** between the **peritoneal cavity** and the **scrotum** promoting the occurrence of an **indirect inguinal hernia**

Gubernaculum testis

- Is **derived** developmentally from the **inguinal ligament of the mesonephros**
- Is the fibrous cord connecting the lower pole of the developing **testis** to the floor of the **scrotum**
- In some way, **guides** the **descent of the testis,** although the details are still hypothetical
- Is **homologous** to the **round ligament of the uterus** and the **ovarian ligament proper** of the **female**
- After the descent of the testis remains as the **scrotal ligament** anchoring the testis to the floor of the scrotum

— **Scrotum**

- Is the **pouch,** in the male, derived from the continuation of the **skin and fascia** of the lower **abdominal wall** into the **perineum**
- Is divided internally into right and left halves by a **median septum;** each half contains

  — A testis
  — An epididymis
  — The lower part of a spermatic cord with its coverings

- Has wall formed by **skin** and the **dartos layer**
- **Dartos layer**

  — Contains **no fat**
  — Contains a large amount of **smooth muscle**
  — Functions to elevate the scrotum to **conserve heat**
  — Is continuous with **Scarpa's fascia** in the abdominal wall, with the **superficial perineal fascia** (Colles' fascia), and with the **superficial fascia of the penis**

- Receives **blood supply** from the

  — **Superficial and deep external pudendal arteries** from the femoral artery

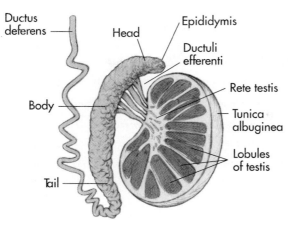

Fig. 5.5 The testis and epididymis.

— **Posterior scrotal arteries** from the internal pudendal artery

• Receives **cutaneous innervation** from the

    — Anterior scrotal branches of the **ilioinguinal nerve**

    — Genital branch of the genitofemoral nerve

    — Posterior scrotal branches of the perineal branch of the **pudendal nerve**

    — Perineal branch of the **posterior femoral cutaneous nerve**

— *Testis (Fig. 5.5)*

• Is a paired ovoid organ measuring approximately 4 by 3 by 2.5 cm

• Lies in the floor of the **scrotal sac**

• Is responsible for the production of **spermatazoa** and **testosterone**

• Is covered by a dense connective tissue capsule, the **tunica albuginea,** which extends inward as fine connective tissue dividing it into 200 to 300 **lobules**

• Is covered anteriorly by the **tunica vaginalis testis,** which

    — Is a **serous sac** derived from the fetal **processus vaginalis**

    — Has a **visceral layer** that covers the epididymis and tunica albuginea of the testis anterolaterally

    — Has a **parietal layer** that is fused externally with the internal spermatic fascia

    — May abnormally accumulate serous fluid (a **hydrocele**) or blood (a **hematocele**)

• Is supplied by the **testicular artery** from the **abdominal aorta**

• Is drained by the **pampiniform plexus** and via the **testicular vein** to the **inferior vena cava** on the right and to the **left renal vein** on the left

Epididymis (see Fig. 5.5)

• Is a **C-shaped** structure formed by the convoluted **duct of the**

epididymis, which is derived from the combined efferent ductules of the testis

- Has a **head** lying at the superior pole of the testis, a **body** along the posterolateral surface, and a **tail** at the inferior pole
    - Is continuous at the tail with the **ductus deferens**

● **Blood vessels of the anterior abdominal wall**

— *Arteries of the anterior abdominal wall*

Superior epigastric artery

- Is a terminal branch of the **internal thoracic artery**
- Enters the rectus sheath to descend **posterior** to the **rectus abdominis muscle**
- Anastomoses with the **inferior epigastric artery** within the rectus abdominis muscle

Inferior epigastric artery

- Arises from the **external iliac artery** proximal to the inguinal ligament
- Ascends **medial to the deep inguinal ring** and pierces the **transversalis fascia** to enter the rectus sheath at the **arcuate line**
- Passes behind the rectus abdominis muscle to anastomose with the **superior epigastric artery**
- Gives rise to the

    — **Cremasteric artery,** which enters the spermatic cord and supplies the cremaster muscle
    — **Pubic branch,** which, when unusually large, may be the source of an **abnormal obturator artery**

Deep circumflex iliac artery

- Is a branch of the **external iliac artery** close to the origin of the inferior epigastric artery
- Runs upward and laterally in the plane between the **transversus abdominis** and **internal abdominal oblique** muscles
- At first parallels the **inguinal ligament** and then the **iliac crest**
- Supplies the lower part of the abdominal wall

Superficial epigastric artery

- Arises from the **femoral artery** just below the inguinal ligament
- Becomes superficial passing through or close to the **saphenous hiatus**
- Passes superiorly and medially, crossing the inguinal ligament toward the umbilicus
- Supplies the **inferior and medial** part of the superficial abdominal wall
- Anastomoses with the **inferior epigastric artery**

Superficial circumflex iliac artery

- Arises from the **femoral artery** just below the inguinal ligament

- Becomes superficial passing through or close to the **saphenous hiatus**
- Passes superiorly and laterally along the **inguinal ligament** toward the **anterior superior iliac spine**
- Supplies the **inferior and lateral** part of the superficial abdominal wall
- Anastomoses with the **deep circumflex iliac artery**

Superficial external pudendal artery

- Arises from the **femoral artery** just below the inguinal ligament
- Becomes superficial passing through or close to the **saphenous hiatus**
- Supplies the external genitalia and the **lower abdominal wall over the pubis** (mons pubis)

Posterior intercostal (7 to 11), subcostal, and lumbar segmental (1 and 2) arteries

- Descend inferiorly and medially between the **transversus abdominis** and **internal abdominal oblique** muscles
- Pierce the rectus sheath to anastomose with the **superior and inferior epigastric arteries**

— *Veins of the anterior abdominal wall*

- Generally drain parallel to their companion artery
- **External iliac vein** receives the

  — Inferior epigastric vein
  — Deep circumflex iliac vein

- **Femoral vein** receives the

  — Superficial circumflex iliac vein
  — Superficial epigastric vein
  — Superficial external pudendal vein

- **Superior epigastric vein**

  — Drains to the **brachiocephalic vein**
  — Through its anastomosis with the inferior epigastric vein provides an **important collateral connection** between the superior and inferior vena caval systems

- **Posterior intercostal veins** (7 to 11), **subcostal vein,** and **lumbar segmental veins** (1 and 2)

  — Drain to the **azygous system** of veins
  — Through their anastomosis with the **inferior epigastric vein** in the **rectus sheath** provide an **important collateral connection** between the superior and inferior vena caval systems

- Thoracoepigastric vein

  — Lies on the lateral abdominal and thoracic walls

— Is a longitudinal connection between the **lateral thoracic vein** and **superficial epigastric vein**

— Provides an **important anastomotic connection** between the **superior and inferior vena cava** in the event of caval blockage

— Enlarges in response to a **blockage** of the **inferior vena cava** by a **tumor** or more commonly in the later stages of **pregnancy**

— May enlarge as part of the collateral drainage accompanying **portocaval anastomoses** and **caput medusae** (see the section on portocaval anastomoses, p. 218)

● **Nerves of the anterior abdominal wall**

• Nerves of the anterior abdominal wall are derived from the **ventral rami of spinal nerves T7 to L1.**

• They pass inferiorly and medially in the plane **between** the **transversus abdominis** and **internal abdominal oblique** muscles.

• They provide **motor innervation** to the **transversus abdominis, internal abdominal oblique, external abdominal oblique, rectus abdominis,** and **pyramidalis** muscles.

• They give rise to **lateral cutaneous branches,** which are analogous to corresponding branches of intercostal nerves, and **anterior cutaneous branches,** which penetrate the rectus sheath along the midline.

• The **ventral rami of T7-T11** are often referred to as **thoracoabdominal nerves.**

• The **ventral ramus of L1** gives rise to the **iliohypogastric** and **ilioinguinal** nerves.

• The ventral ramus of T7 ends cutaneously in the epigastrium over the **xiphoid process.**

• The ventral ramus of T10 ends cutaneously at the level of the **umbilicus.**

• The ventral ramus of L1 ends cutaneously over the **symphysis pubis.**

• The **ilioinguinal nerve** is derived from the **ventral ramus of L1.** It becomes cutaneous at the **superficial inguinal ring** and descends onto the thigh. It supplies the **medial thigh** and the anterior **scrotum** or **labium majora.**

■ **Peritoneum (Fig. 5.6)**

• Is the **serous membrane** that lines the abdominal and pelvic cavities

• Forms a potential space, the **peritoneal cavity,** between the visceral and parietal layers

• **Parietal peritoneum**

— **Lines the walls** of the abdominal cavity, the pelvic cavity, and the inferior surface of the diaphragm

— Is innervated by the **somatic nerves** supplying the abdominal and pelvic walls and the respiratory diaphragm

• **Visceral peritoneum**

— **Covers the abdominal organs,** which have invaginated the peritoneal sac

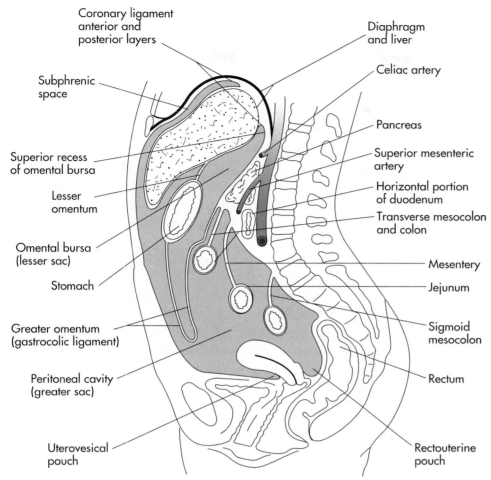

Fig. 5.6 Schematic sagittal section of the abdominal cavity.

Labels on figure:
Coronary ligament anterior and posterior layers
Subphrenic space
Superior recess of omental bursa
Lesser omentum
Omental bursa (lesser sac)
Stomach
Greater omentum (gastrocolic ligament)
Peritoneal cavity (greater sac)
Uterovesical pouch
Diaphragm and liver
Celiac artery
Pancreas
Superior mesenteric artery
Horizontal portion of duodenum
Transverse mesocolon and colon
Mesentery
Jejunum
Sigmoid mesocolon
Rectum
Rectouterine pouch

    — Is innervated by the abdominal **autonomic plexuses**

- Reflects off the body wall as **ligaments** and **mesenteries,** which

    — Are double-layered sheets of **parietal peritoneum**
    — **Suspend organs** within the abdominal cavity
    — **Transmit vessels and nerves** between the body wall and organ

- Peritoneal ligaments and mesenteries

    — *Greater omentum (see Fig. 5.6)*

      - Is the **dorsal mesentery** of the **stomach**
      - Extends from the **greater curvature of the stomach** to the **posterior abdominal wall**
      - Hangs as an **apronlike fold** from greater curvature of the stomach covering the **transverse colon** and small intestine
      - Can prevent the spread of infection by adhering to and localizing areas of inflammation
      - Is composed of the **gastrocolic, gastrolienal, lienorenal,** and **gastrophrenic** ligaments

  - Is derived from the embryonic **dorsal mesentery**

Gastrocolic ligament

  - Is the portion of the **greater omentum** attached to the distal two thirds of the **greater curvature of the stomach** and the first part of the duodenum
  - Drapes over the **transverse colon** and its mesentery but attaches to the posterior body wall
  - Is derived from the embryonic **dorsal mesentery**

Gastrolienal (gastrosplenic) ligament

  - Is the portion of the **greater omentum** extending from the greater curvature of the **stomach** to the hilus of the **spleen**
  - Contains the **short gastric** arteries and veins
  - Is derived from the embryonic **dorsal mesentery**

Lienorenal ligament

  - Is the portion of the **greater omentum** extending from the hilus of the **spleen** to the **left kidney**
  - Contains the **splenic vessels** and the **tail of the spleen**
  - Is derived from the embryonic **dorsal mesentery**

Gastrophrenic ligament

  - Is the small part of the **greater omentum** connecting the **esophagus** and fundus of the **stomach** to the undersurface of the **diaphragm** above the left kidney
  - Is derived from the embryonic **dorsal mesentery**

— *Lesser omentum (see Fig. 5.6)*

  - Is the **ventral mesentery** of the stomach
  - Extends from the **lesser curvature of the stomach** and the first part of the duodenum to the **porta hepatis** of the liver
  - Is **derived** from the embryonic **septum transversum**
  - Includes the **hepatogastric** and **hepatoduodenal** ligaments
  - Forms the anterior wall of the **lesser peritoneal sac**

Hepatogastric ligament

  - Is the portion of the **lesser omentum** between the **lesser curvature of the stomach** and the **liver**
  - Contains the **right and left gastric** arteries and veins near the stomach

Hepatoduodenal ligament

  - Is the portion of the **lesser omentum** between the **first part of the duodenum** and the **liver**
  - Is the **free edge** of the lesser omentum and the **anterior border of the epiploic foramen**
  - Contains the **common bile duct, proper hepatic artery,** and **portal vein**

— *Other peritoneal ligaments*

Phrenicocolic ligament

  - Connects the **left colic flexure** to the **diaphragm**
  - Limits the **left paracolic gutter** superiorly

- Is related superiorly to (and supports) the **spleen**
- Is derived from the embryonic **dorsal mesentery**

Falciform ligament

- Is the part of the ventral mesentery that connects the liver to the anterior abdominal wall above the umbilicus
- Is continuous with the parietal peritoneum of the anterior abdominal wall and the visceral peritoneum of the liver
- In its free edge contains the **ligamentum teres hepatis,** the remnant of the **left umbilical vein** of the fetus
- Is **derived** from the embryonic **septum transversum**

— *Other mesenteries*

Mesentery proper (see Fig. 5.6)

- Attaches to the **small intestine** from the **duodenojejunal flexure** to the **ileocecal junction**
- At its **root** is attached **diagonally** along the **posterior body wall** from the upper left to the lower right
- Is composed of **two layers** of **parietal peritoneum** between which pass the vessels, nerves, and lymphatics supplying the **jejunum** and **ileum**
- Is derived from the embryonic **dorsal mesentery**

Transverse mesocolon (see Fig. 5.6)

- Attaches to the **transverse colon** from the left to the right colic flexures
- Attaches to the posterior body wall across the **anterior surface of the pancreas**
- Normally fuses with the **gastrocolic ligament** to form the **definitive transverse mesocolon**
- Contains the **middle colic artery and vein**
- Is derived from the embryonic **dorsal mesentery**

Sigmoid mesocolon

- Attaches to the sigmoid colon, and along an inverted V-shaped line from the left iliac fossa and across the pelvic brim to descend into the pelvis
- Contains the **sigmoidal arteries and veins**
- Is derived from the embryonic **dorsal mesentery**

Mesoappendix

- Reflects off the posterior body wall at the lower border of the terminal ileum to suspend the **vermiform appendix**
- Transmits the appendicular artery and vein

- **Peritoneal cavity (see Fig. 5.6)**
  - Is a **potential space** between the visceral peritoneum and the parietal peritoneum
  - Is an **empty sac** except for a small amount of lubricating **serous fluid** and the minute **ovum** in the ovulating female
  - Is a completely **closed** cavity in the **male** but is **open** in the **female** through the uterine tube, uterus, and vagina

- Is divided into a **greater sac** and a **lesser sac**
— *Greater sac (see Fig. 5.6)*
  - Is the main part of the peritoneal cavity extending from the diaphragm into the pelvis
  - Communicates with the lesser sac through the epiploic foramen (of Winslow)

Subphrenic recess

  - Is the potential peritoneal space **between** the anterior and superior surfaces of the **liver** and the inferior surface of the **diaphragm**
  - Is divided into **right** and **left** recesses by the **falciform ligament**

Hepatorenal recess

  - Is the potential space **between** the right lobe of the **liver** and the right **kidney**
  - Is limited above by the **right coronary ligament** and below by the **right colic flexure**
  - Opens laterally into the **right paracolic gutters**
  - Is also known as **Morison's pouch**
  - In the **supine position** is the **lowest point** of the peritoneal cavity

Paracolic gutters

  - Lie lateral to the ascending and descending colons
  - Extend over the pelvic brim into the pelvis
  - On the right communicate superiorly with the hepatorenal recess
  - On the left are limited superiorly by the phrenicocolic ligament
  - Provide a potential pathway for the spread of infection within the peritoneal cavity

— *Lesser sac (see Fig. 5.6)*
  - Is also called the **omental bursa**
  - Is the minor part of the peritoneal cavity lying **posterior** to the **stomach, liver,** and **lesser omentum**
  - Communicates with the greater sac through the **epiploic foramen** (of Winslow)
  - Develops as an **evagination** of the **dorsal mesentery** of the **stomach**
  - Has an **inferior recess,** which extends downward behind the stomach into the layers of the **greater omentum**
  - Has a **splenic recess,** which extends to the left behind stomach and between the **gastrosplenic** and **lienorenal** ligaments
  - Has a **superior recess,** which extends on the diaphragm behind the **left lobe of the liver** and between the **inferior vena cava** and **esophagus**

— *Epiploic foramen (of Winslow)*
  - Is the **communication** between the **greater** and **lesser** peritoneal sacs

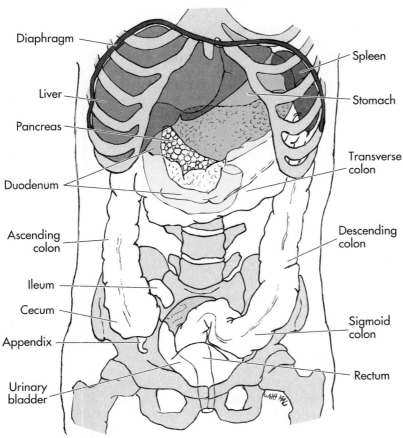

Fig. 5.7 Surface projections of the abdominal viscera.

- Is not uncommonly the site of an internal **hernia**
- Is bounded

   — **Anteriorly** by the **hepatoduodenal ligament** containing the common bile duct, proper hepatic artery, and portal vein
   — **Posteriorly** by the **inferior vena cava**
   — **Superiorly** by the **caudate lobe** of the liver
   — **Inferiorly** by the **first part of the duodenum**

■ Gastrointestinal Viscera (Fig. 5.7)

● Stomach (Fig. 5.8)

- Lies between and is anchored by the **esophagus** proximally and the **duodenum** distally
- Is a highly **distensible,** muscular organ
- Is completely covered by **visceral peritoneum**
- Is located in the **epigastric** and **left hypochondriac regions** of the abdomen
- Has a **lesser curvature,** which

   — Is the short concave **right border**
   — Is attached to the **lesser omentum**

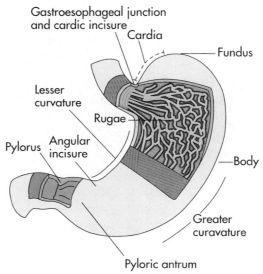

Fig. 5.8 Features of the stomach.

- Has a **greater curvature**, which

  — Is the long convex **left border**
  — Is attached to the **greater omentum**

- Has longitudinal folds in the mucosal lining called **rugae**
- Is divided into a **cardia, fundus, body,** and **pylorus**
- **Cardiac portion**

  — Lies adjacent to the junction with the esophagus
  — Has a physiologic **cardiac sphincter** (not an anatomical sphincter), which prevents regurgitation into the esophagus

- **Fundus**

  — Is **dome shaped** and lies above the entry of the esophagus
  — Often contains gas

- **Body**

  — Extends from the **fundus** to the **incisura angularis**

- **Pylorus**

  — Extends from the **incisura angularis** to the **pyloric orifice** opening into the duodenum
  — Is the most tubular part of the stomach
  — May be divided into a proximal **pyloric antrum** and a distal **pyloric canal**
  — Has an anatomical **pyloric sphincter,** which surrounds the pyloric orifice and controls the emptying of the stomach into the duodenum

Important relationships of the stomach (see Fig. 5.7)

- **Anteriorly** to the

  — Left lobe of the liver
  — Anterior abdominal wall

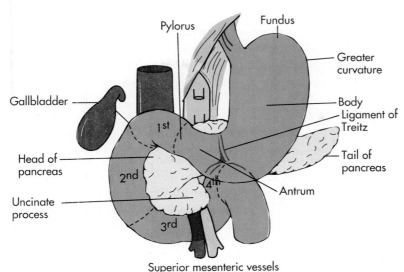

Fig. 5.9 The duodenum.

— Diaphragm

- On the **left** to the spleen
- On the **right** to the quadrate and left lobes of the liver
- **Posteriorly** to the structures of the **bed of the stomach**, including the

    — Spleen
    — Diaphragm
    — Pancreas
    — Upper pole of the left kidney
    — Left suprarenal gland
    — Duodenojejunal flexure
    — Celiac trunk
    — Superior mesenteric vessels

— *Blood supply to the stomach*

- Left and right **gastric arteries**
- Left and right **gastroepiploic arteries**
- **Short gastric arteries**
- Has accompanying veins that drain to the **portal vein** or its tributaries

● Small intestine

- Consists of the **duodenum, jejunum,** and **ileum**

— *Duodenum (Fig. 5.9)*

- Is a **C-shaped tube** extending from the **pylorus** to the **jejunum**
- Surrounds the **head of the pancreas**
- Is **retroperitoneal** except for its most proximal and most distal parts
- **Begins** to the right of the midline at the level of the body of the **first lumbar vertebra**

- **Ends** to the left of midline at the level of the body of the **second lumbar vertebra**
- Is derived from both the **foregut** and the **midgut,** the point of union being approximately the middle of the second part
- Has a thick mucosa arranged in irregular circular folds, the **plicae circulares**
- Is divided into **four parts**
- First part
  - Is also called the **superior** part
  - Lies at the level of the **transpyloric plane** to the right of the body of the **first lumbar vertebra**
  - Is called the **duodenal cap,** or **duodenal bulb,** because of its smooth-walled appearance in radiographs using barium contrast (this part has no plicae circulares)
  - Is joined to the **liver** by the free edge of the **lesser omentum,** the hepatoduodenal ligament
  - Is the most common site for a **duodenal ulcer**
  - Is crossed **posteriorly** by the **portal vein, common bile duct,** and **gastroduodenal artery**

- Second part
  - Is also called the **descending part**
  - Descends vertically to the right of the **bodies of vertebrae L1, L2, and L3**
  - Includes the junction of the **foregut** and the **midgut**
  - Receives the termination of the **common bile duct** and the **main pancreatic duct** at the **hepatopancreatic ampulla** (of Vater), which opens at the **major duodenal papilla**
  - Receives the termination of the **accessory pancreatic duct,** which opens at the **minor duodenal papilla**
  - Is related **posteriorly** to the **right renal vein** and the **hilus of the right kidney,** medially to the **head of the pancreas,** and **laterally** to the **right colic flexure**

- Third part
  - Is also called the **horizontal** or **transverse** part
  - Crosses **anterior** to the body of the **third lumbar vertebra**
  - Is crossed **anteriorly** by the **root of the small intestine** and by the **superior mesenteric vessels**
  - Is crossed **posteriorly** by the **inferior vena cava** and **aorta**

- Fourth part
  - Is also called the **ascending** part
  - Ascends on the left side of the body of the second lumbar vertebra to end at the **duodenojejunal flexure**
  - At the duodenojejunal flexure is attached to the right crus of the diaphragm by a fibromuscular band, the **suspensory ligament of the duodenum** (ligament of Treitz)
  - Is crossed **anteriorly** by the **root of the small intestine**

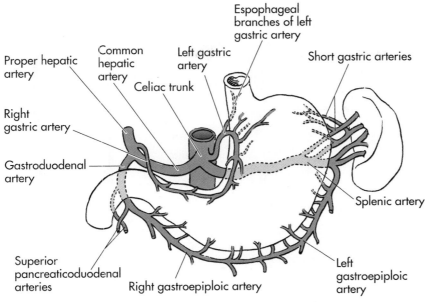

Fig. 5.10 Arteries of the stomach.

> — May have an associated peritoneal recess, the **superior or inferior duodenal fossa,** which may trap a section of small intestine as an **internal hernia**

Blood supply to the duodenum (Figs. 5.10 and 5.11)

- Anterior and posterior **superior pancreaticoduodenal arteries** from the gastroduodenal artery
- Anterior and posterior inferior **pancreaticoduodenal arteries** from the superior mesenteric artery
- **Supraduodenal** and **retroduodenal arteries** from the gastroduodenal artery

— *Jejunum and ileum*

- Are derived from the embryonic **midgut**
- Begin at the **duodenojejunal flexure** in the **upper left quadrant** of the abdominal cavity
- End at the **ileocecal junction** in the **lower right quadrant** of the abdominal cavity
- Are approximately **20 feet in length** with the first 8 feet being jejunum and the last 12 feet being ileum
- Are attached to the **posterior abdominal wall** by the **mesentery of the small intestine** along a line only **15 cm in length**
- Are supplied by the anastomosing branches of the **superior mesenteric artery** (Fig. 5.12)
- Are drained by the **superior mesenteric vein,** which joins the **portal vein** (Fig. 5.13)
- Jejunum

  — Generally occupies the area above the umbilicus
  — Is **larger** and has a **thicker wall** than the ileum

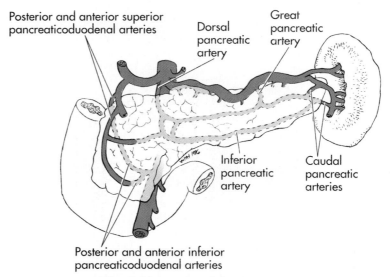

Fig. 5.11 Arteries of the pancreas.

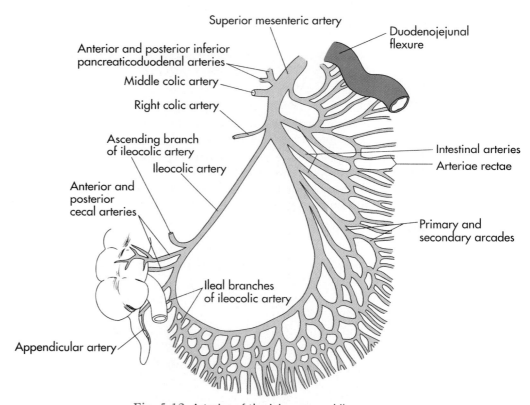

Fig. 5.12 Arteries of the jejunum and ileum.

— Has **abundant plicae circulares**
— Has diffuse lymphoid tissue rather than Peyer's patches
— Has **less fat** in its mesentery than does the ileum leaving translucent "windows" between the blood vessels

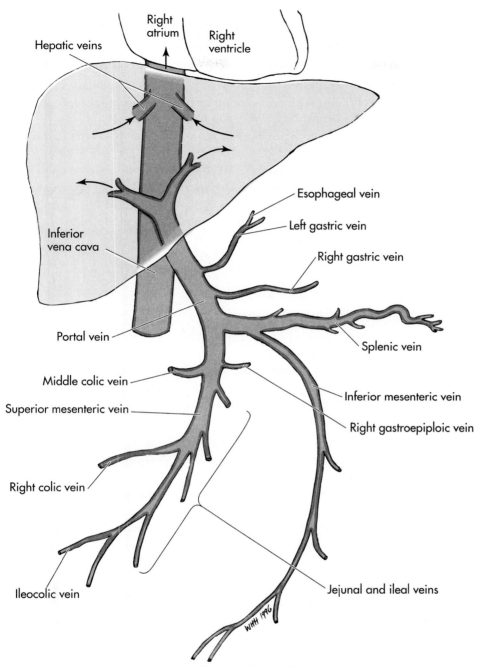

Fig. 5.13 The hepatic portal system.

—— Has **fewer arterial arcades** in its mesentery than does the ileum

• Ileum

—— Generally occupies the area below the umbilicus and extends into the pelvis

—— Is **smaller** and **thinner walled** than the jejunum

— Has **fewer plicae circulares**
— Has **numerous Peyer's patches** (lymphoid aggregations) along its antimesenteric border
— Has **abundant fat** and **numerous arcades** in its mesentery

Meckel's diverticulum

- Is a **fingerlike diverticulum** from the antimesenteric side of the ileum about 2 to 3 feet from the ileocecal junction
- Represents a **persistence** of the **vitelline duct** (vitellointestinal duct)
- Is present in about **2% of the population**
- May contain **stomach** or **pancreatic** tissue
- May retain a **connection** to the **umbilicus** of a newborn, allowing **feces** to leak from the umbilicus (**Meckel's fistula**)

● **Large intestine** (see Fig. 5.7)

- Consists of the **cecum, vermiform appendix, colon, rectum,** and **anal canal**
- Is **4 to 5 feet** long
- Is characterized by the presence of

  — **Tenia coli,** which are **three narrow bands** of longitudinal smooth muscle
  — **Haustra coli,** which are **sacculations** of the wall
  — **Appendices epiploicae,** which are small sacs of fat covered by peritoneum and suspended from the tenia coli

— *Cecum (see Fig. 5.7)*

  - Is a **blind pouch** located at the beginning of the large intestine
  - Is usually completely **covered by peritoneum** and **lies free** in the peritoneal cavity
  - Is joined by the terminal part of the **ileum** at its junction with the ascending colon
  - Receives the **ileocecal orifice** on the inside of the medial wall
  - Has an **ileocecal valve,** which

    — Lies on the posteromedial wall of the cecum
    — Consists of two **transverse folds of mucosa** on either side of the ileocecal orifice
    — Is a **rudimentary valve** and does not prevent reflux of the cecal contents back into the ileum

  - Is attached posteriorly and medially to the **vermiform appendix**
  - Is supplied by the **anterior and posterior cecal arteries** from the ileocolic artery (Fig. 5.14)
  - Is drained by the superior mesenteric vein to the portal vein (see Fig. 5.13)

— *Appendix (see Fig. 5.7)*

  - Arises from the posteromedial side of the cecum just below the **ileocecal valve**
  - Varies considerably in length but is usually **10 to 12 cm**

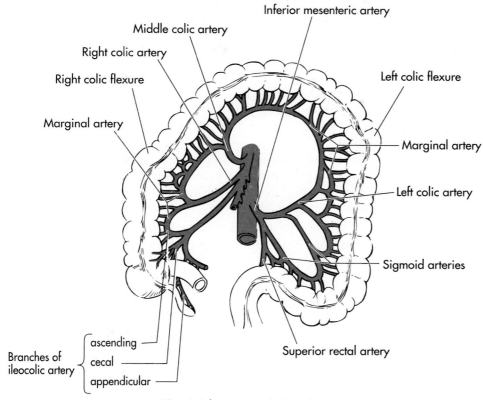

Fig. 5.14 Arteries of the colon.

- Is completely covered by **peritoneum**
- Is suspended from the terminal ileum by its own mesentery, the **mesoappendix**
- Has a mucosa, which is completely infiltrated with **lymphoid tissue**
- Has a complete layer of **longitudinal muscle** derived from the convergence of the **tenia coli**
- When inflamed as in **acute appendicitis,** may involve the parietal peritoneum with pain referred to **McBurney's point** on the anterior abdominal wall (located at the junction of the lateral and middle thirds of a line drawn between the umbilicus and the anterior superior iliac spine)
- Is supplied by the **appendicular artery** from the posterior cecal branch of the ileocolic artery (see Fig. 5.14)

— *Colon (see Fig. 5.7)*

Ascending colon

- Extends from the **ileocecal valve** to the **right colic flexure** just below the liver
- Is covered by peritoneum on its anterior, medial, and lateral sides, but its **posterior side is fused** to the posterior abdominal wall
- Is related on its **right** to the **right paracolic gutter**

- Is related **posteriorly** to the **iliacus and quadratus lumborum muscles** and to the lower pole of the **right kidney**
- Is supplied by the **ileocolic artery** and **right colic artery** from superior mesenteric artery (see Fig. 5.14)

Transverse colon

- Extends from the **right colic flexure** (hepatic flexure) to the more posterior and superior **left colic flexure** (splenic flexure)
- Is suspended from the posterior body wall by the **transverse mesocolon**
- Is attached at its anterior border to the posterior layer of the **greater omentum** which fuses with the transverse mesocolon
- Is suspended at the **left colic flexure** by the **phrenicocolic ligament**
- Is related on the right to the **liver** and on the left to the **spleen**
- Is supplied by the **middle colic artery** from the superior mesenteric artery (with anastomoses with the right and left colic arteries via the marginal artery) (see Fig. 5.14)

Descending colon

- Extends from the **left colic flexure** (hepatic flexure) to the **pelvic brim**, where it becomes continuous with the sigmoid colon
- Is covered by peritoneum on its anterior, medial, and lateral sides, but its **posterior side is fused** to the posterior abdominal wall
- Is related on its **left** to the **left paracolic gutter**
- Is related **posteriorly** to the **iliacus and quadratus lumborum muscles** and to the lower pole of the **left kidney**
- Is crossed **posteriorly** at the pelvic brim by the **external iliac vessels**
- Is supplied by the **left colic artery** from the inferior mesenteric artery (see Fig. 5.14)

Sigmoid colon

- Begins in the **iliac fossa** at the pelvic brim as a continuation of the **descending colon**
- Becomes continuous with the **rectum** in front of the **third sacral vertebra**
- Is suspended from the posterior body wall by the **sigmoid mesocolon**
- Is supplied by the **sigmoidal arteries** from the inferior mesenteric artery (see Fig. 5.14)

■ **Liver, Biliary System, Pancreas, and Spleen**

● **Liver (Figs. 5.7 and 5.15)**

- Is the **largest visceral organ** of the body, weighing about **1.5 kg**
- Is relatively **larger** in the **newborn and child** than in the adult
- Lies mostly in the upper right portion of the abdominal cavity beneath the right dome of the **diaphragm**
- Extends across the midline to the **left midclavicular line**
- Is completely enclosed by a fibrous capsule and is covered by **vis-**

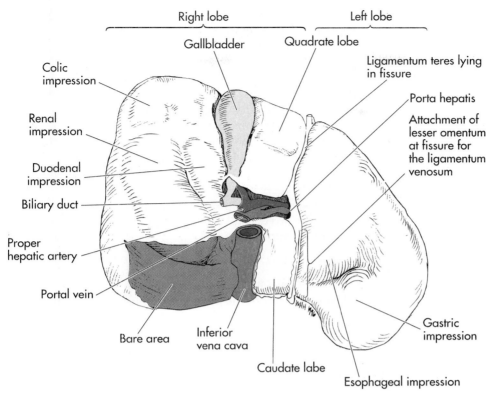

Fig. 5.15 The visceral surface of the liver.

ceral peritoneum except where it directly contacts the underside of the diaphragm

— **Surfaces and borders of the liver**

- **Diaphragmatic surface**

  — Consists of **anterior, superior,** and **posterior** surfaces, which are molded to the underside of the diaphragm
  — Has a **bare area,** which directly contacts the diaphragm with no intervening peritoneum

- **Visceral surface**

  — Is the **inferior surface** which faces inferiorly, posteriorly, and to the left
  — Is in contact with other **abdominal organs**

- **Inferior border**

  — Is where the visceral and diaphragmatic surfaces meet inferiorly

— **Lobes of the liver (see Fig. 5.15)**

- Are clearly seen only on the **visceral surface**
- Are useful **landmarks** but do **not** correspond to the **functional lobes** of the liver
- **Right lobe**

— Is the largest lobe
— Lies to the right of the fossae for the gallbladder and the inferior vena cava

- **Left lobe**

  — Is the small tongue-shaped extension to the left of midline
  — Lies to the left of the **falciform ligament** on the diaphragmatic surface and the fissures for the **ligamentum venosum** and **ligamentum teres** on the visceral surface

- **Caudate lobe**

  — Is **functionally** a part of the **left lobe**
  — Lies posterior to the **porta hepatis** between the groove for the **inferior vena cava** and the **fissure for the ligamentum venosum**

- **Quadrate lobe**

  — Is functionally a part of the **left lobe**
  — Lies to anterior to the **porta hepatis** between the fossa for the **gallbladder** and the fissure for the **ligamentum venosum**

— *Features of the visceral surface of the liver (see Fig. 5.15)*

- **Porta hepatis**

  — Is the **hilus** of the liver
  — Is the transverse fissure **separating** the **caudate** and **quadrate** lobes
  — **Transmits** the right and left **hepatic ducts,** the right and left **hepatic arteries,** the right and left branches of the **portal vein,** branches of the **autonomic plexus,** and **lymphatics**

- **Groove for the inferior vena cava**

  — Lies between the **caudate lobe** and the upper part of the **right lobe**
  — Lies within the **bare area** against the diaphragm
  — Contains the terminations of **hepatic veins** into the inferior vena cava

- **Fossa for the gallbladder**

  — Lies between the **quadrate lobe** and the lower part of the **right lobe**
  — Extends from the **inferior border** of the liver to the **porta hepatis**
  — **Lacks a peritoneal covering** because the gallbladder fuses with the surface of the liver

- **Fissure for the ligamentum venosum**

  — Lies between the **caudate lobe** and the **left lobe**
  — Contains the **ligamentum venosum,** the remnant of the fetal **ductus venosus,** which **bypasses the liver sinu-**

soids by shunting blood from the portal and umbilical veins directly to the hepatic veins

- **Fissure for the ligamentum teres**

  — Lies between the **quadrate lobe** and the **left lobe**
  — Contains the **ligamentum teres hepatis,** the remnant of the **left umbilical vein,** which carries blood returning to the fetus from the placenta

— *Peritoneal ligaments of the liver*

- **Falciform ligament**

  — Is a double layer of **peritoneum**
  — Attaches the liver to the **anterior abdominal wall** and to the undersurface of the **diaphragm**
  — Is derived from the embryonic **septum transversum**
  — In its free margin contains the **ligamentum teres hepatis,** the remnant of the **left umbilical vein**

- **Coronary ligament**

  — Is the reflection of the visceral **peritoneum** of the **liver** onto the undersurface of the **diaphragm**
  — Has **anterior** and **posterior layers,** which are separated by the **bare area,** which lies directly against the diaphragm and is devoid of peritoneum

- **Right triangular ligament**

  — Is the right extremity of the **coronary ligament**
  — Joins the **right lobe** to the undersurface of the diaphragm

- **Left triangular ligament**

  — Is the left extremity of the **coronary ligament**
  — Joins the **left lobe** to the undersurface of the diaphragm
  — Lies **anterior** to the abdominal portion of the **esophagus**

— *Important relationships of the liver*

- **Diaphragmatic surface** is related through the diaphragm to

  — The **costodiaphragmatic recess** of the **right pleural cavity**
  — The base of the **right lung**
  — A lesser degree to the **left pleural cavity and lung**
  — The **pericardial cavity and heart**

- **Bare area** of the liver is in **direct contact** with the

  — Diaphragm
  — Inferior vena cava
  — Right suprarenal gland
  — Superior pole of the right kidney

- **Visceral surface** of the **right lobe** is related to the

  — Gallbladder

— Right kidney
— Right colic flexure
— Second part of the duodenum

- **Visceral surface** of the **left lobe** is related to the

   — Esophagus
   — Fundus and body of the stomach

- **Visceral surface** of the **caudate lobe** is related to the

   — Superior recess of the lesser peritoneal sac
   — Epiploic foramen

- **Visceral surface** of the **quadrate lobe** is related to the

   — Pyloric part of the stomach

— *Blood supply of the liver*

- The liver receives blood from the **proper hepatic artery** and the **portal vein** and is drained by the **hepatic veins**

Proper hepatic artery (see Fig. 5.11)

- Is a branch of the **common hepatic artery** from the celiac trunk
- Reaches the liver through the **hepatoduodenal ligament** (the free edge of the lesser omentum)
- At the porta hepatis divides into a **right hepatic artery** and a **left hepatic artery**
- Carries about 20% of the blood delivered to the liver

Right hepatic artery

- Is a branch of the **proper hepatic artery**
- Supplies the **right lobe**
- Usually gives rise to the **cystic artery** (to the gallbladder) in the angle between the **cystic duct** and the **common hepatic duct** known as the **hepatocystic triangle (of Calot)**
- May arise, not uncommonly, as an aberrant branch of the **superior mesenteric artery**

Left hepatic artery

- Is a branch of the **proper hepatic artery**
- Supplies the **left, quadrate, and caudate lobes**
- May arise, not uncommonly, as an aberrant branch of the **left gastric artery**

Portal vein (see Fig. 5.13)

- Is formed posterior to the neck of the pancreas by the union of the **superior mesenteric vein** and the **splenic vein**
- Reaches the liver through the **hepatoduodenal ligament** (the free edge of the lesser omentum)
- At the porta hepatis divides into **right** and **left** branches
- Delivers **venous blood** from the **gastrointestinal tract**
- Carries about 80% of the blood delivered to the liver

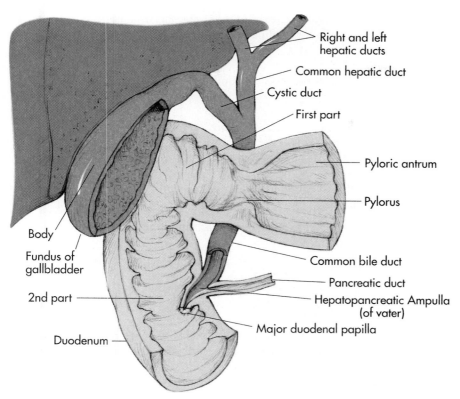

Fig. 5.16 Ducts of the liver, gallbladder, and pancreas.

Hepatic veins

- Are usually **three** in number
- Drain the **hepatic sinusoids**
- Emerge from the posterior surface and empty **directly** into the **inferior vena cava**

● **Biliary system**

— *Gallbladder (Fig. 5.16)*

- Is a pear-shaped organ that functions as part of the excretory apparatus of the liver
- Stores and concentrates bile
- Has a volume of about 30 ml
- Lies in a shallow depression on the visceral surface of the liver **between** the **right lobe** and the **quadrate lobe**
- Is covered by **peritoneum** except where it is closely applied to the liver
- Is divided into a **fundus, body,** and **neck**
- **Fundus**

    — Is the expanded **blind** inferior **end** of the sac
    — Protrudes **below** the **inferior border** of the liver
    — Is completely covered by peritoneum

— Lies against the anterior abdominal wall deep to the **ninth right costal cartilage**

- **Body**

    — Lies between the fundus and the narrow neck

- **Neck**

    — Bends to turn medially and downward into the **porta hepatis**

    — Is continuous with the **cystic duct**

— *Bile ducts (see Fig. 5.16)*

Common hepatic duct

- Is formed in the porta hepatis by union of the **right and left hepatic ducts**
- Is accompanied by the portal vein and the proper hepatic artery

Cystic duct

- Connects the **neck of the gallbladder** to the **common hepatic duct**
- Is lined by a mucous membrane organized into spirally arranged folds (the **spiral valve**), which function to keep the lumen always open

Common bile duct

- Is formed by the union of the **common hepatic duct** and the **cystic duct**
- Descends in the **hepatoduodenal ligament** to the right of the proper hepatic artery and anterior to the portal vein
- Passes behind the **first part of the duodenum** to the right of the gastroduodenal artery
- Pierces the **head of the pancreas** and joins with the **main pancreatic duct** to form the **hepatopancreatic ampulla** (of Vater) within the wall of the duodenum
- Opens into the second part of the duodenum at the **major duodenal papilla**

● **Pancreas (see Figs. 5.7 and 5.9)**

- Is both an **exocrine organ** producing **enzymes** that are discharged into the duodenum to aid **digestion** and an **endocrine organ** producing **hormones** that are discharged into the vascular system to regulate **carbohydrate metabolism**
- Develops from **two** separate **outgrowths** of the **caudal foregut**
- Lies in the bed of the stomach behind the peritoneum of the posterior body wall
- Is an elongated organ lying in the **epigastric** and **left hypochondriac** regions
- Lies at the level of the body of the **first lumbar vertebra**
- Is supplied by branches of the splenic artery and the superior and inferior pancreaticoduodenal arteries (see Fig. 5.11)
- Has a **head, neck, body,** and **tail**

- Head
  - Lies in the **curvature** formed by the **duodenum**
  - Lies anterior to the **inferior vena cava** and the terminations of the renal veins
  - Is traversed by the **common bile duct** as it passes to the second part of the duodenum
  - Has a hooklike **uncinate process,** which projects behind the **superior mesenteric vessels**

- Neck
  - Joins the head and body
  - Is **constricted** where it is crossed posteriorly by the **superior mesenteric vessels** and the origin of the **portal vein**

- Body
  - Is **triangular** in cross section
  - Lies above and to the left of the **duodenojejunal flexure**
  - Extends across the midline overlying the **aorta,** the **left renal vein,** the **splenic artery and vein,** and the termination of the **inferior mesenteric vein**
  - Is crossed anteriorly by the root of the **transverse mesocolon**

- Tail
  - Lies in the **lienorenal ligament** and ends at the **hilus** of the spleen

— *Main pancreatic duct (of Wirsung) (see Fig. 5.16)*
  - Traverses the length of the pancreas from **left to right** receiving tributary ducts in a herringbone pattern
  - In the head turns downward and then to the right to join with the **common bile duct** to form the **hepatopancreatic ampulla** (of Vater) within the wall of the duodenum
  - Opens into the second part of the duodenum at the **major duodenal papilla**

— *Accessory pancreatic duct (of Santorini)*
  - Drains the **uncinate process** and the **lower part of the head**
  - Opens independently into the second part of the duodenum at the **minor duodenal papilla** above the major papilla

● Spleen (see Fig. 5.7)
  - Is **not** an accessory **organ** of the **digestive system**
  - Is the largest **lymphatic organ**
  - Is covered by **visceral peritoneum**
  - Develops in situ in the **dorsal mesentery** of the **stomach** and is not an embryologic derivative of the foregut
  - Lies against the **diaphragm** in the **left hypochondriac region** along the long axis of **ribs 9 through 11**
  - Is related through the diaphragm to the **costodiaphragmatic recess** of the **left pleural cavity**

- Is suspended in the **dorsal mesentery,** attached to the stomach by the **gastrosplenic ligament** and to the posterior body wall by the **lienorenal ligament**
- Is supported inferiorly by the **phrenicocolic ligament,** the peritoneal fold connecting the left colic flexure to the diaphragm
- Is supplied by the **splenic artery** from the **celiac trunk** (see Fig. 5.10)
- **Lienorenal ligament** contains the

    — Tail of the pancreas
    — Splenic artery and vein

- **Gastrosplenic ligament** contains the

    — Left gastroepiploic artery and vein
    — Short gastric arteries and veins

- **Visceral surface** of the spleen is related to the

    — **Left colic flexure** anteriorly
    — **Stomach** superiorly
    — **Left kidney** inferiorly

■ Posterior Abdominal Wall

- ● Lumbar plexus (Fig. 5.17)

    - Is formed by the **ventral rami** of the **upper four lumbar spinal nerves**
    - Is the upper part of the larger **lumbosacral plexus,** which supplies the **lower extremities**
    - Forms within the substance of the **psoas muscle**
    - Largely supplies the **extensor** and **adductor** compartments of the thigh

    — *Subcostal nerve (T12)*

        - Is **not a branch of the lumbar plexus** but does lie in the abdominal wall just above the upper branches of the lumbar plexus
        - Is the **ventral ramus of T12** and is analogous to an intercostal nerve
        - Emerges from beneath the **lateral arcuate ligament** of the diaphragm
        - Runs obliquely downward between the **transversus abdominis** and **internal abdominal oblique** muscles
        - Supplies the **internal abdominal oblique,** the **external abdominal oblique,** the **transversus abdominis,** the **rectus abdominis,** and the **pyramidalis** muscles

    — *Iliohypogastric nerve (L1)*

        - Arises from the **ventral ramus of L1** within the psoas muscle
        - Runs on the anterior surface of the **quadratus lumborum** posterior to the **kidney**
        - Passes forward in the anterior abdominal wall at **first** between the **transversus abdominis** and **internal abdominal oblique**

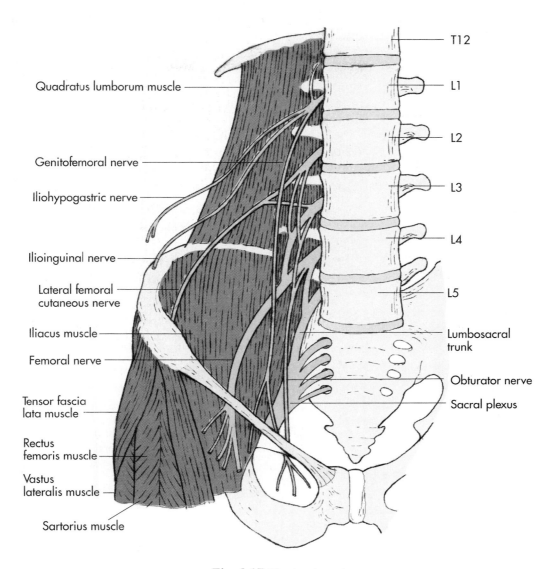

Fig. 5.17 The lumbar plexus.

muscles and **then** between the **internal** and **external abdominal oblique** muscles

• Supplies the **transversus abdominis, internal abdominal oblique,** and **external abdominal oblique** muscles

• Has an **anterior cutaneous branch,** which enlarges over the superficial inguinal ring and supplies **skin** over the **pubis**

• Has a **lateral cutaneous branch,** which supplies skin over the **gluteal region** and **upper lateral thigh**

— *Ilioinguinal nerve (L1)*

• Arises from the **ventral ramus of L1** within the psoas muscle

• Runs on the anterior surface of the **quadratus lumborum** posterior to the **kidney**

• Passes forward in the anterior abdominal wall in the plane between the **transversus abdominis** and **internal abdominal oblique** muscles

- Enters the **inguinal canal** to accompany the **spermatic cord** (or **round ligament** of the uterus) through the **superficial inguinal ring**
- Supplies the **transversus abdominis, internal abdominal oblique,** and **external abdominal oblique** muscles
- Gives **cutaneous branches** to the upper medial thigh and **anterior scrotal or labial branches,** which are cutaneous to the **scrotum** or **labia majora**

— *Genitofemoral nerve (L1, L2)*

- Arises from the **ventral ramus of L1** within the psoas muscle
- Emerges and passes distally on the **anterior** surface of the **psoas muscle**
- Passes **posterior** to the **ureter**
- Divides into a genital and a femoral branch
- **Genital branch**

    — Enters the **deep inguinal ring** to pass with the **spermatic cord** in the male or the **round ligament of the uterus** in the female
    — Supplies the skin of the **scrotum** or the **labia majora**
    — In the male supplies the **cremaster muscle**

- **Femoral branch**

    — Enters the thigh **deep** to the **inguinal ligament** with the femoral artery and within the femoral sheath
    — Supplies a small area of skin just below the **inguinal ligament**

— *Lateral femoral cutaneous nerve (L2, L3)*

- Emerges from the **lateral** side of the psoas muscle
- Passes obliquely across the **iliacus muscle** to pass deep to the **inguinal ligament** just medial to the **anterior superior iliac spine**
- Supplies a large area of the lateral thigh down to the knee

— *Femoral nerve (L2, L3, L4)*

- Is the largest branch of the lumbar plexus
- Emerges from the **lateral** side of the psoas muscle to descend in the gutter between the psoas major and iliacus muscles
- Enters the thigh **deep to** the **inguinal ligament** and **lateral to** the **femoral artery**
- Divides into its **terminal branches** just below the **inguinal ligament**
- Supplies the **muscles** of the **anterior** (extensor) **compartment** of the **thigh** and the **skin of the anterior thigh and medial leg**

— *Obturator nerve (L2, L3, L4)*

- Emerges from the **medial** side of the **psoas major** muscle to enter the **pelvis**

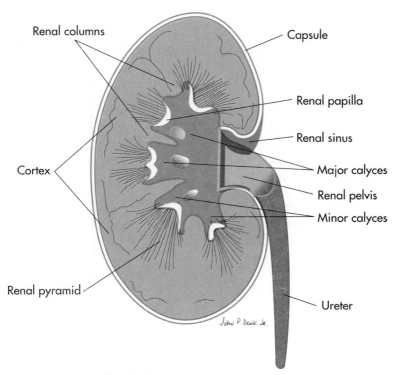

Fig. 5.18 Coronal section of the kidney

- Passes forward with the **obturator artery and vein** on the medial surface of the **obturator internus muscle**
- Enters the **medial thigh** through the **obturator foramen**
- Supplies **muscles** of the **medial** (adductor) **compartment** of the **thigh** and the **skin** of the **lower medial thigh**

— *Accessory obturator nerve (L3, L4)*

- Is present in about 10% of individuals
- Descends along the medial border of the **psoas major** and over the superior pubic ramus deep to the inguinal ligament
- Supplies the pectineus muscle and the hip joint

— *Lumbosacral trunk (L4, L5)*

- Emerges from the medial side of the psoas major muscle
- Descends into the **pelvis** anterior to the **sacroiliac joint**
- Contributes to the **sacral plexus** in the pelvis

● **Kidney (Fig. 5.18)**

- Is a bean-shaped **retroperitoneal** organ lying against the **posterior body wall,** one on each side of the vertebral column
  - In general lies adjacent to the **upper three lumbar vertebrae**
- **Moves** superiorly or inferiorly as much as one inch with movement of the diaphragm **during respiration**
- On the **right side** extends superiorly to the level of the **twelfth rib** and on the **left side** to the level of the **eleventh rib**
- Has a **hilus** on its medial concave surface, which opens into the renal

sinus and transmits the **renal artery, renal vein, renal pelvis,** and **autonomic nerves**

- Is covered by a **fibrous capsule** that is closely applied to its outer surface

- Has a **parenchyma** divided into **cortex** and **medulla**

- **Cortex**

  — Is **lighter** in color and lies immediately **beneath** the **capsule**
  — Extends inward as **renal columns** between the renal pyramids of the medulla

- **Medulla**

  — Is **darker** in color and forms the **inner part** of the kidney
  — Is composed of 8 to 16 **renal pyramids,** the apices of which are directed into the **renal sinus** as **renal papillae**

— *Renal pelvis and ureter (see Fig. 5.18)*

  - **Renal pelvis**

    — Is the expanded **upper end** of the **ureter** lying within the **renal sinus**
    — Gives rise to three or four **major calyces,** each of which gives rise to several **minor calyces**

  - Each **minor calyx**

    — Is associated with a single **renal pyramid**
    — Is **cup shaped** and surrounds a **renal papilla**
    — Receives **urine** from the **renal papilla** for transmission down the ureter to the bladder

  - **Ureter**

    — Is a **muscular tube** that transports urine from the renal pelvis to the urinary bladder
    — Begins at the **lower pole** of the **kidney** as a continuation of the **renal pelvis**
    — Descends **retroperitoneally** on the anterior surface of the **psoas major** muscle
    — Passes anterior to the **bifurcation** of the **common iliac artery** and descends into the **pelvis**
    — Is most likely to become **obstructed** where it **joins the renal pelvis, crosses** the **pelvic brim,** or **enters the bladder wall**
    — Receives its **blood supply** primarily from the **renal** and **vesical arteries** but also from other vessels in proximity during its course
    — Receives its **innervation** from autonomic and afferent fibers in the **ureteric plexus,** which is derived from the **aortic plexus**
    — Is associated with **pain** referred to the cutaneous distribution of **T11-L2,** particularly to the lower abdominal wall, external genitalia, and medial thigh

— *Renal fat and fascia*

- **Support** and **cushion** the kidney
- Provide **compliance** for the movement occurring during **respiration**
- **Renal fascia**

  — Is the condensation of fibrous connective tissue that **surrounds** the **kidney** and **suprarenal gland**
  — **Medially** extends **anterior** and **posterior** to the **renal vessels** but does not cross midline
  — **Inferiorly** extends **anterior** and **posterior** to the **ureter**

- **Perirenal fat**

  — Lies **between** the **capsule** of the kidney and the **renal fascia**
  — Is continuous at the hilus with the fat of the renal sinus

- **Pararenal fat**

  — Lies **outside** the renal fascia
  — Is thickest posteriorly where it lies against the **transversalis fascia**

— *Important relationships of the kidney*

Right kidney

- Is related **anteriorly**

  — To the right **suprarenal gland**
  — To the second part of the **duodenum**
  — To the **right colic flexure**
  — Through the peritoneum to the visceral surface of the **liver**
  — Through the peritoneum to the loops of **small intestine**

Left kidney

- Is related **anteriorly**

  — To the left **suprarenal gland**
  — To the **pancreas**
  — To the **left colic flexure**
  — Through the peritoneum to the **stomach**
  — Through the peritoneum to the **spleen**
  — Through the peritoneum to the loops of **small intestine**

Left and right kidneys

- Are related **posteriorly** to the

  — **Psoas major, quadratus lumborum,** and **transversus abdominis** muscles
  — **Subcostal, ilioinguinal,** and **iliohypogastric** nerves
  — **Diaphragm**
  — Eleventh and twelfth ribs on the left and the twelfth rib only on the right

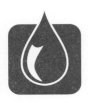

— *Blood vessels of the kidney*

Renal arteries

- Are paired branches of the abdominal **aorta,** one to each kidney
- At the hilus divide into **anterior** and **posterior** branches, which give rise to **segmental arteries,** one to each kidney segment
- **Anterior branch**
    - Typically divides into **upper, middle,** and **lower segmental arteries**
- **Posterior branch**
    - Typically divides into several **posterior** segmental arteries
- **Apical segmental artery**
    - Arises variably from the anterior or posterior branch or from the upper segmental artery
- **Segmental arteries**
    - Are essentially **end arteries** and do not anastomose with other segmental arteries
    - **If occluded,** will result in **death** (avascular necrosis) of that kidney **segment**
- **Right renal artery**
    - Is longer than the left and passes **posterior** to the **inferior vena cava**
- **Accessory renal arteries**
    - Are **segmental arteries** that do not reach the kidney through the **renal hilus**
    - Are **not truly accessory** in that they are the **only** blood **supply to** a single renal **segment**
    - Typically arise directly from the **aorta** or the **renal artery**
    - Present a **hazard** for an unsuspecting surgeon

Renal veins

- Are paired tributaries to the **inferior vena cava,** one from each kidney
- Are **intersegmental** in their distribution (in contrast to the renal arteries)
- Pass **anterior** to the **renal pelvis** and the **renal arteries**
- **Left renal vein**
    - Is longer than the right
    - Passes **anterior** to the **aorta** just below the origin of the superior mesenteric artery
    - Receives the terminations of the **left suprarenal vein** and the **left gonadal vein**
- **Right renal vein**
    - Is shorter than the left

— Passes posterior to the second part of the duodenum and head of the pancreas

● Suprarenal gland

- Is a paired **retroperitoneal** organ lying on the upper pole of the kidney against the **posterior body wall**
- Is surrounded by **perirenal fat**
- Is covered by a dense fibrous **capsule**
- Has an outer **cortex** and an inner **medulla**
- Is supplied by

 — **Superior suprarenal arteries** arising from the **inferior phrenic artery**
 — **Middle suprarenal artery** arising from the **abdominal aorta**
 — **Inferior suprarenal arteries** arising from the **renal artery**

- Has a single **suprarenal vein,** which terminates on the **right** into the **inferior vena cava** and on the **left** into the **left renal vein**
- Adrenal medulla

 — Consists of modified **postganglionic sympathetic neurons** known as **chromaffin cells**
 — **Secretes** the catecholamine hormones, **epinephrine** and **norepinephrine**
 — Receives direct innervation from **preganglionic sympathetic fibers**

- Adrenal cortex

 — Secretes **steroid hormones** under the influence of adrenocorticotropic hormone (ACTH) secreted by the anterior lobe of the pituitary

● **Respiratory diaphragm**

- See Chapter 4.

● **Muscles of the posterior abdominal wall (Table 5.2)**

■ **Aorta and Inferior Vena Cava**

● Abdominal aorta (Fig. 5.19)

- Enters the abdomen through the **aortic hiatus** in the diaphragm anterior to the body of the **twelfth thoracic vertebra**
- Descends on the bodies of the upper four lumbar vertebrae
- Divides over the body of the fourth lumbar vertebra into the right and left **common iliac arteries**
- Gives rise to three **unpaired visceral** branches

 — Celiac trunk
 — Superior mesenteric artery
 — Inferior mesenteric artery

- Gives rise to three **paired visceral** branches

 — Middle suprarenal artery
 — Renal arteries

Table 5.2 *Muscles of the Posterior Abdominal Wall*

NAME	ORIGIN	INSERTION	ACTION	INNERVATION
Psoas major	Body of the twelfth thoracic vertebra; body, transverse processes and intervertebral discs of the five lumbar vertebra	Lesser trochanter of the femur	Flexes and medially rotates the thigh; flexes the trunk on the thigh if the thigh is fixed	Ventral rami of L2 and L3
Psoas minor (when present)	Bodies and intervertebral disc of the twelfth thoracic and first lumbar vertebrae	Pectineal line of the iliopubic ramus	Flexes the trunk	Ventral ramus of L1
Iliacus	Iliac fossa	Lesser trochanter of femur with the psoas	Flexes and medially rotates the thigh; flexes the trunk on the thigh if the thigh is fixed	Femoral nerve
Quadratus lumborum	Medial part of the iliac crest, the iliolumbar ligament	Lower border of the twelfth rib, transverse processes of upper four lumbar vertebra	Depresses the twelfth rib, laterally flexes the vertebral column	Ventral rami of T12 and L1-L3

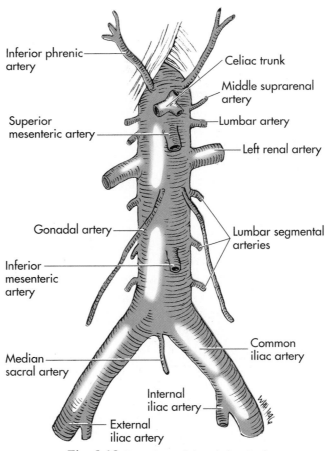

Fig. 5.19 Branches of the abdominal aorta.

    — Gonadal arteries (to the testis or ovary)

   • Gives rise to five **paired somatic** branches (to the body wall)

    — Inferior phrenic artery
    — Four pairs of lumbar segmental arteries

● **Branches of the abdominal aorta**

  — *Celiac, superior mesenteric, and inferior mesenteric arteries*

    • See pp. 218-219.

  — *Inferior phrenic arteries*

    • Arise from the aorta immediately below the aortic hiatus
    • Pass posterior to the esophagus and supply the inferior surface of the diaphragm
    • Give rise to the **superior suprarenal arteries**

  — *Middle suprarenal arteries*

    • Arise from the lateral aorta just above the renal arteries (vertebral level L1)
    • Supply the **suprarenal gland**
    • Anastomose with the superior suprarenal artery from the inferior phrenic artery and the inferior suprarenal artery from the renal artery

  — *Renal arteries*

    • Arise from the aorta below the superior mesenteric artery (vertebral level L1-L2)
    • Give rise to the **inferior suprarenal arteries**
    • Are large arteries carrying about **20%** of the **resting cardiac output**
    • **Right renal artery**

     — Arises a little lower and is a little longer than the left
     — Passes posterior to the inferior vena cava and the right renal vein

    • **Left renal artery**

     — Is shorter than the right
     — Passes posterior to the left renal vein

  — *Gonadal arteries*

    • Arise from the front of the aorta below the renal arteries (vertebral level L2)
    • Descend downward and laterally on the **psoas major muscle** under the peritoneum of the posterior body wall
    • Supply the **testes** in the male and the **ovaries** in the female
    • **Testicular artery**

     — Joins the **spermatic cord** at the deep inguinal ring and traverses the inguinal canal
     — Passes into the **scrotum** to supply the testis

- Ovarian artery

  — Passes into the pelvis
  — Traverses the **suspensory ligament of the ovary** to supply the ovary

— *Lumbar segmental arteries*

- Are usually **four pairs** and are analogous to **intercostal arteries**
- Arise from the **dorsal** surface of the **aorta**
- Pass laterally between the **vertebral bodies** and the **psoas major muscle**
- Pass **behind** the **sympathetic trunks** and on the right behind the **inferior vena cava**
- Supply the crura of the **diaphragm** and the muscles of the **posterior abdominal wall**
- Give rise to

  — A **dorsal branch** that accompanies the dorsal ramus of the spinal nerve
  — A **spinal branch** that supplies the nerve roots and enters the vertebral canal

— *Median sacral artery*

- Is a small unpaired parietal branch
- Arises from the **dorsal** surface of the **aorta** at its bifurcation
- Descends into the pelvis on the front of the **sacrum**
- May give rise to a fifth pair of small lumbar segmental arteries

— *Common iliac arteries*

- Are the **terminal branches** of the **aorta**
- Arise over the front of the body of the **fourth lumbar vertebra**
- Run downward and laterally along the medial border of the **psoas major muscle**
- Terminate opposite the **sacroiliac joint** by dividing into **external and internal iliac** arteries
- Near their termination are crossed anteriorly by the **ureter**
- Normally have **no branches** other than their terminal ones

● Inferior vena cava

- Is formed by the union of the **common iliac veins** just below and to the right of the aortic bifurcation
- Ascends on the posterior abdominal wall to the **right** of the abdominal aorta
- Passes **posterior** to the **liver** and enters the thorax by piercing the **central tendon of the diaphragm**
- Ends in the **right atrium**
- Receives blood from the **lower extremities, pelvis and perineum,** and the **abdomen,** excluding the gastrointestinal tract
- Retroperitoneally is crossed **anteriorly** by the

  — Right gonadal vessels

— Root of the mesentery
— First and third parts of the duodenum
— Head of the pancreas

- Retroperitoneally is crossed **posteriorly** by the

— Right renal artery

- Receives the terminations of the

— Common iliac veins
— Renal veins
— Lumbar segmental veins
— Hepatic veins
— Right gonadal vein (the left ends in the left renal vein)
— Right suprarenal vein (the left ends in the left renal vein)
— Right inferior phrenic vein (the left ends in the left suprarenal vein)

- **Hepatic portal venous system (see Fig. 5.13)**

— *Portal vein*

- Is formed by the union of the **superior mesenteric vein** and the **splenic vein** behind the neck of the pancreas
- Receives the veins corresponding to the branches of the **celiac trunk** and the **superior** and **inferior mesenteric arteries**
- Drains the **gastrointestinal tract, spleen, pancreas,** and **gallbladder**
- Ascends behind the **first part of the duodenum** and passes into the free edge of the lesser omentum, the **hepatoduodenal ligament**
- Within the hepatoduodenal ligament lies posterior to the **common bile duct** and the **common hepatic artery**
- Receives the terminations of the

— Splenic vein
— Superior mesenteric vein
— Right and left gastric veins
— Superior pancreaticoduodenal vein
— Paraumbilical veins

— *Splenic vein (see Fig. 5.13)*

- Forms at the **hilus** of the spleen and enters the **lienorenal ligament**
- Courses along the upper border of the **pancreas**
- Ends behind the neck of the pancreas by joining the **superior mesenteric vein** to form the **portal vein**
- Receives the terminations of the

— Inferior mesenteric vein
— Short gastric veins
— Left gastroepiploic (gastroomental) vein
— Pancreatic veins

— *Superior mesenteric vein (see Fig. 5.13)*

- Ascends to the right of the superior mesenteric artery in the root of the mesentery of the small intestine
- Crosses anterior to the **third part** of the **duodenum** and the **uncinate process** of the **pancreas**
- Ends behind the neck of the pancreas by joining the **splenic vein** to form the **portal vein**
- Receives the terminations of the

    — Tributaries corresponding to the branches of the superior mesenteric artery
    — Right gastroepiploic (gastroomental) vein
    — Inferior pancreaticoduodenal vein

— *Inferior mesenteric vein (see Fig. 5.13)*

- Forms near the pelvic brim by union of the superior rectal and sigmoidal veins
- Ascends on the left side of the posterior body wall
- Diverges from the inferior mesenteric artery to end behind the body of the pancreas in the **splenic vein**
- Receives the terminations of the

    — Superior rectal vein
    — Sigmoidal veins
    — Left colic vein

— *Left gastric vein*

- Is also known as the **coronary vein**
- Drains the left side of the lesser curvature of the **stomach** and the **lower esophagus**
- Terminates directly into the **portal vein**
- **Anastomoses** through its esophageal tributaries with esophageal tributaries of the **azygous system** of veins

— *Right gastric vein*

- Drains the right side of the lesser curvature of the **stomach**
- Terminates directly into the **portal vein**

— *Paraumbilical veins*

- Accompany the **ligamentum teres hepatis** (the obliterated left umbilical vein) in the free edge of the **falciform ligament**
- Connect the left branch of the **portal vein** to the **superficial veins** around the **umbilicus** (the systemic system)

● Portocaval (portosystemic) anastomoses

- Are the points of anastomoses between tributaries of the **portal vein** and tributaries of the **systemic system** (the vena caval system)
- May become distended when flow through the portal system is obstructed, as in cirrhosis
- Occur at the

    — **Lower end of the esophagus** between esophageal tributaries of the left gastric vein (portal) and esophageal tributaries of the azygous system (systemic); engorgement of these veins may result in **esophageal varices**

— **Anal canal** between the superior rectal veins (portal) and the inferior rectal veins (systemic); engorgement of these veins may result in **hemorrhoids**

— **Umbilicus** between the paraumbilical veins (portal) and the superficial veins of the anterior abdominal wall (systemic); engorged veins radiate from the umbilicus in a pattern known as a **caput medusae**

— **Bare areas** where retroperitoneal parts of the gastrointestinal tract (portal) are in contact with the body wall (systemic)

● **Arteries of the gastrointestinal tract**

— *Celiac artery (see Fig. 5.10)*

• Arises from the ventral surface of the aorta anterior to the body of the **T12** vertebra

• Is said to be the **artery of the foregut** but in fact supplies only the caudal part of the embryonic foregut (and the spleen)

• Supplies the gastrointestinal tract from the **lower esophagus** to the middle of the **second part of the duodenum**

• Is related laterally to the paired **celiac ganglia** and is invested by the **celiac plexus**

• Is a **short trunk** that divides into three **terminal branches,** the **splenic artery,** the **common hepatic artery,** and the **left gastric artery**

— *Splenic artery (see Fig. 5.10)*

• Is the **largest branch** of the **celiac trunk**

• Lies against the **posterior body wall** in the **bed of the stomach**

• Follows a tortuous course to the left along the upper border of the **pancreas**

• Reaches the hilum of the spleen through the **lienorenal ligament**

• Gives rise to

— A number of pancreatic branches, including the **dorsal, great,** and **caudal** pancreatic arteries

— Several **short gastric arteries** that reach the fundus of the stomach through the **gastrosplenic ligament**

— The **left gastroepiploic (gastroomental) artery,** which reaches the stomach through the **gastrosplenic ligament** and courses along the **greater curvature** to anastomose with the right gastroepiploic artery

— *Left gastric artery (see Fig. 5.10)*

• Is the **smallest branch** of the **celiac trunk**

• Ascends to the **gastroesophageal junction** and then descends along the **lesser curvature** in the lesser omentum

• Anastomoses with the right gastric artery

- Supplies the lesser curvature of the stomach and the lower esophagus

— *Common hepatic artery (see Fig. 5.10)*

- Passes forward and to the right to lie above the first part of the duodenum
- Gives rise to the **gastroduodenal artery** and continues as the **proper hepatic artery**

Proper hepatic artery (see Fig. 5.10)

- Ascends in the **hepatoduodenal ligament** anterior to the **portal vein** and to the left of the **common bile duct**
- Near the porta hepatis divides into **left** and **right hepatic arteries**
- Gives rise to the **cystic artery** to the gallbladder (usually from the **right hepatic artery**)

Gastroduodenal artery (see Fig. 5.10)

- Arises from the **common hepatic artery** above the first part of the duodenum
- Descends behind the first part of the duodenum
- Gives rise to the

    — **Supraduodenal artery**
    — **Retroduodenal artery**
    — **Posterior superior pancreaticoduodenal artery**

- Terminates by dividing into the

    — **Anterior superior pancreaticoduodenal artery**
    — **Right gastroepiploic artery**

Superior pancreaticoduodenal arteries (see Fig. 5.11)

- Arise as independent **anterior and posterior** superior pancreaticoduodenal branches from the **gastroduodenal artery**
- **Rarely** arise from a common trunk
- Supply the **head** of the pancreas and the **first and second parts** of the duodenum (which arise embryologically from the **caudal foregut**)
- Posterior *superior* pancreaticoduodenal artery

    — Arises from the **gastroduodenal** artery behind the first part of the duodenum
    — Descends along the left side of the common bile duct
    — Anastomoses with the posterior *inferior* pancreaticoduodenal artery

- Anterior *superior* pancreaticoduodenal artery

    — Arises as a **terminal branch** of the **gastroduodenal artery** below the first part of the duodenum
    — Descends as an arcade along the head of the pancreas as it lies in the curvature of the duodenum
    — Anastomoses with the anterior *inferior* pancreaticoduodenal artery

Right gastroepiploic (gastroomental) artery (see Fig. 5.11)

- Arises as a **terminal branch** of the **gastroduodenal artery** below the first part of the duodenum
- Passes to the left along the **greater curvature** of the stomach to anastomose with the **left gastroepiploic artery** (from the splenic artery)

— *Superior mesenteric artery (see Fig. 5.12)*

- Arises from the ventral surface of the aorta behind the **neck of the pancreas** and anterior to the body of the L1 vertebra
- At its origin is crossed posteriorly by the **left renal vein**
- Descends anterior to the **third part of the duodenum** and the **uncinate process of the pancreas**
- Enters the root of the mesentery
- Is said to be the **artery of the midgut**
- Supplies the head of the pancreas and the gastrointestinal tract from the **second part of the duodenum** to approximately the **left colic flexure**
- Is related laterally to the paired **superior mesenteric ganglia** and is invested by the **superior mesenteric plexus**
- Gives rise to the

    — **Inferior pancreaticoduodenal artery**
    — **Middle colic artery**
    — **Right colic artery**
    — **Ileocolic artery**
    — **Intestinal arteries** to the jejunum and ileum

Inferior pancreaticoduodenal artery (see Figs. 5.11 and 5.12)

- Arises as the **first branch** of the **superior mesenteric artery** or often from its **first jejunal branch**
- Divides into **anterior** and **posterior** *inferior* pancreaticoduodenal arteries that embrace the head of the pancreas
- Anastomoses through the arcade on the head of the pancreas with the **anterior and posterior** *superior* **pancreaticoduodenal arteries** (from the gastroduodenal artery)

Middle colic artery (see Fig. 5.12)

- Arises from the **superior mesenteric artery** anterior to the **uncinate process** as it is crossed by the root of the **transverse mesocolon**
- Enters the **transverse mesocolon** to supply the **transverse colon**
- Divides into a **right branch,** which anastomoses with the **right colic artery,** and a **left branch,** which anastomoses with the **left colic artery**
- Contributes to the **marginal artery**

● Right colic artery (see Fig. 5.12)

- Usually arises from the proximal part of the **superior mesenteric artery** but often arises from the proximal part of the **ileocolic artery**

- Crosses to the **right** behind the **peritoneum** of the posterior abdominal wall
- Divides into **ascending** and **descending** branches, which supply the **ascending colon**
- Contributes to the **marginal artery**

Ileocolic artery (see Fig. 5.12)

- Arises from the right side of the **superior mesenteric artery**
- Crosses to the **right** behind the **peritoneum** of the posterior abdominal wall to reach the right iliac fossa
- Gives rise to the

   — **Ascending colic branch,** which anastomoses with the **right colic artery** along the ascending colon
   — **Ileal branch,** which anastomoses with the **terminal ileal branch** of the superior mesenteric artery
   — **Anterior and posterior cecal arteries,** which supply the cecum
   — **Appendicular artery** (often a branch of the posterior cecal artery), which descends posterior to the ileum to enter the **mesoappendix** and supply the **vermiform appendix**

— *Inferior mesenteric artery (see Fig. 5.14)*

- Is said to be the **artery of the hindgut**
- Arises from the ventral surface of the aorta anterior to the body of the **L3** vertebra
- At its origin lies **behind** or just below the **third part of the duodenum**
- Descends behind the **peritoneum** of the posterior abdominal wall to the left side of the aorta
- Supplies the **descending colon, sigmoid colon, rectum,** and upper half of the **anal canal**
- Gives rise to the

   — **Left colic artery**
   — **Sigmoid arteries**
   — **Superior rectal artery**

Left colic artery (see Fig. 5.14)

- Arises from the **inferior mesenteric artery** and passes behind the peritoneum to the left
- Divides into **ascending** and **descending** branches, which join the **marginal artery**
- Supplies the left colic flexure and the descending colon

Sigmoidal arteries (see Fig. 5.14)

- Arise from the **inferior mesenteric artery** and pass into the sigmoid mesocolon
- Form a series of **anastomosing arcades** that supply the **sigmoid colon** and communicate with the **marginal artery**

Superior rectal artery (see Fig. 5.14)

- Is the continuation of the **inferior mesenteric artery** after giving off the sigmoidal arteries

- Descends into the **pelvis** and divides into two or three branches that supply the **rectum** and the **upper half of the anal canal**
- Anastomoses with the **middle rectal artery** (from the internal iliac artery) and the **inferior rectal arteries** (from the internal pudendal artery)

Marginal artery (of Drummond) (see Fig. 5.14)

- Is a **composite artery** that runs along the **mesenteric border** of the **colon** from the ileocecal junction to the junction of the sigmoid colon and rectum
- Is formed from branches of the **ileocolic, right colic, middle colic, left colic,** and **sigmoidal arteries**

■ Nerves of the Abdomen

● Vagus nerves

- Vagus nerves enter the abdomen on the surface of the esophagus as **anterior** and **posterior vagal trunks.**
- They supply **parasympathetic** and **general visceral afferent** innervation to the abdominal viscera.
- They break up into branches on the anterior and posterior **stomach** and end by joining the **aortic, celiac,** and **superior mesenteric plexuses.**
- They supply the gastrointestinal tract as far distally as the **left colic flexure.**
- **Parasympathetic preganglionic** cell bodies are located in the **dorsal motor nucleus** in the brain stem.
- **Parasympathetic postganglionic** cell bodies are located in **terminal ganglia** located in the autonomic plexuses or in the wall of the organ supplied.
- **Visceral afferent fibers** in the vagus nerves are from cell bodies in the **inferior vagal (nodose) ganglia.**

● Thoracic splanchnic nerves

- Thoracic splanchnic nerves are visceral branches of the T5-T12 thoracic sympathetic ganglia.
- They supply abdominal organs rather than thoracic organs.
- They contain mostly preganglionic sympathetic fibers, which synapse in abdominal prevertebral ganglia, and visceral afferent fibers.
- The **greater splanchnic** nerve arises from the T5-T9 sympathetic ganglia and ends in the celiac ganglion.
- The **lesser splanchnic** nerve arises from the T10-T11 sympathetic ganglia and usually ends in the superior mesenteric ganglion or aorticorenal ganglion.
- The **least splanchnic** nerve arises from the T12 sympathetic ganglion and enters the aorticorenal ganglion.

● Lumbar splanchnic nerves

- Are visceral branches of the four **lumbar sympathetic ganglia**
- Branches of the **upper two** lumbar sympathetic ganglia

  — Join the **celiac** and **superior mesenteric plexuses**
  — Contain mostly **preganglionic sympathetic fibers,** which synapse in **celiac** and **superior mesenteric ganglia**

— Contain **visceral afferent fibers** from cell bodies in the **L1-L2 dorsal root ganglia**

- Branches of the **lower two** lumbar sympathetic ganglia

  — Join the **intermesenteric** and **inferior mesenteric plexuses**
  — Contain mostly **postganglionic sympathetic fibers**
  — Contain **visceral afferent fibers** from cell bodies in the **L1-L2 dorsal root ganglia**

● **Pelvic splanchnic nerves**

- Are also known as **nervi erigentes**
- Are visceral branches of the ventral rami of the second, third, and fourth **sacral spinal nerves**
- Comprise the sacral parasympathetic outflow
- Join the **inferior hypogastric (pelvic) plexus**
- Contain **preganglionic parasympathetic fibers,** which synapse on **terminal ganglia** in the inferior hypogastric plexus or in the wall of the organ to be innervated
- Contain **visceral afferent fibers** from cell bodies in the **dorsal root ganglia** at S2-S4
- Reach the **inferior mesenteric plexus** to be distributed to the **descending and sigmoid colon** (caudal to the left colic flexure)

● **Autonomic plexus of the abdomen**

- The autonomic plexus of the abdomen consists of an extensive **aortic (prevertebral) plexus** lying over the front of the abdominal aorta.
- It is divided into **parts** named according to the **vessel** to which it is related (thus the **celiac, superior mesenteric, intermesenteric,** and **inferior mesenteric** plexuses).
- It supplies the abdominal organs and the gastrointestinal tract as far distally as the **sigmoid colon.**
- It contains **sympathetic and parasympathetic fibers** of the autonomic nervous system and their accompanying **general visceral afferent fibers.**
- **Sympathetic and parasympathetic fibers** are motor to smooth muscle and glands of the abdominal viscera and generally function below the level of consciousness.

- **General visceral afferent fibers** accompanying the vagal **parasympathetic** fibers generally function as the sensory limb of the **autonomic reflex arc** and are from cell bodies in the **inferior vagal ganglion** at the base of the skull.
- **General visceral afferent fibers** accompanying the **sympathetic** fibers generally **conduct** the modality of **pain** and are from cell bodies in the **dorsal root ganglia** of the T5-L2 spinal nerves.

— *Celiac plexus*

- Lies against the aorta at the root of the **celiac trunk**
- Receives

  — **Parasympathetic fibers** and accompanying visceral afferent fibers from the **vagus nerve**

— **Sympathetic fibers** and accompanying visceral afferent fibers from the **greater splanchnic nerve**

- Is distributed along the branches of the **celiac trunk** as hepatic, **gastric,** and **splenic** plexuses
- Has an associated prevertebral ganglion, the **celiac ganglion,** which contains the cell bodies of **postganglionic sympathetic neurons** for synapse with **preganglionic sympathetic fibers**

— *Superior mesenteric plexus*

- Lies against the aorta at the root of the **superior mesenteric artery**
- Receives

— **Parasympathetic fibers** and accompanying visceral afferent fibers from the **vagus nerve**

— **Sympathetic fibers** and accompanying visceral afferent fibers from the **lesser splanchnic nerve**

- Is distributed along the branches of the superior mesenteric artery as the **superior mesenteric plexus**
- Has an associated prevertebral ganglion, the **superior mesenteric ganglion,** which contains the cell bodies of **postganglionic sympathetic neurons** for synapse with **preganglionic sympathetic fibers**

— *Inferior mesenteric plexus*

- The inferior mesenteric plexus lies against the aorta at the root of the **inferior mesenteric artery.**
- It receives **parasympathetic fibers** and accompanying visceral afferent fibers from the **pelvic splanchnic nerves** via the inferior and superior hypogastric plexuses. It also receives **sympathetic fibers** and accompanying visceral afferent fibers from the **lumbar splanchnic nerves.**
- It is distributed along the branches of the inferior mesenteric artery.
- It has no associated prevertebral ganglion.
- *Remember* that the structures supplied by the **inferior mesenteric artery** (and the inferior mesenteric plexus) receive **parasympathetic** innervation from the **pelvic splanchnic nerves** and not the vagus nerve.

● **Lumbar sympathetic trunk**

- Passes from the thorax to the abdomen behind the medial arcuate ligament of the diaphragm
- Lies on the bodies of the lumbar vertebrae along the medial border of the psoas major muscle
- Typically has **four** segmentally arranged **ganglia**

— Which contain the cell bodies of **sympathetic postganglionic neurons**

— All of which give a **grey ramus communicans** to the corresponding spinal nerve

— The first two of which give a **white ramus communicans** to the corresponding spinal nerve

- Gray ramus communicans

  — Connects each **ganglion** to a corresponding **lumbar spinal nerve**

  — Contains **postganglionic sympathetic fibers** that are distributed through the lumbar spinal nerves to **sweat glands,** vascular **smooth muscle,** and **arrector pili muscles** of the abdominal wall and lower extremity

- **White ramus communicans**

  — Connects the ganglion at L1 and L2 to the corresponding lumbar spinal nerve

  — Is found only above L2 because this represents the caudal extent of the intermediolateral cell column

  — Contains preganglionic sympathetic fibers and visceral afferent fibers

MULTIPLE CHOICE
REVIEW QUESTIONS

1. Which of the following is *true* of the hepatic portal vein?

   a. It forms by union of the superior mesenteric and inferior mesenteric veins.
   b. It receives venous blood from most of the gastrointestinal tract.
   c. It passes to the liver through the falciform ligament.
   d. It forms anterior to the head of the pancreas.
   e. It terminates directly into the inferior vena cava.

2. Branches of the superior mesenteric artery typically supply all *except* which of the following?

   a. Duodenum
   b. Pancreas
   c. Spleen
   d. Appendix
   e. Transverse colon

3. The deep inguinal ring is best described by which of the following?

   a. It is a diverticulum of the parietal peritoneum.
   b. It is the site of a direct inguinal hernia.
   c. It is located immediately medial to the inferior epigastric artery.
   d. It transmits the round ligament of the uterus in the female.
   e. It lies just lateral to the rectus sheath at the level of the umbilicus.

4. The aponeurosis of the external oblique muscle contributes to all *except* which of the following?

   a. Inguinal ligament
   b. Superficial inguinal ring
   c. Anterior wall of the inguinal canal
   d. Conjoint tendon
   e. Anterior lamina of the rectus sheath

5. Which of the following is *true* of the falciform ligament?

   a. It is also known as the lesser omentum.
   b. It is an inward extension of the linea alba from the anterior abdominal wall.
   c. It contains the ligamentum teres hepatis.
   d. It separates the caudate and quadrate lobes of the liver.
   e. It connects the bladder to the umbilicus.

6. A surgeon's finger placed in the epiploic foramen (of Winslow) will be related superiorly to which of the following?

   a. First part of the duodenum
   b. Caudate lobe of the liver
   c. Head of the pancreas
   d. Common bile duct
   e. Hepatic veins

7. Which of the following best describes the left renal vein?

   a. It is shorter than the right renal vein.
   b. It receives the left gonadal vein.
   c. It lies posterior to the renal pelvis.
   d. It is part of the hepatic portal system.
   e. It terminates in the cysterna chyli.

8. The suprarenal gland is supplied by branches of all *except* which of the following?

   a. Inferior phrenic artery
   b. Renal artery
   c. Abdominal aorta
   d. Splenic artery

9. Which of the following describes the duodenum?

   a. It begins at the pylorus of the stomach.
   b. It develops entirely from the embryonic foregut.
   c. It receives the common bile duct in its first part.
   d. It is entirely retroperitoneal.
   e. It has a horizontal part that passes anterior to the superior mesenteric vessels.

10. Derivatives of the hindgut are typically supplied by which of the following?

    a. Celiac trunk
    b. Superior mesenteric artery
    c. Inferior mesenteric artery
    d. Internal iliac artery
    e. External iliac artery

Chapter 6

Pelvis and Perineum

■ **Pelvis**

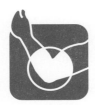

● Bony pelvis (Fig. 6.1; see also Chapter 3, pp. 75-77)

- Is composed of the paired **hip bones**, the **sacrum**, and the **coccyx**
- Is tilted so that in the anatomical position

    — The **anterior superior iliac spines** and the **pubic tubercles** lie in the same coronal plane
    — The **coccyx** and the upper margin of the **pubic symphysis** lie in the same horizontal plane

- Is divided by the **pelvic brim** into an upper **greater pelvis** (false pelvis or major pelvis) and a lower **lesser pelvis** (true pelvis or minor pelvis)

    ● **Pelvic brim**

    — Is also called the **superior pelvic aperture** or the **pelvic inlet**
    — Is bounded by the **promontory** of the sacrum, the **arcuate line** of the ilium, and the **iliopectineal line** of the pubis (the arcuate line and iliopectineal line together make up the **linea terminalis**)

    ● **Pelvic outlet**

    — Is a diamond-shaped area
    — Is bounded by the coccyx, sacrotuberous ligaments, ischial tuberosities, ischiopubic rami, and pubic symphysis
    — Is narrower in all dimensions than the inlet

    ● **Greater pelvis**

    — Is the expanded portion of the bony pelvis **above** the pelvic brim
    — Forms the lowest part of the **abdominal cavity**

    ● **Lesser pelvis**

    — Is the narrowed portion of the bony pelvis **below** the pelvic brim
    — Is open to the abdominal cavity above
    — Is closed below by the **pelvic diaphragm** (the levator ani and coccygeus muscles)

● Joints of the pelvis

- See Chapter 3, pp. 85-87.

● **Sex differences in the bony pelvis (Table 6.1)**

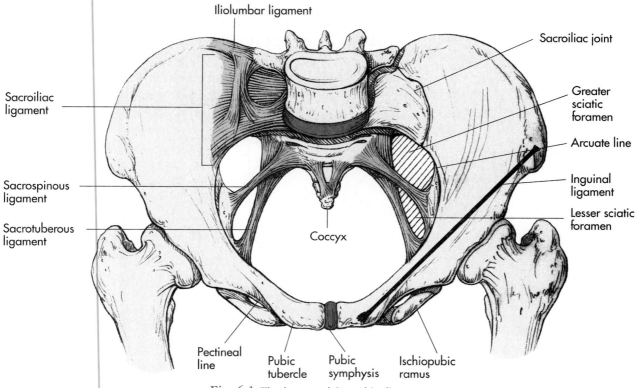

Fig. 6.1 The bony pelvis and its ligaments.

Table 6.1   *Sex Differences in the Bony Pelvis*

FEATURE	MALE	FEMALE
False pelvis	Deep	Shallow
Pelvic inlet	Narrow and heart shaped	Wide and almost oval
Pelvic cavity	Longer, noticeably tapered, cone shaped	Shorter, cylindrical, roomier
Pelvic outlet	Smaller	Larger due to eversion of the ischial tuberosities
Subpubic angle	Less than 70°	Greater than 80°
Greater sciatic notch	Narrower, about 70°	Wider, about 90°
Shape of sacrum	Longer, narrower, more curved	Shorter, wider, and flatter
Muscular markings	Pronounced	Light
Ischiopubic rami	Rough and everted for attachment of the crura of the penis and the ischiovcavernosus muscle	No eversion and only light markings
Anterior pelvic wall	Longer	Shorter
Ischial spines	Inverted, closer together	More widely separated
Acetabulum	Larger, equal in diameter to the distance between the acetabulum and the pubic symphysis	Smaller, diameter considerably less than the distance between the acetabulum and the pubic symphysis

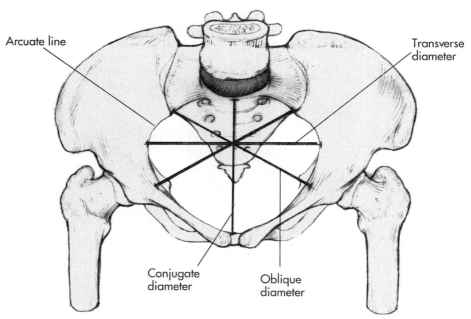

Fig. 6.2 Diameters of the superior pelvic aperture.

● **Measurements of the pelvic inlet and outlet (Fig. 6.2)**

- The **conjugate diameter** is the **anteroposterior** measurement of the superior pelvic aperture.

  — It is between the upper border of the **pubic symphysis** and the **sacral promontory.**

  — It is also called the **obstetric conjugate diameter** or **true conjugate diameter.**

- The **oblique diameter** is the **oblique** measurement of the superior pelvic aperture between the **iliopubic eminence** and the opposite **sacro-iliac joint.**

- The **transverse diameter** can be determined for both the pelvic inlet and the pelvic outlet.

  — At the **pelvic inlet** it is the **maximum distance** between the opposing **arcuate lines.**

  — At the **pelvic outlet** it is the distance between the **ischial spines.**

- The **diagonal conjugate diameter** is between the **lower border** of the **pubic symphysis** and the **sacral promontory.**

  — It may be estimated manually during a vaginal examination.

  — It is approximately 2 cm greater than the **conjugate diameter.**

- The **anteroposterior diameter of the pelvic outlet** is the distance between the lower border of the **pubic symphysis** and the **tip of the coccyx.**

- Note that the **smallest diameter** of the pelvic outlet is the **transverse diameter** between the ischial spines.

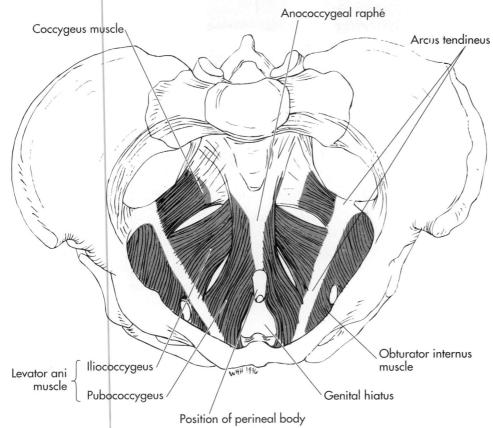

Fig. 6.3 The pelvic diaphragm view from above.

- Note also that the **maximum measurement** of **pelvic inlet** is the **transverse diameter** and the maximum diameter of the **pelvic outlet** is the **anteroposterior diameter.** Thus, during childbirth, the head must rotate 90 degrees between the pelvic inlet and outlet.
- **Pelvic cavity**
  - The pelvic cavity consists of a bony frame covered with muscles, fascia, and peritoneum.
  - It is described as having paired **lateral walls,** a **posterior wall,** and a **floor.**
  - The **lateral wall** is formed by the
    — Hip bone below the pelvic brim
    — Obturator membrane
    — Obturator internus muscle and fascia
    — Sacrotuberous and sacrospinous ligaments
  - The **posterior wall** is formed by the sacrum and coccyx and the piriformis muscle.
  - The **floor** is formed by the **pelvic diaphragm.**
  — *Pelvic diaphragm (Fig. 6.3)*
    - Consists of the **levator ani** and **coccygeus** muscles

- Forms a **muscular sling** that supports the **pelvic organs**
- Is **incomplete anteriorly** to allow for passage of the **urethra** and **vagina**
- Forms the medial wall of the **ischiorectal fossa**
- Functions as a unit to raise the **pelvic floor**
- **Coccygeus** muscle

  — Is also called the **ischiococcygeus muscle**
  — Parallels and blends with the **sacrospinous ligament**
  — Is innervated by branches of the ventral rami of the fourth and fifth sacral spinal nerves

- **Levator ani** muscle

  — Maintains the integrity of the pelvic floor
  — Is susceptible to damage during childbirth
  — Is functionally important in maintaining **urinary continence** and preventing **prolapse** of the uterus
  — Arises from the **arcus tendineus of the levator ani**, a condensation of the fascia of the obturator internus muscle
  — Consists of the **pubococcygeus** and **iliococcygeus** muscles
  — Is innervated by branches of the ventral ramus of the fourth sacral spinal nerves

- **Pubococcygeus** muscle

  — Has an anterior component that surrounds the base of the prostate in the male (the **levator prostatae** muscle) or the lower end of the vagina in the female (the **pubovaginalis** muscle) and anchors to the perineal body
  — Has a posterior component that fuses with the opposite muscle at the **anococcygeal ligament** and **coccyx**
  — Has an inferior component, the **puborectalis** muscle

- **Puborectalis** muscle

  — Is formed from the inferior fibers of the pubococcygeus muscle
  — Forms a **sling** around the **anorectal junction**
  — Is responsible for the **angle** formed between the rectum and the anal canal
  — Functions as a **sphincter** to maintain anal continence
  — Relaxes during **defecation**

● Other features of the pelvic walls and floor
  — *Obturator membrane*
      - Is a dense fibrous sheet that closes the **obturator foramen** except at the **obturator canal** where the obturator nerve and vessels pass into the thigh
      - On its inner surface provides attachment for the **obturator internus** muscle
      - On its outer surface provides attachment for the **obturator externus** muscle

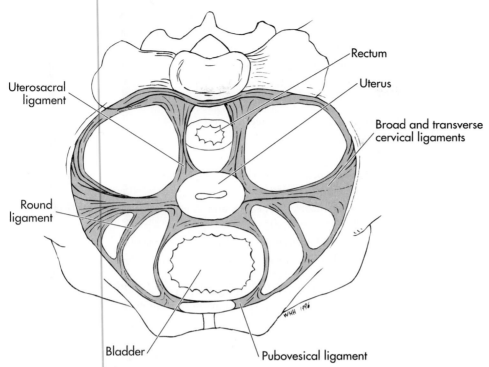

Rectum

Uterus

Uterosacral ligament

Broad and transverse cervical ligaments

Round ligament

Bladder

Pubovesical ligament

Fig. 6.4 The pelvic fascia and supporting ligaments of the uterus.

— *Sacrotuberous ligament (see Fig. 6.1)*

• Extends from the posterior surface of the **sacrum** to the **ischial tuberosity**

• Forms the inferior boundary of the **lesser sciatic foramen**

• Lies in a plane posterior to the **sacrospinous ligament**

• **Stabilizes** the sacroiliac joint and **prevents rotation** of the sacrum resulting from the downward force of the weight of the body

— *Sacrospinous ligament (see Fig. 6.1)*

• Extends from the **sacrum and coccyx** to the **ischial spine**

• Separates the **greater sciatic foramen** from the **lesser sciatic foramen**

• Lies in a plane anterior to the **sacrotuberous ligament**

• **Stabilizes** the sacroiliac joint and **prevents rotation** of the sacrum resulting from the downward force of the weight of the body

● Pelvic fascia (Fig. 6.4)

• Lines the floor and walls of the pelvic cavity

• Is continuous with the extraperitoneal **transversalis fascia** of the abdomen

• Is condensed in some locations to form **fascial ligaments**

— *Puboprostatic (male) or pubovesical (female) ligament (see Fig. 6.4)*

• Is a condensation of the superior fascia of the pelvic diaphragm

- Fills the anterior gap in the levator ani (the **genital hiatus**)
- Attaches the neck of the **bladder** to the posterior surface of the **pubis**
- In the female, may be called the **pubocervical ligament** because it extends behind the bladder to the cervix of the uterus

— *Transverse cervical ligament (see Fig. 6.4)*

- Is also known as the cardinal ligament or Mackenrodt's ligament
- Is a **fibromuscular** thickening of the pelvic fascia in the base of the **broad ligament**
- Extends from the **cervix** and lateral fornix of the **vagina** to the lateral pelvic wall
- Is crossed superiorly by the **uterine vessels**
- Functions to **stabilize** and **support** the uterus and vagina

— *Sacrogenital (male) or uterosacral (female) ligament (see Fig. 6.4)*

- Is a fibromuscular condensation of the pelvic fascia
- In the **female** extends from the **cervix** and **vagina** to the **sacrum**
- In the **male** extends from the **prostate** and neck of the **bladder** to the **sacrum**
- Passes lateral to the **rectum** where it is covered by the **sacrogenital** or **uterosacral fold** of peritoneum
- Functions to **stabilize** and **support** the pelvic organs

● **Pelvic organs**

— *Rectum*

- Is the part of the large intestine between the **sigmoid colon** and the **anal canal**
- Begins at the level of the **third sacral vertebra**
- Is not straight as its name implies but is **curved** along the anterior surface of the sacrum and coccyx as the **sacral flexure**
- In its **proximal third** is covered by peritoneum on the **anterior** and **lateral** sides
- In its **middle third** is covered by peritoneum only on the **anterior** surface
- In its **distal third** has no peritoneal covering
- Has a complete longitudinal layer of muscle instead of teniae coli
- Does not have **haustra** or **appendices epiploicae**
- On its inner surface has **three** shelflike **transverse folds,** which

    — Are called the **valves of Houston**
    — Include the mucosa, submucosa, and the circular layer of smooth muscle
    — Are more obvious when the rectum is distended and may serve to support the fecal material

- Accumulates feces pending evacuation through the anal canal
- Is supplied primarily by the **superior rectal artery** from the **inferior mesenteric artery** but also by the **middle and inferior rectal arteries**
- Is drained primarily by the **superior rectal vein,** a tributary of the **inferior mesenteric vein,** which anastomoses with the middle and inferior rectal veins (an example of a **portocaval anastomosis)**
- Receives parasympathetic innervation from the **pelvic splanchnic nerves** and sympathetic postganglionic innervation from the **inferior hypogastric plexus**

— *Ureter*

- Is a muscular tube that propels urine from the **renal pelvis** to the **urinary bladder** by peristaltic contractions
- Crosses the **pelvic brim** at the bifurcation of the **common iliac artery**
- Descends behind the peritoneum on the **lateral pelvic wall** passing medial to the **umbilical artery** and the **obturator nerve and vessels**
- Reaches the **pelvic floor** near the **ischial spine**
- In the female, lies in the base of the **broad ligament** where it is crossed **anteriorly and superiorly** by the **uterine artery** (an important relationship because the ureter may be mistakenly ligated when performing a hysterectomy)

- In the male, is crossed **superiorly** by the **ductus deferens** near the bladder
- Is **constricted** as it crosses the **pelvic brim** and as it enters the bladder

— *Urinary bladder (Figs. 6.5 and 6.6)*

- Is a **highly distensible** muscular organ, the size, shape, and position of which change as it fills with urine
- When empty has the shape of a **three-sided pyramid** with a base, an **apex,** a **superior surface,** and **two inferolateral surfaces**
- Apex
  - Points anteriorly and is attached to the umbilicus by the **median umbilical ligament,** a remnant of the **urachus** (this connection may remain patent resulting in a leakage of urine from the umbilicus of a newborn)
- Base
  - Faces posteriorly
  - Is related to the **seminal vesicles** and **rectum** in the male
  - Is related to the **uterus** and **vagina** in the female
  - Receives the **ureters** at the superolateral angles
  - Opens into the **urethra** at the inferior angle
- Superior surface
  - Is completely covered by **peritoneum**

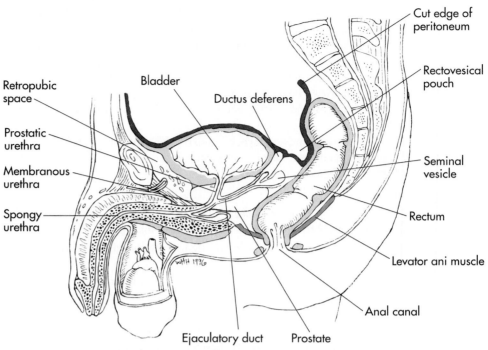

Retropubic space

Prostatic urethra

Membranous urethra

Spongy urethra

Bladder

Ductus deferens

Cut edge of peritoneum

Rectovesical pouch

Seminal vesicle

Rectum

Levator ani muscle

Anal canal

Ejaculatory duct   Prostate

Fig. 6.5 Sagittal section through the male pelvis.

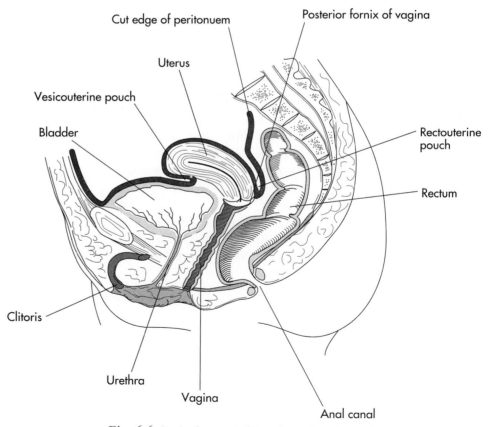

Cut edge of peritonuem

Uterus

Vesicouterine pouch

Bladder

Clitoris

Urethra

Vagina

Posterior fornix of vagina

Rectouterine pouch

Rectum

Anal canal

Fig. 6.6 Sagittal section through the female pelvis.

— Forms the dome of the bladder, which rises into the abdominal cavity as the bladder fills

- **Neck**

  — Surrounds the **urethra** at the **inferior angle**
  — Is relatively immobile, especially in the male where it is firmly attached to the **prostate**

- **Muscle of the bladder wall**

  — Is collectively known as the **detrusor muscle**
  — Consists of an **inner and outer longitudinal layer** and a **middle circular layer**
  — At the neck surrounds the urethra as the circularly arranged **sphincter vesicae**

- Is supplied by the **superior** and **inferior vesical arteries** from the internal iliac arteries

- Is drained by the **vesical** and **prostatic venous plexuses** to the internal iliac veins

- Is innervated by the **vesical** and **prostatic plexuses,** which are extensions of the inferior hypogastric plexus

Internal features of the urinary bladder

- The **trigone** is the smooth internal surface of the **triangular base** of the bladder. It remains smooth and does not contract or stretch with emptying or filling of the bladder.

- The **ureteric orifices** open at the superolateral angles of the trigone.

- The **internal urethral orifice** lies at the inferior angle of the trigone.

- The **interureteric fold** is the fold of mucosa connecting two ureteric orifices.

— *Seminal vesicle (Fig. 6.7)*

- Is a blind-ending, coiled, and sacculated **tube** embedded in the pelvic **fascia**
- Lies **posterior** to the base of the **bladder** and **lateral** to the ampulla of the **ductus deferens**
- Lies **anterior** to the **rectum** through which it normally can be palpated
- Unites with the **ductus deferens** near the base of the prostate to form the **ejaculatory duct**
- Does not store spermatozoa
- Produces **seminal fluid,** which

  — Imparts an **alkalinity** to the ejaculate protecting the **spermatazoa** from the acidic environment of the vagina
  — Contains **fructose,** which is **nutritive** to spermatazoa
  — Adds **bulk** to the ejaculate facilitating the mechanics of **ejaculation**

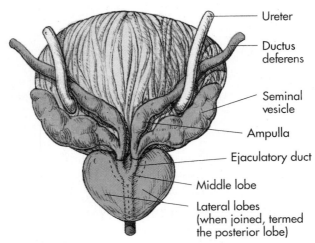

Fig. 6.7 Posterior view of the relationships of the ureter, ductus deferens, and seminal vesicle.

— *Ductus deferens (see Fig. 6.7)*

- Is a thick-walled **muscular tube** that begins at the lower pole of the testis as a continuation of the **epididymis**
- Ascends in the **spermatic cord** and traverses the **inguinal canal** to enter the abdomen at the **deep inguinal ring**
- Passes lateral to the **inferior epigastric vessels** and crosses the **external iliac vessels** to reach the pelvic brim
- Descends on the lateral wall of the pelvis passing medial to the **ureter, umbilical artery,** and **obturator nerve and vessels**
- Is dilated at its distal end to form the **ampulla**
- Ends by joining the **duct of the seminal vesicle** to form the **ejaculatory duct**

— *Ejaculatory duct (see Fig. 6.7)*

- Is formed by the union of the **ductus deferens** and the **duct of the seminal vesical**
- Passes through the posterior part of the **prostate**
- Opens into the **prostatic urethra** on the **colliculus seminalis** lateral to the **prostatic utricle**

— *Prostate gland (see Fig. 6.7)*

- Lies between the **neck of the bladder** and the **urogenital diaphragm**
- Lies **anterior** to the **rectum** through which it normally can be palpated
- Surrounds the first part of the male **urethra**
- Surrounds the **ejaculatory ducts** as they pass to terminate in the urethra
- Consists of numerous **branched glands** supported by a dense **smooth muscle** and **connective tissue** stroma
- Opens by 25 to 30 ducts into the **prostatic sinus**, a recess in the **prostatic urethra** alongside the **colliculus seminalis**

- Secretes a whitish fluid, which has a **characteristic odor** and contains **enzymes** that liquefy semen
- Is **cone-shaped** with its **base** directed toward the **bladder** and its **apex** resting on the superior fascia of the **urogenital diaphragm**
- Is supported laterally by the **pubococcygeus** muscles
- Is bound to the pubic symphysis by the **puboprostatic ligament**
- Is surrounded by a connective tissue **capsule** and a separate condensation of **pelvic fascia** (the false capsule), which are separated by the **prostatic venous plexus**
- Is divided by clinicians into five poorly defined lobes

  — **Anterior lobe** (lies anterior to the urethra and is mostly fibromuscular containing little glandular tissue)
  — **Posterior lobe** (lies posterior to the urethra and inferior to the plane of the ejaculatory ducts)
  — Paired **lateral lobes** (lie between the anterior and posterior lobes lateral to the urethra and form the bulk of the gland)
  — **Middle lobe** (median lobe) (lies posterior to the urethra and superior to the plane of the ejaculatory ducts and when **enlarged** results in **obstruction of the urethra** at the neck of the bladder)

Internal features of the prostatic urethra (Fig. 6.8)

- The **urethral crest** is the longitudinal ridge in the posterior wall of the prostatic urethra.
- The **colliculus seminalis** is a smooth enlargement of the **urethral crest**.

  — It receives the openings of the paired **ejaculatory ducts** and the **prostatic utricle.**
  — It is also called the **verumontanum.**

- The **prostatic sinus** is the depression on each side of the colliculus seminalis that receives the openings of the **prostatic ducts.**
- The **prostatic utricle** is a blind pouch that opens at the apex of the **colliculus seminalis.** It is thought to be the **remnant** of the fused **paramesonephric ducts** and, as such, is the **male homologue** of the **uterus** and **upper vagina.**

— *Ovary (Fig. 6.9)*

- Has a thin fibrous capsule called the **tunica albuginea**
- Is covered by a modified peritoneum called the **germinal epithelium**
- Is attached to the **posterior** aspect of the **broad ligament** by the **mesovarium**
- Is related at its **upper pole** to the fimbriated end of the **uterine tube**
- Is suspended from the lateral pelvic wall by the **suspensory ligament of the ovary,** which

  — Is an extension of the **broad ligament** to the pelvic brim

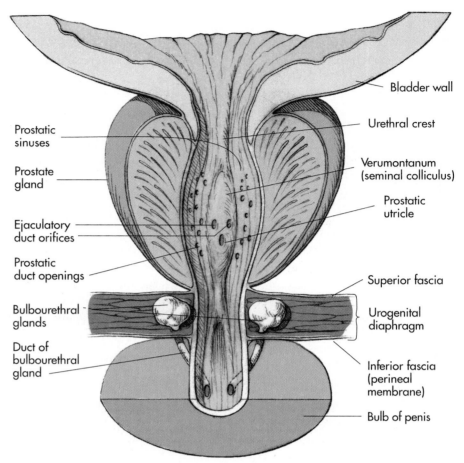

Bladder wall

Urethral crest

Prostatic sinuses

Verumontanum (seminal colliculus)

Prostate gland

Prostatic utricle

Ejaculatory duct orifices

Prostatic duct openings

Superior fascia

Bulbourethral glands

Urogenital diaphragm

Duct of bulbourethral gland

Inferior fascia (perineal membrane)

Bulb of penis

Fig. 6.8 The prostatic and membranous urethrae.

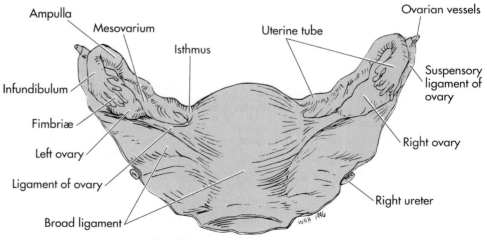

Ampulla

Mesovarium

Isthmus

Uterine tube

Ovarian vessels

Infundibulum

Suspensory ligament of ovary

Fimbriæ

Left ovary

Right ovary

Ligament of ovary

Broad ligament

Right ureter

Fig. 6.9 The female pelvic organs.

—— Contains the **ovarian vessels**

• Lies against the lateral wall of the pelvis in the **ovarian fossa,** a depression between the **ureter** posteriorly and the **umbilical artery** anteriorly

• Is joined to the side of the uterus below the uterotubal junction by the **ligament of the ovary (proper),** which

—— Is continuous through the wall of the uterus with the **round ligament of the uterus**

—— Is a remnant of the **inguinal ligament of the mesonephros** (the genitoinguinal ligament)

• Is supplied mainly by the **ovarian artery** from the abdominal aorta but also through anastomoses by the **uterine artery**

• Is drained by the **ovarian vein,** which ends in the **inferior vena cava** on the right and the **left renal vein** on the left

—— *Uterine tube (Fig. 6.9)*

• Is also called the **fallopian tube** or **oviduct**

• Lies in the upper border of the **broad ligament** extending from the ovary to the uterus

• Connects the **uterine cavity** to the **peritoneal cavity**

• Functions to

—— Convey the ovum, fertilized or not, to the uterine cavity

—— Serve as a conduit for spermatozoa traveling to meet the ovum

—— Provide the appropriate environment for fertilization to occur

• May be divided into four parts

• **Infundibulum**

—— Is the **trumpetlike** expansion of the lateral end

—— Has fingerlike processes called **fimbriae** that embrace the ovary, one of which attaches to the ovary (the **ovarian fimbria**)

—— Opens into the **peritoneal cavity** and receives the egg at ovulation

• **Ampulla**

—— Is the medial continuation of the infundibulum; makes up about one half of the uterine tube

—— Is the site where **fertilization** normally occurs

• **Isthmus**

—— Is the medial third of the tube lying between the ampulla and the uterine wall

• **Intramural part**

—— Is the narrowest part of the uterine tube

—— Passes through the **uterine wall** to open into the uterine cavity

— *Uterus (see Fig. 6.9)*

- Is the organ in which the embryo and fetus develops and is nourished until birth
- Is a pear-shaped and thick-walled muscular organ
- Lies in the middle of the **lesser pelvis** with the **uterine tubes** and **ovaries** on either side
- Is divided into the **fundus, body,** and **cervix**
- Is **anteverted** (angled forward at the junction of the cervix and vagina) **and anteflexed** (angled forward at the junction of the body and cervix)
- Is covered on its **anterior surface** by peritoneum, which reflects forward onto the superior surface of the bladder forming the **uterovesical pouch**
- Is covered on its **posterior surface** by peritoneum, which extends over the **posterior fornix** of the vagina and then reflects onto the anterior surface of the rectum forming the **rectouterine pouch** (of Douglas)
- Is supported by the

  — Transverse cervical ligaments
  — Uterosacral ligaments
  — Pubocervical ligaments

- **Body**

  — Is the expanded **upper two thirds** of the uterus
  — Is continuous below with the **cervix**

- **Fundus**

  — Is the rounded **upper part of the body** lying above the entrances of the uterine tubes

- **Cervix**

  — Is the cylindrical **lower one third** of the uterus
  — Projects inferiorly into the **vagina**

- **Cervical canal**

  — Is the **cavity** of the cervix
  — Communicates with the cavity of the body at the **internal os** and with the cavity of the vagina at the **external os**

Broad ligament (see Fig. 6.9)

- Is formed by the **two layers of peritoneum,** which come together at the lateral border of the **uterine body** and extend laterally to the **pelvic wall**
- Provides little support for the uterus
- Contains the

  — Uterine tube in its upper free border
  — Round ligament of the uterus
  — Ligament of the ovary (proper)
  — Uterine vessels

- — Ovarian vessels
- — Uterine and ovarian nerves and lymphatics

- Forms the **suspensory ligament of the ovary** at the lateral pelvic wall
    - Includes the **mesometrium, mesosalpinx,** and **mesovarium**
    - **Mesometrium**
        - — Reflects from the lateral border of the uterus and lies below the mesovarium
    - **Mesosalpinx**
        - — Lies between the uterine tube and the base of the mesovarium
    - **Mesovarium**
        - — Uterine tube in its upper free border

- — *Vagina (see Fig. 6.6)*
    - Is the female organ of **copulation** receiving the penis during coitus
    - Forms the lower end of the **birth canal**
    - Serves as the **excretory duct** for the products of **menstruation**
    - Communicates with the **uterus** above and opens into the **vestibule** of the external genitalia below
        - Is a highly distensible fibromuscular tube
        - At its upper extent forms a recess around the cervix called the **fornix of the vagina,** which, although continuous, is often divided into **anterior, posterior,** and **lateral fornices**
        - In most virgins is partially closed at its opening into the vestibule by a thin fold of skin called the **hymen**
        - In its **upper half** lies in the **pelvis** and in its **lower half** lies in the **perineum**
        - Is supplied primarily by the **vaginal artery** from the **internal iliac artery** and by **vaginal branches of the uterine artery,** also from the internal iliac artery
            - Is drained by **vaginal veins** into the **internal iliac veins**
        - Is **relatively insensitive** to stimulus being supplied by the **uterovaginal plexus,** an extension of the inferior hypogastric plexus, except in its lowest part where it is supplied by the **pudendal nerve**
            - Is **supported** by the
                - — Levator ani muscle
                - — Urogenital diaphragm
                - — Perineal body
                - — Transverse cervical, uterosacral, and pubosacral ligaments
            - Is **related anteriorly** to the
                - — Uterine cervix
                - — Base of the bladder
                - — Urethra

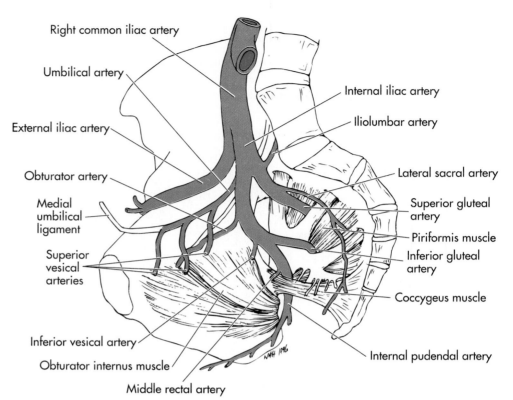

Fig. 6.10 Branches of the internal iliac artery.

- Is **related posteriorly** to the
    — Anal canal
    — Rectum
    — Rectouterine pouch (of Douglas)

- **Arteries of the pelvis (Fig. 6.10)**
    — *Internal iliac artery (see Fig. 6.10)*
        - Arises at the bifurcation of the **common iliac artery** anterior to the **sacroiliac joint**
        - Crosses the **pelvic brim** to descend into the pelvis
        - At the pelvic brim is crossed anteriorly by the **ureter**
        - Lies anterior to the **internal iliac vein** and the **lumbosacral trunk**
        - Supplies the **perineum**, the **gluteal region**, and the **pelvic organs and walls**
        - Ends opposite the upper margin of the greater sciatic notch by dividing into **anterior and posterior divisions**

        Anterior division of the internal iliac artery (see Fig. 6.10)

        - Has a **variable pattern** of branching so that specific vessels are best **identified** on the **basis of their distribution**

        UMBILICAL ARTERY

        - Usually arises from the anterior division near its origin
        - Passes anteriorly along the **lateral wall** of the pelvis

- Gives rise to

  — Two or three **superior vesical arteries** to the superior sur-face of the bladder
  — The artery to the ductus deferens (either directly or from one of the superior vesical arteries), which supplies the ductus deferens, bladder, and seminal vesicle

- Is obliterated (not patent) distally and continues onto the lower abdominal wall as the medial umbilical ligament (see Fig. 5.3)

OBTURATOR ARTERY

- Passes anteriorly along the **lateral wall** of the pelvis with the **obturator nerve**
- Exits the pelvis through the **obturator canal**
- In the thigh supplies the **obturator externus muscle** and the **hip joint**
- In 30% of people may arise from the **inferior epigastric artery** as an **abnormal obturator artery,** which is susceptible to injury in an inguinal hernia repair

INFERIOR GLUTEAL ARTERY

- Passes **between** the **ventral rami** of the **first and second** or the second and third **sacral spinal nerves**
- Leaves the pelvis by passing through the **greater sciatic fora-men** below the **piriformis muscle**
- Supplies the **gluteal region**

INTERNAL PUDENDAL ARTERY

- Leaves the pelvis by passing through the **greater sciatic fora-men** below the **piriformis muscle**
- In the **gluteal region** courses around the posterior surface of the **ischial spine**
- Enters the **perineum** through the **lesser sciatic foramen**
- Passes forward in the **pudendal canal** with the **pudendal nerve**
- Is distributed to the **perineum**

INFERIOR VESICAL ARTERY

- Usually arises from the distal part of the anterior division of the internal iliac artery
- In the male supplies the fundus and base of the **bladder,** the **prostate,** and the **seminal vesicle**
- In the female is replaced by the **vaginal artery**

MIDDLE RECTAL ARTERY

- Arises from the terminal part of the anterior division, often in common with the **inferior vesical artery**
- Supplies the **lower rectum**
- Anastomoses with the **superior and inferior rectal arteries**

UTERINE ARTERY (FIGS. 6.10 AND 6.11)

- Passes medially across the pelvic floor in the base of the **broad ligament**
- Near the uterus passes **above** and **anterior** to the **ureter,** which

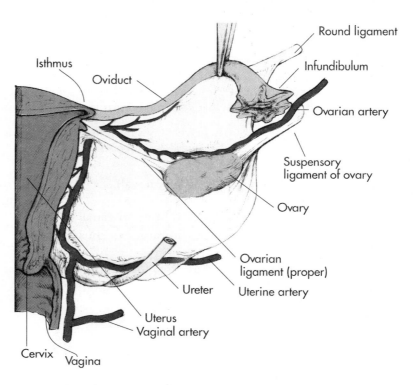

Fig. 6.11 Blood supply to the ovary, uterus, and vagina.

is at risk when ligating the uterine artery during a hysterectomy procedure

- Passes above the **lateral fornix of the vagina** to ascend along the lateral wall of the **uterus** between the layers of the **broad ligament**
- Gives a vaginal branch, which anastomoses with the vaginal artery
- Ends by giving a **tubal branch** and an **ovarian branch**, which **anastomoses** with the **ovarian artery**
- Supplies the **uterus, vagina, uterine tubes,** and **ovary**

Vaginal artery (see Figs. 6.10 and 6.11)

- Usually **arises** from the distal part of the anterior division of the **internal iliac artery** but may arise from the **uterine artery**
- Supplies the **vagina** and the base of the bladder
- In the male is replaced by the **inferior vesical artery**

Posterior division of the internal iliac artery (see Fig. 6.10)

Superior gluteal artery

- Passes **between** the **lumbosacral trunk** and the **ventral ramus** of the **first sacral spinal nerve**
- Leaves the pelvis by passing through the **greater sciatic foramen** above the **piriformis muscle**
- Supplies the **gluteal region**

ILIOLUMBAR ARTERY

- Ascends anterior to the sacroiliac joint across the pelvic brim into the **iliac fossa**
- Divides along the lateral margin of the **psoas** muscle into a branch to the **iliacus** and a **lumbar branch** (which replaces the fifth lumbar segmental artery)
- Supplies the **iliacus, psoas,** and **quadratus lumborum** muscles

LATERAL SACRAL ARTERY

- Usually arises as two separate vessels that **ascend** and **descend** along the **anterior sacrum**
- Gives branches that enter the **anterior sacral foramina**

Other arteries of the pelvis

OVARIAN ARTERY (SEE FIG. 6.11)

- Arises from the **abdominal aorta** just below the renal artery and in front of the **body of the second lumbar vertebra**
- Descends on the **psoas major muscle** behind the peritoneum
- Crosses anterior to the **external iliac vessels** to enter the **suspensory ligament of the ovary** at the pelvic brim
- Reaches the ovary through the **mesovarium** of the broad ligament
- Supplies the **ovary** and **uterine tube**
- Anastomoses with the ovarian branch of the **uterine artery**

SUPERIOR RECTAL ARTERY

- Is a direct continuation of the **inferior mesenteric artery**
- Supplies the **rectum** and the upper half of the **anal canal**
- Anastomoses with the **middle rectal artery** (from the internal iliac artery) and the **inferior rectal artery** (from the internal pudendal artery)

MEDIAN SACRAL ARTERY

- Is a small artery arising as an unpaired branch of the **aorta** at its bifurcation
- Descends **retroperitoneally** on the front of the **sacrum** with the **hypogastric plexus**
- May give rise to the fifth lumbar segmental artery

— *Lymphatic drainage of the pelvis*

- Is closely related to the blood supply of the organ
- Mostly follows the internal iliac vessels to the **internal iliac nodes** and subsequently to the external iliac and aortic nodes
- From the **ovary or testis** is along the ovarian/testicular vessels directly to the **aortic nodes**
- From the **rectum** is largely along the superior rectal vessels to the **inferior mesenteric nodes** and subsequently to the aortic nodes

■ **Nerves of the Pelvis**

● Sacral plexus

- Is formed by the **fourth** and **fifth lumbar ventral rami** (the lumbosacral trunk) and the **first four sacral ventral rami**

- Is the lower part of the larger **lumbosacral plexus,** which supplies the **pelvis, perineum, and lower extremities**
- Forms on the ventral surface of the **piriformis muscle**

— *Sciatic nerve (L4, L5, S1, S2, S3)*

- Is the largest branch of the sacral plexus and the largest nerve in the body
- Consists of two separate nerves, the **common peroneal nerve** and the **tibial nerve**
- Leaves the pelvis through the **greater sciatic foramen** below the piriformis muscle

— *Superior gluteal nerve (L4, L5, S1)*

- Leaves the pelvis through the greater sciatic foramen **above the piriformis** muscle with the superior gluteal artery and vein
- In the gluteal region supplies the **gluteus medius,** the **gluteus minimus,** the **tensor fasciae latae,** and the **hip joint**

— *Inferior gluteal nerve (L5, S1, S2)*

- Leaves the pelvis through the greater sciatic foramen **below the piriformis** muscle with the inferior gluteal artery and vein
- In the gluteal region supplies the **gluteus maximus** muscle

— *Posterior femoral cutaneous nerve (S1, S2, S3)*

- Leaves the pelvis through the greater sciatic foramen **inferior to the piriformis**
- In the gluteal region descends on the posterior surface of the sciatic nerve
- Supplies the skin of the **buttocks, posterior thigh, popliteal fossa,** and **external genitalia**

— *Nerve to the obturator internus (L5, S1, S2)*

- Leaves the pelvis through the greater sciatic foramen **below the piriformis** muscle
- In the gluteal region descends on the **superior gemellus** muscle to pass below the **ischial spine** and enter the **lesser sciatic foramen**
- Supplies the **superior gemellus** and **obturator internus** muscles

— *Nerve to the quadratus femoris (L4, L5, S1)*

- Leaves the pelvis through the greater sciatic foramen **below the piriformis** muscle and deep to the sciatic nerve
- In the gluteal region runs anterior to the **superior and inferior gemellus** and **obturator internus** muscles
- Supplies the **inferior gemellus** and **quadratus femoris** muscles

— *Pudendal nerve (S2, S3, S4)*

- Leaves the pelvis through the greater sciatic foramen **inferior to the piriformis** muscle along with the **internal pudendal artery and vein**

- In the gluteal region descends posterior to the **ischial spine** and enters the **lesser sciatic foramen**
- Is distributed to the **perineum** and has **no branches in the gluteal region**

● **Branches of the lumbar plexus in the pelvis**

— *Lumbosacral trunk (L4, L5)*

- Is formed from part of the fourth lumbar ventral ramus and all of the fifth lumbar ventral ramus
- Emerges from the medial side of the psoas major muscle
- Descends into the **pelvis** anterior to the **sacroiliac joint**
- Contributes to the **sacral plexus** in the pelvis

— *Obturator nerve (L2, L3, L4)*

- Emerges from the **medial** side of the **psoas major** muscle to enter the **pelvis**
- Passes forward with the **obturator artery and vein** on the medial surface of the **obturator internus muscle**
- Enters the **medial thigh** through the **obturator foramen**
- Supplies **muscles** of the **medial** (adductor) **compartment** of the **thigh** and the **skin** of the **lower medial thigh**

● **Autonomic nerves of the pelvis**

— *Sacral sympathetic trunk*

- Is continuous with the **lumbar sympathetic trunk** over the sacral promontory posterior to the common iliac vessels
- Descends on the ventral surface of the sacrum with the pair converging over the coccyx to form the **ganglion impar**
- Contains descending **sympathetic preganglionic fibers,** which

  — Have entered the sympathetic trunk from **white rami communicantes** associated with the **upper lumbar spinal nerves**
  — Arise from the cell bodies of **preganglionic sympathetic neurons** in the **intermediolateral cell column (IMLCC)** of the lumbar spinal cord

- Contains descending **general visceral afferent (GVA)** fibers, which

  — Have entered the sympathetic trunk from **white rami communicantes** associated with the **upper lumbar spinal nerves**
  — Arise from the cell bodies in the **dorsal root ganglia** of the **upper lumbar spinal nerves**

- Typically has **four** segmentally arranged **ganglia**
  — Which contain the cell bodies of **sympathetic postganglionic neurons**
  — All of which give a **gray ramus communicans** to the corresponding spinal nerve

- **Gray ramus communicans**

    — Connects each **ganglion** to a corresponding **sacral spinal nerve**

    — Contains **postganglionic sympathetic fibers**, which are distributed through the sacral spinal nerves to **sweat glands**, vascular **smooth muscle**, and **arrector pili muscles** of the perineum and lower extremity

— *Sacral splanchnic nerves*

  - Are visceral branches of the four **sacral sympathetic ganglia**
  - Contain mostly **postganglionic sympathetic fibers** from cell bodies in the **sacral sympathetic ganglia**
  - Contain **visceral afferent fibers** from cell bodies in the **L1-L2 dorsal root ganglia**
  - Join the **inferior hypogastric (pelvic) plexus**

— *Pelvic splanchnic nerves*

  - Are also known as **nervi erigentes**
  - Are visceral branches of the ventral rami of the S2, S3, S4 spinal nerves
  - Comprise the sacral parasympathetic outflow
  - Mediate the parasympathetic influences on **defecation, micturition, and erection**
  - Join the **inferior hypogastric (pelvic) plexus**
  - Contain **preganglionic parasympathetic fibers**, which

    — Arise from the cell bodies of parasympathetic neurons located in the sacral **parasympathetic nucleus** in spinal cord segments S2, S3, and S4

    — Synapse on **terminal ganglia** in the inferior hypogastric plexus or in the wall of the organ to be innervated

  - Contain **visceral afferent fibers** from cell bodies in the **dorsal root ganglia** at S2-S4
  - Reach the **inferior mesenteric plexus** to be distributed to the **descending and sigmoid colon** (caudal to the left colic flexure)

- **Autonomic plexus of the pelvis**

  - Is the **inferior hypogastric plexus** (also called the **pelvic plexus**)
  - Supplies the pelvic organs and the gastrointestinal tract distal to the **left colic flexure**
  - Is formed by contributions from the

    — Hypogastric nerves
    — Pelvic splanchnic nerves
    — Sacral splanchnic nerves

  - Contains

    — Parasympathetic preganglionic fibers
    — Parasympathetic postganglionic fibers
    — Sympathetic postganglionic fibers
    — Terminal ganglia

— A few sympathetic preganglionic fibers and sympathetic ganglia

— Visceral afferent fibers (accompanying both parasympathetic and sympathetic fibers)

- Is divided into **parts** named according to the **organ** to which the part is related (thus the **vesical, prostatic, rectal,** and **uterovaginal** plexuses)

— *Superior hypogastric plexus*

- Is a direct continuation of the **aortic plexus** over the body of the fifth lumbar vertebra below the aortic bifurcation
- Contains

— **Parasympathetic preganglionic fibers** and accompanying **visceral afferent fibers,** which have ascended in the hypogastric nerves from the inferior hypogastric plexus

— **Sympathetic postganglionic fibers** and accompanying **visceral afferent fibers** from the aortic plexus and the visceral branches of the third and fourth lumbar sympathetic ganglia

- Divides into **left and right hypogastric nerves,** which descend into the pelvis to join the inferior hypogastric plexus
- Has no associated prevertebral ganglion

— *Hypogastric nerve*

- The hypogastric nerve is a direct continuation of the **superior hypogastric plexus.**
- It ends by joining the **inferior hypogastric plexus.**
- It contains the same fibers found in the superior hypogastric plexus.
- Remember that the structures supplied by the **inferior mesenteric artery** (and the inferior mesenteric plexus) receive **parasympathetic** innervation from the **pelvic splanchnic nerves,** which have ascended from the inferior hypogastric plexus through the hypogastric nerves to the superior hypogastric plexus.
- Remember also that the **sympathetic fibers** in the hypogastric nerve originate in the **T10 to L2** spinal cord segments and are accompanied by **visceral afferent fibers** from the dorsal root ganglia at this same level. Thus **pain** from the pelvis may be **referred** to the cutaneous distribution of these segments.

Perineum

- Is the diamond-shaped area below the **pelvic diaphragm**
- Has the same boundaries as the **inferior pelvic aperture**
- Is bounded

— **Anteriorly** by the **pubic symphysis**

— **Anterolaterally** by the **ischiopubic rami**

— **Laterally** by the **ischial tuberosities**

— **Posterolaterally** by the **sacrotuberous ligaments**

— **Posteriorly** by the **coccyx**

- Has a **roof** formed by the **pelvic diaphragm**

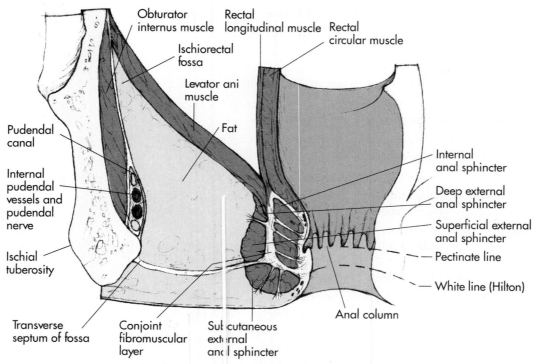

Fig. 6.12 Coronal section of the rectum and anal canal.

- Has a **floor** formed by the **skin and fascia** of the perineum
- Is divided by a line between the **ischial tuberosities** into an anterior **urogenital triangle** and a posterior **anal triangle**

● Anal triangle

— *Anal canal (Fig. 6.12)*

- Is continuous with the **rectum** at the **pelvic diaphragm**
- At its junction with the rectum bends posteriorly (the **perineal flexure**) because of the forward pull of the **puborectalis muscle**
- Opens externally at the **anus**
- Is kept **closed** by the **levator ani** and the **internal** and **external anal sphincters** except during defecation
- **Internal anal sphincter**

  — Is formed by a thickened ring of **circular smooth muscle**
  — Surrounds the upper part of the **anal canal** terminating at the level of the **white line** (of Hilton)
  — Is controlled **reflexly** and **involuntarily** with the parasympathetic system promoting relaxation and the sympathetic system promoting contraction

- **External anal sphincter**

  — Is composed of three adjacent rings of skeletal muscle, the **subcutaneous**, the **superficial**, and the **deep** parts
  — Surrounds the entire length of the **anal canal**

— Is controlled **voluntarily** by the **inferior rectal nerves** from the pudendal nerve

Internal features of the anal canal (see Fig. 6.12)

- **Anal columns:** 5 to 10 longitudinal ridges of mucosa in the upper half of the anal canal
- **Anal valves:** crescentric folds of mucosa that join the bases of adjacent anal columns
- **Anal sinuses:** pocketlike recesses above the anal valves
- **Pectinate line**

    — Is the **serrated line** joining the lower margins of the **anal valves**
    — Marks the **junction** between the embryonic hindgut lined by **endoderm** and the proctodeum lined by **ectoderm**
    — Marks the **transition** from the **columnar epithelium** of the gut tube to the **stratified squamous epithelium** of the skin
    — Marks the **divide** between visceral and somatic **arterial supply, venous drainage, lymphatic drainage, and innervation**

- **White line**

    — Is also known as the **anocutaneous line**
    — Lies below the pectinate line
    — Marks the palpable **intersphincteric groove** separating the lower border of the **internal anal sphincter** and the subcutaneous part of the **external anal sphincter**

- **Internal hemorrhoids**

    — Occur **above** the pectinate line
    — Are relatively **insensitive to pain** because they are supplied by **visceral afferent fibers**

- **External hemorrhoids**

    — Occur **below** the pectinate line
    — Are very **sensitive to pain** because they are supplied by **somatic afferent fibers**

— *Ischiorectal fossa (ischioanal fossa) (see Figs. 6.12 and 6.13)*

- Is the **wedge-shaped** perineal space lying between the **anal canal** medially, the **obturator internus muscle and fascia** laterally, the **pelvic diaphragm** superiorly, and the **skin** inferiorly
- Extends anteriorly between the **urogenital diaphragm** and pelvic diaphragm as the **anterior recess**
- Extends posteriorly deep to the **gluteus maximus muscle** to the **sacrotuberous ligament** as the **posterior recess**
- Is filled with the tough, fibrous **ischiorectal fat pad,** which cushions the perineum and allows distention of the rectum
- Communicates between sides deep to the **anococcygeal ligament** providing a route for the potential spread of infection

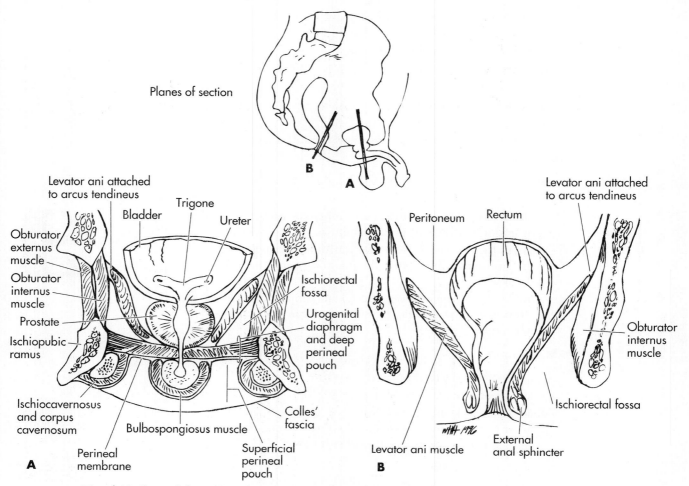

Fig. 6.13 Floor of the male pelvis. The inset shows the planes of the two coronal sections **A** and **B**.

- Contains the

  — Ischiorectal fat pad
  — Pudendal nerve and internal pudendal vessels
  — Inferior rectal nerve and vessels
  — Perineal branch of the posterior femoral cutaneous nerve

Pudendal canal (Alcock's canal) (see Fig. 6.12)

- Is a tunnel in the **fascia** of the **obturator internus muscle** on the lateral wall of the **ischiorectal fossa**
- Lies against the medial surface of the **ischial tuberosity and ramus**
- Contains the **pudendal nerve** and **internal pudendal vessels**, which supply the perineum

● **Urogenital triangle**

— *Urogenital diaphragm (see Fig. 6.13)*

- Consists of a layer of skeletal muscle between two layers of fascia

- Connects the paired **ischiopubic rami** below the pelvic diaphragm
- Is penetrated by the **membranous urethra** in the male and by the **membranous urethra and vagina** in the female
- From superior to inferior is composed of the

    — **Superior fascia** of the urogenital diaphragm
    — **Deep transverse perineal** and **sphincter urethrae** muscles
    — **Inferior fascia** of the urogenital diaphragm (commonly called the **perineal membrane**)

— *Deep perineal pouch (see Fig. 6.13)*

- Is the closed space lying between the **superior fascia** and the **inferior fascia** of the urogenital diaphragm
- Contains

    — Deep transverse perineal muscles
    — Sphincter urethrae
    — Membranous urethra
    — Internal pudendal vessels
    — Dorsal nerve of the penis or clitoris
    — Part of the vagina (female)
    — Bulbourethral glands (male)

Deep transverse perineal muscle

- Consists of transversely arranged fibers extending between the **ischiopubic rami**
- Inserts into the **perineal body**
- In the female, anterior fibers insert into the lateral wall of the **vagina**
- Supports the pelvic viscera and fixes the perineal body
- Is innervated by the **deep perineal nerve** (from the perineal branch of the pudendal nerve)

Sphincter urethrae muscle

- Consists of circularly arranged skeletal muscle fibers that lie in the same plane and are inseparable from the **deep transverse perineal** muscles
    - In the female lies anterior to the vagina
    - Surrounds and compresses the **membranous urethra** helping to maintain urinary continence
    - Provides **voluntary control** of the micturition reflex
    - Is innervated by the **deep perineal nerve** (from the perineal branch of the pudendal nerve)

— *Superficial perineal pouch (see Fig. 6.13)*

- Is the space lying between the **inferior fascia of the urogenital diaphragm** (perineal membrane) and the **membranous layer of the superficial perineal fascia** (Colles' fascia)
- Is a closed space except anteriorly where it communicates over

the pubis with the potential space deep to the membranous layer of the superficial abdominal fascia (Scarpa's fascia)

- Contains the

    — Crura and bulb of the penis (male)
    — Crura of the clitoris and bulbs of the vestibule (female)
    — Greater vestibular (Bartholin's) glands (female)
    — Ischiocavernosus muscles
    — Bulbospongiosus muscles
    — Branches of the internal pudendal vessels
    — Branches of the perineal nerves (from the internal pudendal nerves)
    — Superficial transverse perineal muscles

Superficial perineal fascia (Colles' fascia) (see Fig. 6.13)

- Is continuous with the **membranous layer of the superfical fascia** of the anterior abdominal wall (Scarpa's fascia)
- Is continuous with the **dartos layer** of the scrotum
- Continues onto the body of the penis as the **superficial fascia of the penis**
- Is **fused** to the **ischiopubic rami** and the posterior margin of the **urogenital diaphragm**
- Is **unattached** anteriorly over the **pubic symphysis and body**
- Forms the superficial boundary of the superficial perineal pouch

Deep perineal fascia

- Has the same attachments as the superficial perineal fascia except that it attaches anteriorly to the **pubic symphysis and body**
- Forms a **closed space** deep to the superficial perineal fascia
- Is **commonly ignored** by many authors because it apparently does not serve as a **barrier** to the passage of urine (as the result of a ruptured urethra) onto the abdominal wall deep to the membranous layer of superficial fascia
- Extends onto the penis as far as the glans as the **deep fascia of the penis**
- Does not extend over the scrotum

Superficial transverse perineal muscle (Fig. 6.14)

- Is a **poorly developed** paired muscle
- Arises from the ischial ramus near the ischial tuberosity
- Inserts into the **perineal body**
- May function to **stabilize** the perineal body (assuming it has a functional significance)
- Is innervated by the **deep perineal nerve** (from the perineal branch of the pudendal nerve)

Ischiocavernosus muscle (see Fig. 6.14)

- Arises from the inner surface of the **ischiopubic ramus** and **ischial tuberosity** and from the **perineal membrane**
- Inserts into and covers the **crus** of the **penis or clitoris**

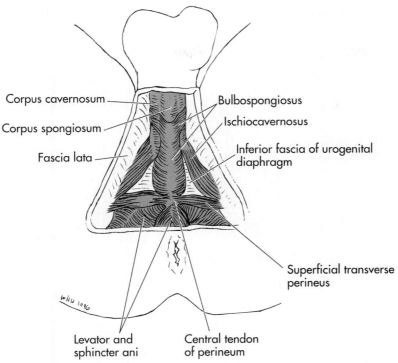

Fig. 6.14 Muscles of the superficial perineal space in the male.

- May help **maintain erection** by compressing the crus and impeding venous flow
- Is innervated by the **deep perineal nerve** (from the perineal branch of the pudendal nerve)

Bulbospongiosus muscle (see Fig. 6.14)

- In the male arises from the **perineal body** and the **median raphe** of the bulb
- In the male invests the **bulb of the penis** and inserts into the **corpus spongiosum** and **perineal membrane**
- In the female arises from the **perineal body**
- In the female invests the **bulb of the vestibule** and inserts into the dorsum of the **clitoris** and the **pubic arch**
- In the male helps **maintain erection** and helps expel urine and semen from the urethra
- In the female helps reduce the vaginal **vestibule**
- Is innervated by the **deep perineal nerve** (from the perineal branch of the pudendal nerve)

— *Perineal body (see Fig. 6.14)*

- Is also called the **central tendon of the perineum**
- Is a **fibromuscular mass** lying in the midline between the **urogenital diaphragm** anteriorly and the **anal canal** posteriorly
    - In the female lies between the **anus** and **vagina**
    - In the male lies between the **anus** and **scrotum**
    - Is an important point of **support** for the **pelvic organs**

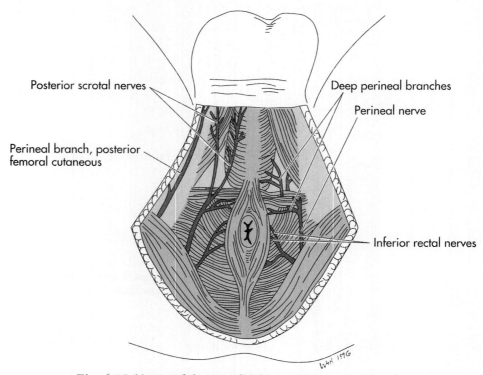

Posterior scrotal nerves

Perineal branch, posterior
femoral cutaneous

Deep perineal branches

Perineal nerve

Inferior rectal nerves

Fig. 6.15 Nerves of the superficial perineal space in the male.

  • Is susceptible to injury during **childbirth** and may be intentionally cut posteriorly from the vagina toward the anus to prevent uncontrolled tearing (an **episiotomy**)

  • Serves as a **central point of attachment** for the

— Superficial and deep transverse perineal muscles
— Bulbospongiosus muscles
— Pubococcygeus muscles (of the levator ani)
— External anal sphincter
— Superior and inferior fascia of the urogenital diaphragm
— Superficial and deep perineal fascia

— *Pudendal nerve (Fig. 6.15)*

  • Arises from the ventral rami of the **second, third, and fourth** sacral spinal nerves

  • Is the principal nerve supply to the perineum

  • Enters the perineum through the **lesser sciatic foramen** adjacent to the **ischial spine**

  • Lies in the **pudendal canal** on the lateral wall of the **ischiorectal fossa**

  • Gives rise to the

— Inferior rectal nerve
— Perineal nerve
— Dorsal nerve of the penis or clitoris

- Inferior rectal nerve
  - Arises from the pudendal nerve in the **pudendal canal**
  - Crosses the **ischiorectal fossa** through the ischiorectal fat pad breaking up into several branches
  - Supplies the **external anal sphincter** (skeletal muscle)
  - Supplies the skin around the anus and the lower part of the anal canal

- **Dorsal nerve of the penis or clitoris**
  - Arises as a terminal branch of the pudendal nerve near the posterior border of the urogenital diaphragm
  - Enters the **deep perineal pouch** with the internal pudendal artery
  - Passes through the deep pouch on the **superior surface** of the **perineal membrane**
  - Passes with the **dorsal artery of the penis or clitoris** through the gap anterior to the urogenital membrane
  - Pierces the **suspensory ligament** to run on the dorsum of the penis or clitoris lateral to the dorsal artery
  - Supplies the body, prepuce, and glans of the penis or clitoris

- **Perineal nerve**
  - Arises as terminal branch of the pudendal nerve
  - Quickly divides into a **deep branch,** which supplies the **muscles of the urogenital triangle,** and a **superficial branch,** which gives off several cutaneous **posterior scrotal or labial branches**

— *Internal pudendal artery (Fig. 6.16)*
  - Arises from the anterior division of the **internal iliac artery**
  - Is the principal blood supply to the perineum
  - Enters the perineum through the **lesser sciatic foramen** adjacent to the **ischial spine**
  - Lies in the **pudendal canal** on the lateral wall of the **ischiorectal fossa**
  - Is accompanied in its course by the **pudendal nerve**
  - Gives rise to the

    - Inferior rectal artery
    - Perineal artery
    - Artery of the bulb of the penis or clitoris
    - Deep artery of the penis or clitoris (a terminal branch)
    - Dorsal artery of the penis or clitoris (a terminal branch)

Inferior rectal artery
  - Arises from the internal pudendal artery in the **pudendal canal**
  - Divides into several branches, which cross the **ischiorectal fossa** through the ischiorectal fat pad
  - Supplies the skin and muscle of the **lower anal canal**
  - Anastomoses with the **middle and superior rectal arteries**

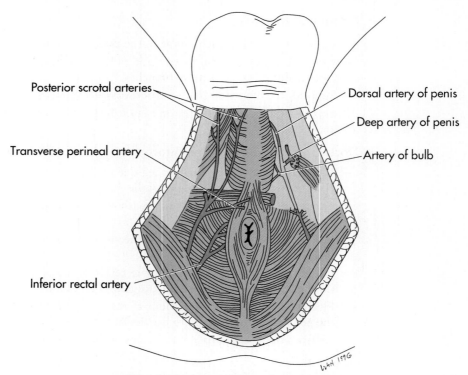

Fig. 6.16 The internal pudendal artery.

Perineal artery

- Arises from the internal pudendal artery at the posterior margin of the **urogenital diaphragm**
- Enters the **superficial perineal pouch**
- Gives rise to the

    — **Transverse perineal artery,** which accompanies the **deep perineal nerve**
    — **Posterior scrotal or labial arteries,** which accompany the **posterior scrotal or labial nerves**

- Supplies the perineal body, the muscles of the superficial perineal pouch, and the scrotum

Artery of the bulb of the penis or clitoris

- Arises from the internal pudendal artery in the **deep perineal pouch**
- Passes medially piercing the **perineal membrane**
- In the **male,** supplies the **bulb of the penis** and the **bulbourethral gland;** in the **female,** supplies the **bulb of the vestibule** and the **greater vestibular gland**

Deep artery of the penis or clitoris

- Arises as a **terminal branch** of the internal pudendal artery
- Arises in the **deep perineal pouch** and pierces the **perineal membrane** to enter the **crus of the penis or clitoris**
- Supplies the erectile tissue of the **corpus cavernosum**

Dorsal artery of the penis or clitoris

- Arises as a **terminal branch** of the internal pudendal artery
- Arises in the **deep perineal pouch** piercing the **perineal membrane** and the **suspensory ligament** of the penis or clitoris to reach the dorsum of the penis or clitoris
- Passes distally on the shaft of the penis or clitoris between the **deep dorsal vein** and the **dorsal nerve**
- Supplies the prepuce, glans, and skin and fascia of the penis or clitoris

— *Venous drainage of the perineum*

- Veins corresponding to the branches of the internal pudendal artery mostly follow the **internal pudendal vein** to the **internal iliac vein.**
- The (superficial) **external pudendal vein** receives the **superficial dorsal vein** of the penis or clitoris and ends in the **great saphenous vein** (a tributary of the femoral vein).
- The **deep dorsal vein of the penis or clitoris** is **unpaired** and lies in the **midline** of the penis or clitoris between the paired dorsal arteries.

    — It enters the **pelvis** through the gap between the **transverse perineal ligament** and the **arcuate pubic ligament.**
    — In the male, it drains into the **prostatic venous plexus;** in the female, it drains into the **vesical venous plexus** (tributaries of the internal iliac veins).

— *Lymphatic drainage of the perineum*

- Is mostly to the **superficial inguinal nodes** along the external pudendal vessels and includes drainage of the lower part of the anal canal
- Is to the **internal iliac nodes** along the internal pudendal vessels for the deep perineal space, membranous urethra, and most of the vagina
- From the body of the penis may drain directly to the **internal iliac nodes** along the deep dorsal vein

— *Male external genitalia (Fig. 6.17)*
Penis (see Fig. 6.17)

- Is the male organ of **copulation**
- Is surrounded by the

    — **Superficial penile fascia,** which is continuous with the **superficial perineal fascia**
    — **Deep penile fascia,** which is continuous with the **deep perineal fascia**

- Is suspended from the

    — **Pubic symphysis** by the **suspensory ligament** of the penis, which fuses with the **deep penile fascia**
    — **Anterior body wall** by the **fundiform ligament,** which is

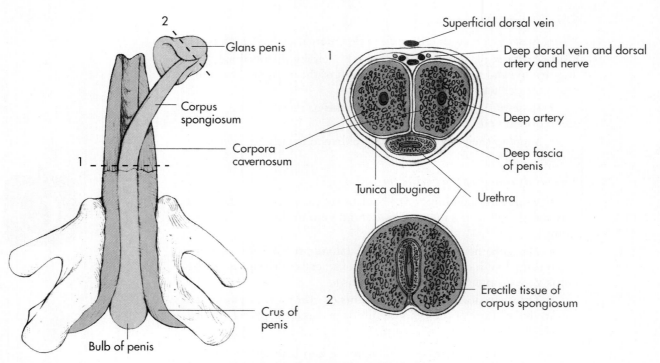

Fig. 6.17 **1,** Cross-section through the shaft of the penis. **2,** Cross-section through the gians of the penis.

continuous with the **membranous layer of superficial fascia** and blends with the **superficial penile fascia**

- Is related on its **dorsal surface** to the

  — Paired **superficial dorsal veins** of the penis
  — Unpaired **deep dorsal vein** of the penis
  — Paired **dorsal arteries** of the penis
  — Paired **dorsal nerves** of the penis

- Consists of a **body** and a **root**
- **Root**

  — Lies in the **superficial perineal pouch**
  — Includes the **two crura** and the **bulb** of the penis

- **Body**

  — Begins at the **pubic symphysis** and ends at the **glans penis**
  — Consists of the two **corpora cavernosa** and the single **corpus spongiosum**
  — Is capped distally by the **glans,** the expanded distal enlargement of the **corpus spongiosum**

- Each **crus of the penis**

  — Is a cylindrical mass of **erectile tissue**
  — Arises from the medial surface of the **ischiopubic ramus** and from the adjacent **perineal membrane**

— Is covered by the **ischiocavernosus muscle**

— Continues onto the body of the penis as the **corpus cavernosa**

- **Bulb of the penis**

    — Lies in the **superficial perineal pouch**

    — Lies on and is firmly attached to the **inferior fascia of the urogenital diaphragm** (perineal membrane)

    — Is covered by the bulbospongiosus muscle

    — Is continuous anteriorly with the **corpus spongiosum** of the body of the penis

    — Contains the **spongy urethra** and the **ducts of the bulbourethral glands**

- **Glans**

    — Is the expanded distal portion of the **corpus spongiosum**

    — Is covered by the **prepuce**, a retractable hood of skin connected to the ventral surface by the **frenulum**

    — At its tip has the external opening of the **urethra**

- **Spongy (penile) urethra**

    — Is the distal continuation of the **membraneous urethra**

    — Traverses the **bulb** and the **corpus spongiosum**

    — Lies in the midline on the **ventral surface** of the body

    — Dilates in the glans penis to form the **fossa navicularis**

Scrotum, testis, and epididymis

- The scrotum, testis, and epididymis are described with the anterior abdominal wall. See Chapter 5.

Bulbourethral glands (Cowper's glands) (see Fig. 6.8)

- Lie on either side of the **membranous urethra** of the **male**
- Are located in the **deep perineal pouch** embedded in the **deep transverse perineal** and **sphincter urethrae** muscles
- Have **long ducts** (2.5 cm) that pierce the inferior fascia of the urogenital diaphragm and end in the **spongy** (penile) **urethra**

— ***Female external genitalia (vulva) (Fig. 6.18)***

Clitoris (see Fig. 6.18)

- Is the **homologue** of the **penis** and consists mainly of **erectile tissue**
- Like the glans of the penis is **highly sensitive**
- Does not contain the urethra
- Arises from the ischiopubic rami by two **crura,** which continue onto the clitoris as the **corpora cavernosa**
- Has a **body** formed by fusion of the paired **corpora cavernosa**
- Ends distally in the **glans,** which is connected to the **bulbs of the vestibule** by two thin threads of erectile tissue
- Is attached to the pubic symphysis by the **suspensory ligament of the clitoris**

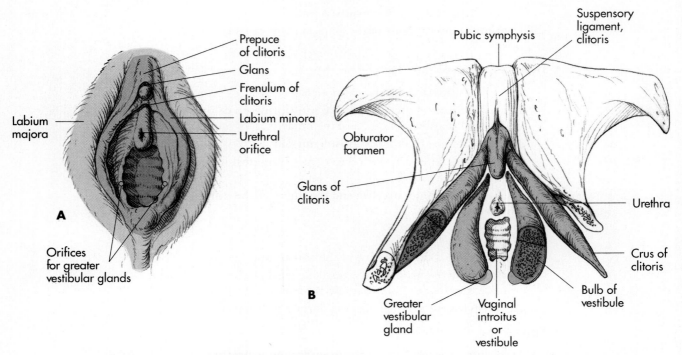

Fig. 6.18 The female pudenda. **A,** External genitalia. **B,** The clitoris and the bulb of the vestibule.

Labia majora (see Fig. 6.18)

- Are **homologous** to the **scrotum** in the male
- Are two prominent fatty folds of skin that extend downward and backward from the **mons pubis**
- Are hairless on the inner surface but, after puberty, are covered by coarse hair on the outer surface
- Are separated by a midline **pudendal cleft**
- Unite anteriorly at the **anterior labial commissure**
- Contain the terminations of the **round ligaments** of the uterus

Labia minora (see Fig. 6.18)

- Are small folds of skin lying in the **pudendal cleft** on either side of the **vaginal opening**
- Are **hairless** and contain **no fat**
- Are separated by the **vestibule of the vagina**
- Join posteriorly to form the **fourchette**
- Divide anteriorly into

  — Lateral folds, which fuse over the dorsum of the clitoris to form the **prepuce of the clitoris**
  — Medial folds, which join below the clitoris to form the **frenulum of the clitoris**

Vestibule of the vagina (see Fig. 6.18)

- Is the midline cleft between the two labia minora
- Contains the openings of the **urethra,** the **vagina,** and the **ducts of the greater vestibular glands**

Bulb of the vestibule (see Fig. 6.18)

- Is the homologue of the **bulb of the penis**
- Is divided into two masses of **erectile tissue** that lie on either side of the **vaginal opening** and are covered by the **bulbospongiosus muscle;** they unite anteriorly and extend as a thin strand to join the **glans of the clitoris**

Greater vestibular glands (Bartholin's glands) (see Fig. 6.18)

- Are paired **mucus-secreting glands** that are homologous to the **bulbourethral glands** in the male
- Lie in the **superficial perineal pouch** deep to the posterior part of the bulbs of the vestibule
- Open into the **vaginal vestibule** at the margins of the vaginal orifice
- Provide **lubrication** for coitus

Multiple Choice Review Questions

1. The urogenital diaphragm includes all *except* which of the following?

    a. Deep transverse perineal muscle
    b. Sphincter urethrae
    c. Colles' fascia
    d. Perineal membrane
    e. Superior fascia of the urogenital diaphragm

2. All *except* which of the following have attachment to the perineal body?

    a. Coccygeus muscle
    b. Pubococcygeus muscle
    c. External anal sphincter
    d. Superficial transverse perineal muscles
    e. Perineal membrane

3. The wall of the vagina has a direct relationship to all *except* which of the following?

    a. Urethra
    b. Bladder
    c. Uterovesical pouch
    d. Rectouterine pouch
    e. Rectum

4. The lymphatics from the ovary drain primarily into which of the following?

    a. Internal iliac nodes
    b. External iliac nodes
    c. Superficial inguinal nodes
    d. Inferior mesenteric nodes
    e. Aortic nodes

5. Which of the following concerning the right and left hypogastric nerves is *false*?

    a. They connect the superior and inferior hypogastric plexuses.
    b. They carry vagal parasympathetic fibers to supply the pelvic viscera.
    c. They have no associated prevertebral ganglion.
    d. They form from a bifurcation of the superior hypogastric plexus.
    e. They carry fibers that supply the descending and sigmoid colon.

6. Each of the following structures normally crosses the pelvic brim *except* which of the following?

    a. Uterine artery
    b. Ovarian artery
    c. Superior rectal artery
    d. Round ligament of the uterus
    e. Ureter

7. The deep perineal pouch of the male contains all *except* which of the following?

    a. Bulbourethral glands (of Cowper)
    b. Deep transverse perineal muscles
    c. Sphincter urethrae muscle
    d. Membranous urethrae
    e. Perineal nerve

8. The duct of the seminal vesicle does which of the following?

    a. Opens directly into the prostatic utricle
    b. Unites with the ductus deferens before opening onto the seminal colliculus
    c. Unites with the prostatic duct before opening into the prostatic sinus
    d. Joins the duct of the bulbourethral gland (of Cowper) before opening into the membranous urethrae
    e. Unites with the opposite duct to form a single ejaculatory duct

9. Parasympathetic fibers that supply the pelvic organs are found in all *except* which of the following?

    a. Nervi erigentes
    b. Inferior hypogastric plexus
    c. Sacral plexus
    d. Vesical plexus
    e. Pelvic plexus

10. Which of the following is *true* of the pectinate line of the anal canal?

    a. It is formed by the upper margins of the anal columns.
    b. It is also known as the anocutaneous line.
    c. It marks the junction of the internal and external anal sphincters.
    d. It approximates the transition from visceral afferent innervation to somatic afferent innervation.

Chapter 7

Back

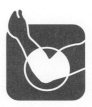

■ Vertebral Column

- Consists of 32 to 34 individual vertebrae and their intervertebral disks
- Protects the spinal cord
- Supports the weight of the head and trunk
- Transmits the body weight to the hip bones and lower extremities

● Typical vertebra (Fig. 7.1)

- Shows features common to all except the few **atypical** vertebrae
- Consists of a **body**, a **vertebral arch**, and **processes** for muscular attachment and articulation with adjacent vertebrae
- **Body**

  — Is a short, anteriorly located cylinder
  — Is covered on its superior and inferior surfaces by **hyaline cartilage** (articular cartilage)
  — Is the **weight-bearing** portion of the vertebra

- **Vertebral arch**

  — Is a U-shaped component attached to the posterior aspect of the body
  — Consists of **two pedicles** joined by **two laminae**
  — With the body forms the **vertebral foramen**
  — Gives rise to the **spinous, transverse,** and **articular processes**

- **Spinous process**

  — Is a posterior projection at the union of the two laminae
  — Provides attachment for muscles and ligaments

- **Transverse process**

  — Is a lateral projection at the union of the pedicle and lamina
  — Provides attachment for muscles and ligaments

- **Articular processes**

  — Consist of two **superior articular processes** and two **inferior articular processes**
  — Arise at the junction of the pedicle and lamina
  — Articulate with the **inferior articular processes** of the vertebra **above** and with the **superior articular processes** of the vertebra **below**

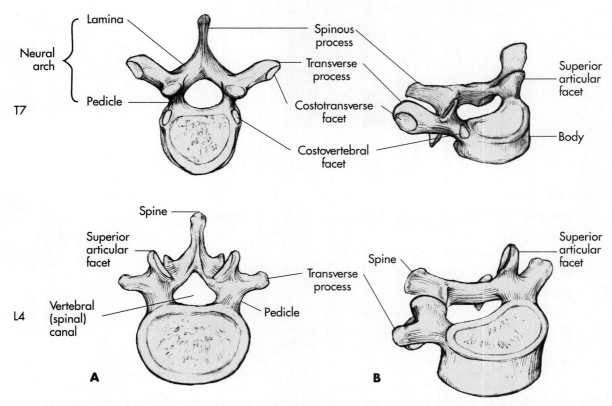

Fig. 7.1 Typical vertebrae. Two views of T7 and L4 vertebrae. **A,** Superoinferior views. **B,** Right anterior oblique views.

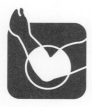

- **Vertebral foramen**

  — Is the space enclosed by **the vertebral arch** and the posterior surface of the **body**

  — With the other vertebral foramina forms the **vertebral canal,** which contains the **spinal cord** and its coverings

- **Intervertebral foramen**

  — Is formed by the approximation of the **superior and inferior vertebral notches** on the pedicles of adjacent vertebrae

  — Transmits the **spinal nerves** and their related blood vessels

- **Cervical vertebrae (Fig. 7.2)**

  - Are usually **seven in number** with numbers **3 through 6 being typical** and numbers **1, 2, and 7 being atypical**

  - **Typical cervical vertebra** has

    — A small, **wide body** that supports relatively little weight

    — A small, **bifid spinous process**

    — A triangular-shaped **vertebral foramen** that is larger than the body

    — A **transverse foramen** in the transverse process for passage of the vertebral artery and vein

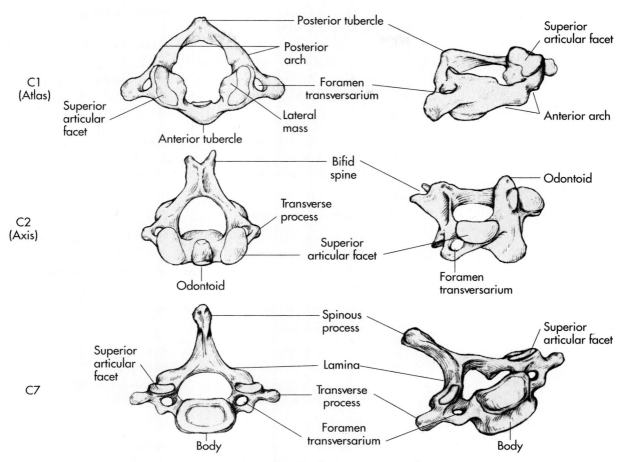

Fig. 7.2 Atypical cervical vertebrae. Two views of C1, C2, and C7 vertebrae.

— **Anterior and posterior tubercles** on the transverse process

— **A sulcus for the spinal nerve,** which lies between the anterior and posterior tubercles

— A **superior articular process** with the articular surface facing **posteriorly and superiorly**

— An **inferior articular process** with the articular surface facing **anteriorly and inferiorly**

• **Atlas** (see Fig. 7.2)

— Is the atypical first cervical vertebra

— Has **no body** and **no spinous process**

— Consists of **anterior and posterior arches,** paired **lateral masses,** and paired **transverse processes**

— Has a **facet** on the posterior surface of the **anterior arch** for articulation with the **dens**

— Has an **anterior tubercle** on the anterior arch and a **posterior tubercle** on the posterior arch

— Has a **sulcus** on the upper surface of the posterior arch for the **vertebral artery**

— Articulates with the skull at the **atlantooccipital joint** and with the axis at the **atlantoaxial joint**

— Allows **flexion and extension of the head** to occur at its joints with the occipital bone

- **Axis** (see Fig. 7.2)

  — Is the atypical second cervical vertebra

  — Has the **dens**, or **odontoid process**, which is a peglike extension from the superior surface of the body of the axis

  — Allows **rotation of the head** to occur at its joints with the atlas

- **Seventh cervical vertebra** (see Fig. 7.2)

  — Is often called the **vertebra prominens** because of its particularly long spinous process, which is readily palpable

  — Has a **small transverse foramen** that does not contain the vertebral artery

— *Other features of the cervical vertebrae*

- **Carotid tubercle**

  — Is the prominent **anterior tubercle** on the transverse process of the **sixth cervical vertebra**

  — Is crossed anteriorly by the **common carotid artery,** which can be compressed against it

- **Cervical rib**

  — When present is related to the **seventh cervical vertebra**

  — Results from the development of the **costal element** of the **transverse process** (the anterior tubercle)

  — May be associated with **compression** of the **brachial plexus** or the **subclavian vessels**

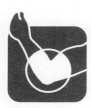

- **Thoracic vertebrae** (Fig. 7.3)

  - Are usually **12 in number**
  - Are characterized by

    — A medium-sized, heart-shaped **body**

    — A long **spinous process** that is angled inferiorly

    — **Costal demifacets** on the **body** for articulation with the **head of the rib** (note that the head of the rib articulates with the **body of the same number and with the body above**)

    — **Costal facets** on the **transverse process** for articulation with the **tubercle of the rib** of the same number

    — A **superior articular process** with the articular surface facing **posteriorly and laterally**

    — An **inferior articular process** with the articular surface facing **anteriorly and medially**

  — *Other features of the thoracic vertebrae*

    - **First thoracic vertebra**

      — Has a **complete facet** on its upper body for articulation with the **entire head** of the first rib

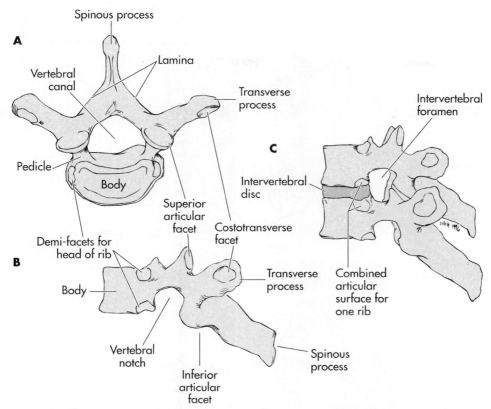

Fig. 7.3 Thoracic vertebrae. **A,** Superior view. **B,** Lateral view. **C,** Articulated pair of thoracic vertebrae; lateral view.

— Has a **demifacet** on its lower body for articulation with the upper part of the **head** of the second rib

- **Tenth, eleventh, and twelfth ribs**

    — Have only **complete facets** on their bodies for articulation with the **entire head** of the corresponding rib

- **Eleventh and twelfth ribs**

    — **Lack facets** on their **transverse processes** for articulation with the corresponding rib

● **Lumbar vertebrae**

- Are usually **five in number**
- Are characterized by

    — A massive, kidney-shaped **body**
    — A short, thick **spine,** which is quadrangular in shape and projects posteriorly
    — A **superior articular process** with the articular surface facing **medially and slightly posteriorly**
    — An **inferior articular process** with the articular surface facing **laterally and slightly anteriorly**
    — An **accessory process** on the posterior base of the **transverse process** for attachment of the **longissimus muscle**
    — A **mamillary process** on the posterior surface of the **superior articular process** for attachment of the **multifidus muscle**

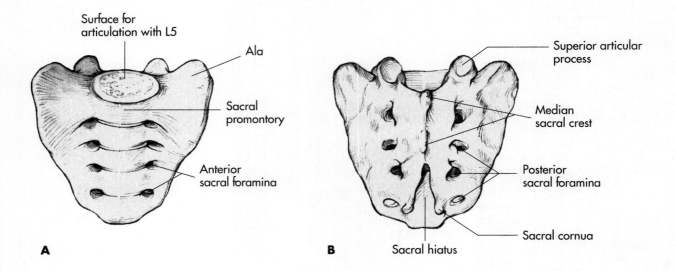

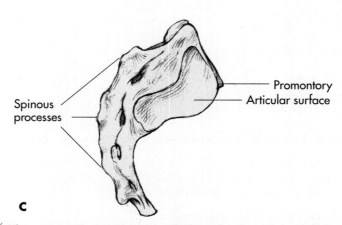

Fig. 7.4 The sacrum. **A,** Anterior view. **B,** Posterior view. **C,** Lateral view.

● **Sacrum (Fig. 7.4)**

- Transfers the weight of the body from the vertebral column to the pelvis
- Is formed by the fusion of the **five sacral vertebrae**
- Is a single wedge-shaped bone with its ventral surface facing inferiorly
- Articulates with the inferior articular processes of the **fifth lumbar vertebra** and with the **hip bones** at the **sacroiliac joints**
- **Anterior sacral foramina**

  — Are the four paired openings that transmit the **ventral rami** of spinal nerves S1-S4

- **Posterior sacral foramina**

  — Are the four paired openings that transmit the **dorsal rami** of spinal nerves S1-S4

- Sacral promontory
  - Is the anteriorly projecting **superior lip** of the body of the **S1 vertebra**
  - Is the posterior boundary of the **superior pelvic aperture**

- Sacral canal
  - Is the **vertebral canal** formed by the **sacral foramina**
  - Contains the **dural sac** and its contents down to the lower border of the **second sacral vertebra**
  - Below S2 contains the **filum of the dura** and the **dorsal and ventral roots** of the lower sacral nerves and the coccygeal nerve

- Ala
  - Is the **winglike projection** of the lateral mass of the **first sacral vertebra**

- Median sacral crest
  - Represents the fused spinous processes of the first four sacral vertebra

- Sacral hiatus
  - Is the defect on the dorsal surface of the sacrum resulting from a deficiency in the **spine and lamina** of the fifth sacral vertebra

- Sacral cornua
  - Represents the rudimentary **pedicle** of the fifth sacral vertebra
  - Is an important **landmark** for locating the sacral hiatus to administer **caudal anesthesia** (a caudal block)

● Coccyx
  - Is a small triangular bone formed from the four rudimentary coccygeal vertebrae
  - Is often in two pieces with the first coccygeal vertebra remaining separate and the last three fusing

● Joints between vertebrae
  - *Intervertebral disc (Fig. 7.5)*

    - Is a **fibrocartilaginous joint** between the bodies of two adjacent vertebrae
    - Corresponds in shape to the **bodies** of the adjacent vertebrae
    - Is separated from each vertebral body by a thin plate of **hyaline cartilage**
    - Accounts for about a **quarter of the length** of the vertebral column
    - Permits a small amount of movement between adjacent vertebra but cumulatively allows considerable flexibility in the vertebral column
    - Functions as a **shock absorber** when distorted by compression
    - Consists of the **annulus fibrosus** and the **nucleus pulposus**
    - None between the first and second cervical vertebrae (the atlas and axis) or between the sacral vertebrae

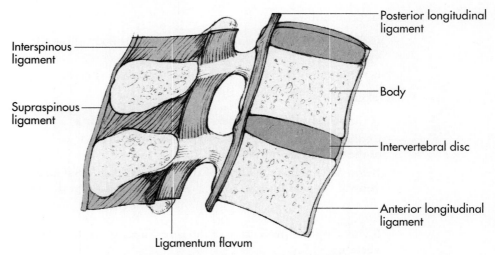

Interspinous ligament

Supraspinous ligament

Ligamentum flavum

Posterior longitudinal ligament

Body

Intervertebral disc

Anterior longitudinal ligament

Fig. 7.5 Ligaments between vertebrae.

- **Annulus fibrosus**

    — Is the **fibrocartilage** outer portion of the disc
    — Forms a strong union between vertebrae
    — Is composed of **concentric rings** of obliquely arranged **collagen,** which attach above and below to the **hyaline cartilage plates**
    — Is firmly attached to the **anterior and posterior longitudinal ligaments**

- **Nucleus pulposus**

    — Is the mucoid center of the intervertebral disc
    — Imparts the shock-absorbing quality to the disc
    — Is a **remnant** of the embryonic **notocord**

Herniated intervertebral disc (ruptured disc)

- Is the **protrusion** of the **nucleus pulposus** through a tear in the annulus fibrosus
- Usually occurs **posteriorly** into the vertebral canal **lateral** to the **posterior longitudinal ligament**
    - May impinge on a **spinal nerve** or its roots
    - Occurs most commonly in the **cervical** and **lumbar** regions
- May be predisposed by **degenerative changes** in the annulus fibrosus or may result from a sudden **increase in the compression forces** on lifting a heavy weight

- Facet joints (zygapophyseal joints)

    - Are the **synovial joints** between the **superior and inferior articular facets** of adjacent vertebrae
    - Depending on the vertebral level, provide varying amounts of flexion, extension, rotation, or lateral flexion

- Ligaments between vertebrae (see Fig. 7.5)
  - **Supraspinous ligament**
    — Connects the **tips** of the **spinous processes**
    — Limits flexion of the vertebral column

  - **Ligamentum nuchae**
    — Is an extension of the **supraspinous ligament** into the cervical region
    — Extends from the tip of the **seventh cervical spinous process** to the **external occipital protuberance**
    — Forms a **fibrous septum** between the neck muscles on each side
    — Limits flexion of the vertebral column

  - **Interspinous ligament**
    — Connects adjacent spinous processes
    — Limits flexion of the vertebral column

  - **Anterior longitudinal ligament**
    — Runs the entire length of the vertebral column
    — Is attached to the anterior surface of the **vertebral bodies** and the **intervertebral discs**
    — Is broad and strong
    — Binds the vertebrae together and supports the annulus fibrosus
    — Limits extension of the vertebral column

  - **Posterior longitudinal ligament**
    — Runs the entire length of the vertebral column
    — Is attached to the posterior surface of the **vertebral bodies** and the **intervertebral discs**
    — Lies within the **vertebral canal**
    — Binds the vertebrae together and supports the annulus fibrosus
    — Limits **flexion** of the vertebral column

  - **Ligamentum flavum**
    — Is a paired ligament that connects the **laminae** of adjacent vertebrae
    — Arises from the deep surface of the lamina above to the superior border of the lamina below
    — Is a **yellowish color** because of the large content of elastic tissue
    — Limits flexion of the vertebral column

- Joints between the skull, atlas, and axis (Fig. 7.6)
  — *Atlantooccipital joint*
    - Is a paired **synovial joint** between the **occipital condyle** and the **superior articular facet** of the **atlas**
    - Allows **flexion, extension,** and some **lateral flexion** of the head but **not rotation**

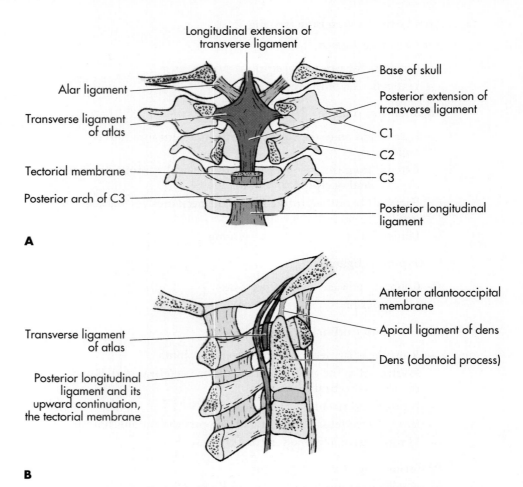

Fig. 7.6 Ligaments connecting the skull and vertebral column. **A,** Posterior view. **B,** Midline sagittal view.

— *Ligaments of the atlantooccipital joint (see Fig. 7.6)*

- **Anterior antlantooccipital membrane**

    — Extends from the anterior margin of the **foramen magnum** to the **anterior arch of the atlas**

    — Is the upward continuation of the **anterior longitudinal ligament**

- **Posterior antlantooccipital membrane**

    — Extends from the posterior margin of the **foramen magnum** to the **posterior arch of the atlas**

    — Is the upward continuation of the paired **ligamenta flava**

    — Is penetrated by the **vertebral artery** and the **suboccipital nerve**

— *Atlantoaxial joint*

- The atlantoaxial joint consists of three separate synovial joints.

- The paired **lateral atlantoaxial joint** is between the **inferior articular facet** of the **atlas** and the **superior articular facet** of the **axis.**
- The **median atlantoaxial joint** is between the **anterior surface of the dens** and the posterior surface of the **anterior arch of the atlas.**
- A **synovial bursa** is also present between the **posterior surface of the dens** and the **transverse ligament of the atlas.**
- The atlantoaxial joint allows **rotation of the head** but not flexion, extension, or lateral flexion.

● Ligaments between the axis and occipital bone (see Fig. 7.6)

- **Tectorial membrane**
  — Is the upward continuation of the **posterior longitudinal ligament**
  — Extends from the posterior surface of the **body of the atlas** to the basilar part of the **occipital bone** anterior to the foramen magnum
  — Covers the posterior surface of the **dens**

- **Apical ligament**
  — Extends from the **apex of the dens** to the **occipital bone** anterior to the foramen magnum

- **Alar ligament**
  — Is a stout ligament connecting the side of the **dens** to a tubercle on the medial aspect of the **occipital condyle**
  — **Limits rotation** at the atlantoaxial joint

- **Cruciform ligament**
  — Consists of the **transverse ligament** and a **vertical ligament**
  — Binds the **dens** tightly against the **anterior arch of the atlas**

- **Transverse ligament of the atlas**
  — Is part of the **cruciate ligament**
  — Runs between the **lateral masses** of the atlas
  — Is separated from the dens by a **synovial bursa**

- **Vertical ligament**
  — Is part of the **cruciate ligament**
  — Has superior and inferior **longitudinal bands**
  — Extends from the back of the body of the **axis** to the anterior margin of the **foramen magnum**

● Curvatures of the vertebral column (Fig. 7.7)

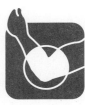

— *Normal curvatures*

  - **Primary curvature** of the spine
    — Exists before birth
    — Is C-shaped and **concave anteriorly**
    — Is retained in the **thoracic** and **sacral** regions of the adult

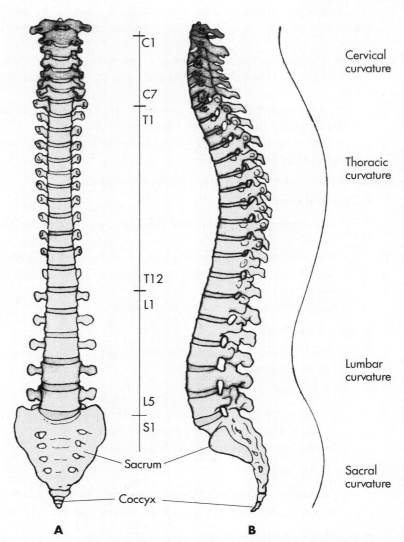

Fig. 7.7 Normal curvatures of the vertebral column. **A,** Anterior view. **B,** Lateral view.

- **Secondary curvature** of the spine

  — Develops after birth in the **cervical** and **lumbar** regions

  — Is **concave posteriorly**

  — Becomes apparent in the **cervical region** when the infant begins to hold up its head

  — Becomes apparent in the **lumbar region** when the infant begins to walk

— *Abnormal curvatures*

  - **Lordosis**

    — Is an abnormal curvature, or the exaggeration of a normal curvature, which is **convex anteriorly**

— Is a normal compensation of the **lumbar region** to the additional weight of pregnancy

- **Kyphosis**

    — Is an abnormal curvature, or the exaggeration of a normal curvature, which is **convex posteriorly**

- **Scoliosis**

    — Is any **lateral curvature** of the spine
    — Is never normal

Muscles of the Back

- Superficial muscles of the back

    - Develop as outgrowths of the limb bud mesoderm and are not true back muscles
    - Are described in Chapter 2 (see Table 2.1)

- Intrinsic muscles of the back (Fig. 7.8)

    - Are the longitudinally arranged **extensor muscles** of the vertebral column
    - Are derived from the **epimere** of the embryo
    - Are innervated by the **dorsal primary rami** of the spinal nerves
    - Lie in the **vertebral gutters** on each side of the spinous processes
    - Include the **splenius** group, the **erector spinae** group, and the **transversospinalis** group

    — *Splenius group*

        - Is also called the **spinotransverse group**
        - Runs obliquely across the back of the neck, covering it similar to **a bandage**
        - Consists of the **splenius capitis** and the **splenius cervicis**
        - Arises from the **upper thoracic spines** and the **ligamentum nuchae**
        - Passes upward and laterally to insert on the **transverse processes** of the upper cervical vertebrae and on the **superior nuchal line** and **mastoid process**
        - Rotates the head and extends and laterally rotates the neck

    — *Erector spinae group (Fig. 7.8)*

        - Is also called the **sacrospinalis** group
        - Is a massive, longitudinally arranged group
        - **Extends** and **laterally flexes** the head and vertebral column
        - Is also active in **flexion** of the vertebral column resisting the downward force of gravity
        - Has an extensive origin from the sacrum, iliac crest, and the lumbar and lower thoracic spinous processes
        - Is divided into **three parallel columns** based on its insertion
        - Iliocostalis

            — **Is the lateral** column

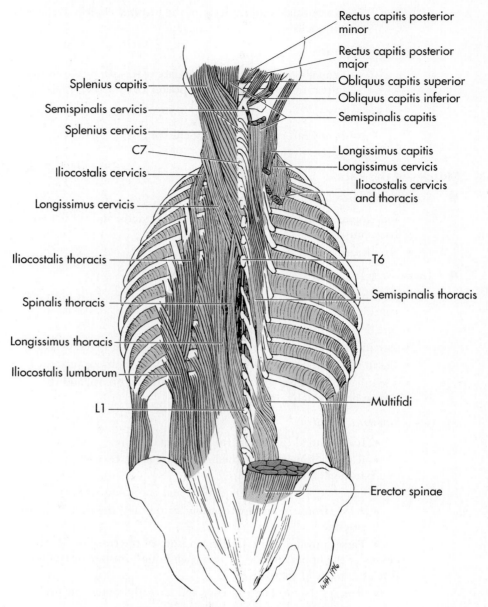

Splenius capitis

Semispinalis cervicis

Splenius cervicis

C7

Iliocostalis cervicis

Longissimus cervicis

Iliocostalis thoracis

Spinalis thoracis

Longissimus thoracis

Iliocostalis lumborum

L1

Rectus capitis posterior minor

Rectus capitis posterior major

Obliquus capitis superior

Obliquus capitis inferior

Semispinalis capitis

Longissimus capitis

Longissimus cervicis

Iliocostalis cervicis and thoracis

T6

Semispinalis thoracis

Multifidi

Erector spinae

Fig. 7.8 Intrinsic muscles of the back.

— Attaches to the **ribs at their angles** and to the **transverse processes** of the **cervical vertebrae**
— Is divided into **lumborum, thoracis,** and **cervicis** components

• **Longissimus**

— Is the **middle** column
— Attaches to the **ribs,** the **transverse processes** of thoracic and cervical vertebrae, and the **mastoid process** of the skull

— Is divided into **thoracis, cervicis,** and **capitis** components

- **Spinalis**

  — Is the **medial** column
  — Attaches to the vertebral **spinous processes**
  — Is best developed as the **thoracis** component (in the thoracic region)

— *Transversospinalis group (see Fig. 7.8)*

- Lies deep to the erector spinae group
- Consists of relatively short bundles, which ascend **superiorly** and **medially**
- Connects **transverse processes** below with **spinous processes** above
- Includes the **semispinalis, multifidus,** and **rotator** muscles
- **Semispinalis** muscle

  — Arises from the **transverse processes** of thoracic and cervical vertebrae
  — Inserts into the **spinous processes** of cervical and thoracic vertebrae and the **occipital bone** of the skull
  — Is divided into **thoracis, cervicis,** and **capitis** components

- **Multifidus** muscle

  — Arises from the **sacrum,** the **ilium,** and the **transverse processes** of lumbar, thoracic, and cervical vertebrae
  — Inserts into the **spinous processes** of lumbar, thoracic, and cervical vertebrae
  — Is best developed in the **lumbar region** where it is covered by the origin of the erector spinae muscle

- **Rotator** muscles

  — Lie deep to the multifidus muscles
  — Extend from the **transverse process** to the **lamina and spine** of the vertebra above
  — Include **short rotator** muscles, which join adjacent vertebrae, and **long rotator** muscles, which attach to the second vertebra above
  — Are found at all levels but are best developed in the **thoracic** region

— *Other intrinsic muscles of the back*

- Belong to the **segmental group** of muscles
- Include the **interspinales** and the **intertransversarii,** which are small muscles between adjacent spinous processes and adjacent transverse processes, respectively

● **Suboccipital region (Fig. 7.9)**

- Lies deep to the **semispinalis capitis** muscle in the upper part of the neck

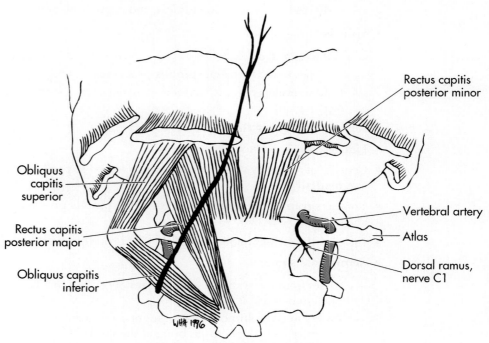

Rectus capitis
posterior minor

Obliquus
capitis
superior

Rectus capitis
posterior major

Obliquus capitis
inferior

Vertebral artery

Atlas

Dorsal ramus,
nerve C1

Fig. 7.9 The suboccipital region.

- Includes the
  — Suboccipital muscles (Table 7.1)
  — Suboccipital nerve
  — Greater occipital nerve
  — Third occipital nerve (least occipital)
  — Vertebral artery

- **Suboccipital muscles** join the atlas, the axis, and the base of the skull and include the
  — Rectus capitis posterior major
  — Rectus capitis posterior minor
  — Obliquus capitis superior
  — Obliquus capitis inferior

- **Suboccipital triangle**
  — Is bounded **medially** by the **rectus capitis posterior major**
  — Is bounded **laterally** by the **obliquus capitis superior**
  — Is bounded **inferiorly** by the **obliquus capitis inferior**
  — Contains the **vertebral artery** and the **suboccipital nerve**

- **Suboccipital nerve**
  — Is the **dorsal ramus** of the first cervical spinal nerve
  — Pierces the **posterior atlantooccipital membrane** to reach the **suboccipital triangle**
  — In the suboccipital triangle lies between the **vertebral artery** and the **posterior arch of the atlas**

Table 7.1	*Muscles of the Suboccipital Region*			
Muscle	**Origin**	**Insertion**	**Action**	**Innervation**
Rectus capitis posterior major	Spine of the axis	Lateral part of the inferior nuchal line	Extension of the head and rotation to the same side	Suboccipital nerve
Rectus capitis posterior minor	Posterior arch of the atlas	Medial part of the inferior nuchal line	Extension of the head	Suboccipital nerve
Obliquus capitis inferior	Spine of the axis	Transverse process of the atlas	Rotation of the head to the same side	Suboccipital nerve
Obliquus capitis superior	Transverse process of the atlas	Occipital bone between the superior and inferior nuchal lines	Extension and lateral flexion of the head	Suboccipital nerve

    — Supplies the **suboccipital muscles**

    — Has no cutaneous component

- **Vertebral artery**

  — Arises from the **subclavian artery** in the neck and ascends through the **transverse foramina** of the cervical vertebrae

  — Emerges from the **transverse foramen** of the **atlas** to enter the **suboccipital triangle**

  — Runs transversely across the **posterior arch of the atlas** to penetrate the **posterior atlantooccipital membrane**

- **Greater occipital nerve**

  — Is the **dorsal ramus** of the **second** cervical spinal nerve

  — Enters the **suboccipital region** at the lower border of the **obliquus capitis inferior** muscle

  — Runs upward across the **suboccipital triangle** to pierce the semispinalis capitis and trapezius muscles

  — Joins the **occipital artery** and supplies **cutaneous** innervation to the **scalp**

- **Third occipital nerve**

  — Is the **dorsal ramus** of the **third** cervical spinal nerve

  — Ascends across the suboccipital region to supply **cutaneous** innervation to the **scalp** of the occipital region

- ● Other features of the back

  - **Triangle of auscultation**

    — Is bounded **medially** by the lateral border of the **trapezius**

    — Is bounded **laterally** by the medial border of the **scapula**

    — Is bounded **inferiorly** by the upper border of the **latissimus dorsi**

    — Has **no intervening muscles** between the skin and the rib cage, allowing the lung sounds to be heard more clearly

    — Is most pronounced when the shoulders are pulled forward

- Lumbar triangle
  - Is bounded **medially** by the lateral border of the **latissimus dorsi**
  - Is bounded **laterally** by the posterior border of the **external abdominal oblique**
  - Is bounded **inferiorly** by the upper border of the **iliac crest**
  - Has a **floor** formed by the **internal abdominal oblique**
- Thoracolumbar fascia
  - Is the **deep fascia** investing the **intrinsic back muscles** in the thoracic and lumbar regions
  - Is thin in the thoracic region and **thick** in the **lumbar** region
  - Has an **anterior layer,** which lies in front of the intrinsic back muscles and attaches to the **transverse processes** of the **lumbar vertebrae**
  - Has a **posterior layer,** which lies behind the intrinsic back muscles and attaches to the **spinous processes** of lumbar and lower **thoracic vertebrae**
  - **Fuses** with the **aponeuroses** of the **internal abdominal oblique, transversus abdominis,** and **latissimus dorsi** muscles
- Topographic landmarks of the back (Fig. 7.10)

● Innervation of the back

- Both the **intrinsic muscles of the back** and the **overlying skin** are supplied in a segmental pattern by the **dorsal primary rami** of the spinal nerves.
- **Dorsal primary rami** (except for the first cervical) divide into **medial** and **lateral** branches.
- **All** medial and lateral branches **supply muscle,** but only **some become cutaneous.**
- In general, **above** the middle thoracic level the **medial branches** become cutaneous and **below** this level the **lateral branches** become cutaneous.

■ **Meninges and Spinal Cord**

● Meninges (Fig. 7.11)

- Consists of three concentric sheaths that surround and enclose the **spinal cord** within the **spinal canal.**

— *Dura mater*

- Is a tough fibrous layer that forms a closed sac around the **brain** and **spinal cord**
- Fuses with the inside of the skull at the **foramen magnum** but lies free within the **vertebral canal** surrounded by the **epidural space**
- In the vertebral canal surrounds the **spinal cord** and the **nerve roots,** including the cauda equina
- Projects around the **spinal nerve roots** and fuses with the **periosteum** at the **intervertebral foramen**
- **Ends** blindly at the level of the **second sacral vertebra**

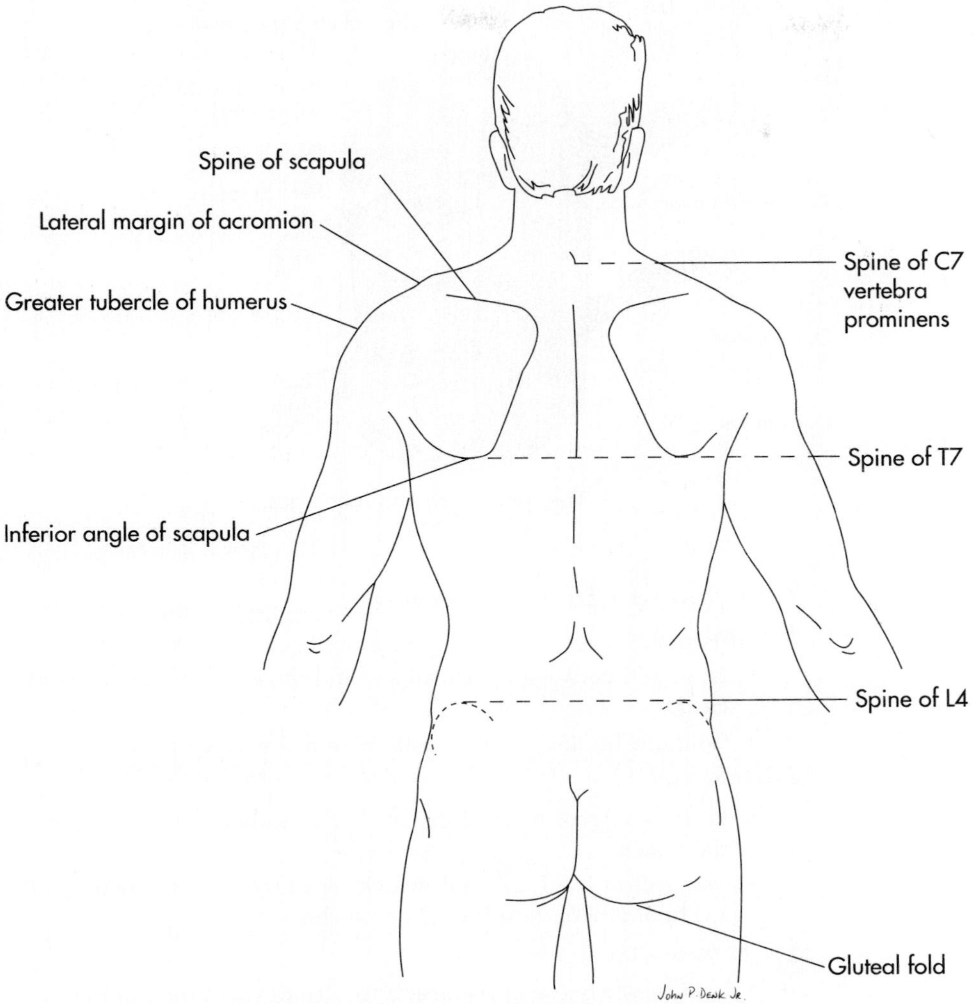

Fig. 7.10 Topographic landmarks of the back.

- Is continuous inferiorly with the **filum of the dura**
— *Arachnoid mater*
    - Is the delicate **intermediate** meningeal layer
    - Is **attached** to the inner surface of the **dura mater**
    - Is **attached** to the **pia mater** by fine strands that traverse the subarachnoid space
    - Is coextensive with the dura mater ending inferiorly at the level of the **second sacral vertebra**
— *Pia mater*
    - Is a fine vascular layer that is **closely applied** to the surface of the **spinal cord**
    - Extends along the **nerve root** to the spinal nerve
    - Extends from the lower end of the spinal cord as the **filum terminale**

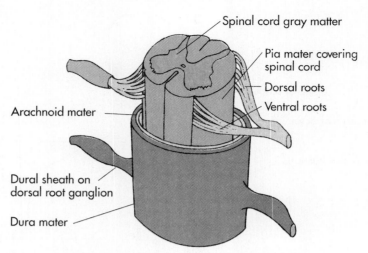

Spinal cord gray matter

Pia mater covering spinal cord

Dorsal roots

Ventral roots

Arachnoid mater

Dural sheath on dorsal root ganglion

Dura mater

Fig. 7.11 The spinal cord and meninges.

— *Other features related to the meninges*
  Epidural space

- Is located between the **dural sac** and the wall of the **vertebral canal**
- Contains **fat** and the **internal vertebral venous plexus**

Subdural space

- Is often referred to by clinicians but in reality is only a **potential space**
- May collect leaking blood, which separates the dura mater and arachnoid mater (a subdural hemorrhage)

Subarachnoid space

- Is the space between the **arachnoid mater** and the **pia mater**
- Contains **cerebrospinal fluid**
- Extends laterally along the **nerve roots** to the **intervertebral foramen**
- Extends caudally to the level of the **second sacral vertebra**
- Below the end of the spinal cord (at the lower border of L1) enlarges to form the **lumbar cistern,** which

  — Contains the **cauda equina,** the dorsal and ventral roots of the lower lumbar and sacral spinal nerves
  — Can be tapped with a long needle to remove a sample of cerebrospinal fluid without the risk of injury to the spinal cord (a **lumbar puncture**)

Denticulate ligament

- Is a flattened, longitudinal extension of the **pia mater** on the lateral sides of the spinal cord
- Lies between the dorsal and ventral rootlets
- Has **toothlike projections** that cross the **subarachnoid space** and pierce the arachnoid mater to **anchor the spinal cord** to the inner surface of the **dural sac**

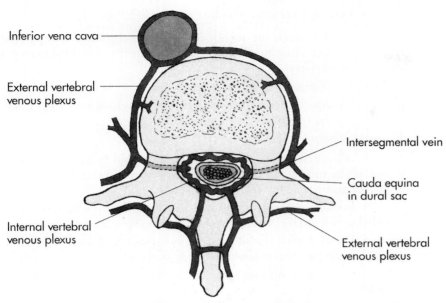

Inferior vena cava

External vertebral
venous plexus

Intersegmental vein

Cauda equina
in dural sac

Internal vertebral
venous plexus

External vertebral
venous plexus

Fig. 7.12 Venous drainage of the vertebral column and spinal cord at L3.

Filum terminale

- Is a threadlike extension of the **pia mater** from the **conus medullaris**
- Is surrounded by the **cauda equina** in the **lumbar cistern**
- Penetrates the **arachnoid mater** and **dura mater** to become continuous with the **filum of the dura,** which attaches to the coccyx

Vertebral venous plexus (Batson's plexus) (Fig. 7.12)

- Is an interconnecting system of veins **without valves**
- Will allow **blood flow in either direction** depending on the pressure gradient
- Extends from the **coccyx** to the **base of the skull**
- **Anastomoses** with the **segmental veins** at all levels and with the **dural venous sinuses**
- Provides a pathway for the **dispersion of malignant tumor cells** from the pelvic, abdominal, and thoracic **viscera** to the **vertebrae, spinal cord,** and **brain**
- Consists of **internal** and **external** vertebral venous plexuses
- **Internal vertebral venous plexus** (see Fig. 7.12)

  — Lies in the **epidural space** within the vertebral canal
  — Is arranged in a **ladderlike** pattern anterior and posterior to the dural sac
  — Drains the vertebral column, meninges, and the spinal cord
  — Anastomoses with the **dural venous sinuses** through the foramen magnum
  — Anastomoses with the **external vertebral venous plexus** via the **intervertebral veins,** which pass through the **intervertebral foramina** and the **sacral foramina**

- **External vertebral venous plexus** (see Fig. 7.12)

    — Surrounds the outside of the vertebral column lying on the **vertebral bodies** anteriorly and on the **vertebral arch** posteriorly

    — Is drained by the segmental veins

    — Anastomoses with the **internal vertebral venous plexus** via the **intervertebral veins**

Lumbar puncture

- Allows the removal of **cerebrospinal fluid** from the lumbar cistern of the subarachnoid space for laboratory testing or the introduction of **anesthetics** or **contrast material**

- Involves the insertion of a needle in the **midline** between the **third and fourth** or **fourth and fifth** lumbar vertebrae

- Involves little risk of injury to the spinal cord because it terminates at the **lower border** of the body of the first lumbar vertebra

- To reach the subarachnoid space, the needle must penetrate in order

    — Skin

    — Fascia

    — Supraspinous ligament

    — Interspinous ligament

    — Ligamentum flavum

    — Epidural space

    — Dura

    — Arachnoid

● Spinal cord

- Begins at the **foramen magnum** where it is continuous with the medulla of the brain stem

- Ends at the level of the **lower border of the first lumbar vertebra** in the adult

- Is only about **two thirds** as long as the vertebral canal

- Has a **cervical enlargement** related to the **brachial plexus** and innervation of the **upper extremity**

- Has a **lumbosacral enlargement** related to the **lumbosacral plexus** and innervation of the **lower extremity**

- Has a tapered lower end known as the **conus medullaris**

- Receives blood from the

    — Single **anterior spinal artery** and the paired **posterior spinal arteries,** which arise from the vertebral arteries or the posterior inferior cerebellar arteries (Fig. 7.13)

    — **Radicular arteries,** which arise from the vertebral, ascending cervical, posterior intercostal, and lumbar segmental arteries and which travel with the spinal nerves through the intervertebral foramina (see Fig. 7.13)

— *Spinal nerves (Fig. 7.14)*

- Consist of **31 pairs** of segmentally arranged nerves: 8 cervical, 12 thoracic, 5 lumbar, 5 sacral, and 1 coccygeal

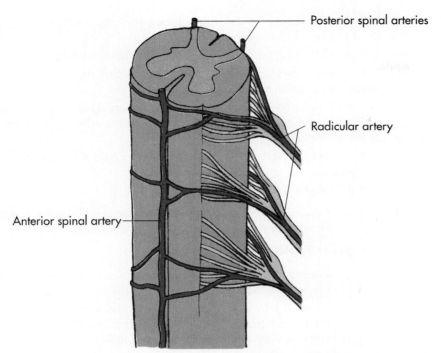

Posterior spinal arteries

Radicular artery

Anterior spinal artery

Fig. 7.13 Blood supply of the spinal cord.

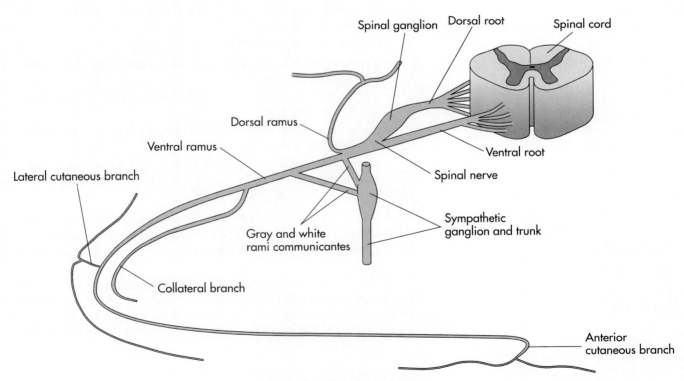

Spinal ganglion

Dorsal root

Spinal cord

Dorsal ramus

Ventral ramus

Lateral cutaneous branch

Gray and white
rami communicantes

Collateral branch

Ventral root

Spinal nerve

Sympathetic
ganglion and trunk

Anterior
cutaneous branch

Fig. 7.14 A typical spinal nerve.

- Are formed by the union of a **dorsal root** and a **ventral root** at the intervertebral foramen
- Exit the vertebral canal through the **intervertebral foramen**
- Outside the intervertebral foramen terminate by dividing into a **dorsal ramus** and a **ventral ramus**
- Each receives a **gray ramus communicans** from the sympathetic trunk, which conveys **postganglionic sympathetic fibers** to the spinal nerve
- Are **mixed nerves** containing all of the **general functional components**
  - **Dorsal root**

    — Contains the axons of **afferent** neuron cell bodies located in the **dorsal root ganglion**

  - **Ventral root**

    — Contains the axons of **efferent** neuron cell bodies located in the **ventral horn** of the spinal cord

    — At the T1-L2 level contains the axons of **efferent** preganglionic sympathetic neuron cell bodies located in the **intermediolateral cell column** of the spinal cord

  - **Dorsal rami**

    — Supply the intrinsic back muscles and the overlying skin

  - **Ventral rami**

    — Supply the muscles and skin of the anterolateral neck and trunk and all of the muscles and skin of the upper and lower extremities

Components of the mixed spinal nerve

- **General somatic afferent (GSA)** fibers from cell bodies in the dorsal root ganglion
- **General visceral afferent (GVA)** fibers from cell bodies in the dorsal root ganglion
- **General somatic efferent (GSE)** fibers from cell bodies in the ventral horn of the spinal cord
- **General visceral efferent (GVE)** fibers **(postganglionic sympathetic)** from cell bodies in the sympathetic chain ganglia

Other components of the mixed spinal nerve

- At the T1-L2 levels, the **trunk** of the spinal nerve (and not the dorsal or ventral ramus) also contains **preganglionic sympathetic fibers (GVE)** from cell bodies in the intermediolateral cell column of the spinal cord.
- At the S2-S4 levels, the **trunk and proximal ventral rami** also contain **preganglionic parasympathetic fibers (GVE)** from cell bodies in the sacral parasympathetic nucleus of the spinal cord. These leave the ventral rami as **pelvic splanchnic nerves** (nervi erigentes).

MULTIPLE CHOICE REVIEW QUESTIONS

1. The unique feature of the first cervical vertebra is that it does *not* have which of the following?

    a. Superior articular facet
    b. Transverse foramen
    c. Transverse process
    d. Body
    e. Vertebral arch

2. The transverse process of the typical thoracic vertebra bears a facet for articulation with which of the following?

    a. Head of the rib
    b. Neck of the rib
    c. Tubercle of the rib
    d. Transverse process of the vertebra below
    e. Bifid spinous process of the vertebra above

3. Which of the following nerves provides the motor innervation to the obliquus capitis inferior muscle?

    a. Lesser occipital
    b. Greater occipital
    c. Least occipital
    d. Suboccipital
    e. The dorsal ramus of C2

4. The ligament that joins the laminae of adjacent vertebrae is which of the following?

    a. Ligamentum nuchae
    b. Supraspinous ligament
    c. Interspinous ligament
    d. Posterior longitudinal ligament
    e. Ligamentum flavum

5. The internal vertebral plexus of veins is located in which of the following?

    a. Spinal cord
    b. Subdural space
    c. Epidural space
    d. Subarachnoid space
    e. Dural sac

6. Which of the following is *true* of the normal lumbar curvature of the vertebral column?

    a. It is present before birth.
    b. It is absent after puberty.
    c. It is convex posteriorly.
    d. It is concave posteriorly.

7. Which of the following is *true* about the medial column of the erector spinae group of muscles?

    a. It is known as the longissimus muscle.
    b. It arises from spinous processes.
    c. It inserts into transverse processes.
    d. It is a flexor of the vertebral column.
    e. It is innervated by ventral rami of spinal nerves.

8. The subarachnoid space typically extends caudally to which vertebral level?

    a. T12
    b. L2
    c. L4
    d. S2
    e. S4

9. The cauda equina consists of which of the following?

    a. Ventral and dorsal roots
    b. Ventral and dorsal rami
    c. Spinal nerves
    d. Ventral rami only

10. The transversospinalis muscle group includes which of the following muscles?

    a. Splenius capitis
    b. Semispinalis capitis
    c. Rectus capitis posterior major
    d. Serratus posterior superior
    e. Iliocostalis lumborum

Chapter 8

Head and Neck

■ **Neck**

● Muscles of the anterior neck (Tables 8.1 and 8.2)

● Muscles of the posterior neck (see Chapter 7)

● Triangles of the neck (Fig. 8.1) The area bounded by the midline of the neck, the clavicle, the anterior border of the trapezius muscle, and the lower border of the mandible and skull is divided by the **sternocleidomastoid muscle** into an **anterior triangle** and a **posterior triangle.**

— *Anterior triangle*

• Is bounded by the anterior midline, the anterior border of the sternocleidomastoid, and the superior border of the clavicle

• Is subdivided by the digastric muscle and the superior belly of the omohyoid muscle into **submandibular, submental, carotid,** and **muscular** triangles

Submandibular triangle

• Is bounded by the inferior border of the **mandible** and the anterior and posterior bellies of the **digastric muscle**

• Has a **floor** formed by the **mylohyoid** and **hyoglossus** muscles

• Contains the

— Submandibular salivary gland (superficial part)
— Facial vein superficial to the gland
— Facial artery deep to the gland
— Submandibular lymph nodes

Submental triangle

• Is an unpaired triangle lying above the **hyoid bone** and between the anterior bellies of the **digastric muscles**

• Has a **floor** formed by the **mylohyoid muscles**

• Contains the

— Submental lymph nodes
— Beginnings of the anterior jugular veins

Carotid triangle

• Is bounded by the anterior border of the **sternocleidomastoid,** the superior belly of the **omohyoid,** and the posterior belly of the **digastric** muscles

• Has a **floor** formed by parts of the middle and inferior **pharyngeal constrictor** muscles and the **thyrohyoid** muscle

292

Table 8.1	**Superficial Muscles of the Anterior Neck**			
NAME	ORIGIN	INSERTION	ACTION	INNERVATION
Trapezius	Occipital bone, ligamentum nuchae, and spines of all thoracic vertebrae	Spine of scapula, acromion, and lateral one third of clavicle	Elevates and rotates scapula	Spinal portion accessory nerve (motor) and C3 and C4 (sensory)
Sternocleido-mastoid	Manubrium sterni and medial one third of clavicle	Mastoid process and lateral part of superior nuchal line	One muscle alone flexes the head and neck rotating the face to the opposite side; both muscles together flex the head and neck	Spinal portion accessory nerve (motor) and C2 and C3 (sensory)
Infrahyoid Muscles				
Sternohyoid	Manubrium sterni and medial end of clavicle	Body of hyoid bone	Depresses hyoid bone and larynx	Ansa cervicalis
Sternothyroid	Manubrium sterni and first costal cartilage	Oblique line of thyroid cartilage	Depresses hyoid bone and larynx	Ansa cervicalis
Thyrohyoid	Oblique line of thyroid cartilage	Body and greater horn of hyoid bone	Depresses hyoid bone or elevates larynx	C1 by way of the hypoglossal nerve
Omohyoid	Superior belly: body of hyoid bone Inferior belly: upper border of scapula medial to suprascapular notch	Intermediate tendon bound to clavicle and first rib	Depresses hyoid bone	Ansa cervicalis
Suprahyoid Muscles				
Stylohyoid	Styloid process of temporal bone	Body of hyoid bone	Elevates hyoid bone	Facial nerve
Digastric	Anterior belly: digastric fossa of mandible Posterior belly: mastoid notch of temporal bone	Intermediate tendon bound to body of hyoid bone	Elevates hyoid bone and tongue; depresses mandible	Anterior belly: mylohyoid nerve (from mandibular division of trigeminal nerve) Posterior belly: facial nerve
Mylohyoid	Mylohyoid line of mandible	Body of hyoid bone and median raphe	Elevates floor of mouth and hyoid bone; depresses mandible	Mylohyoid nerve (from mandibular division of trigeminal nerve)
Geniohyoid	Inferior genial tubercle of mandible	Body of mandible	Elevates hyoid bone and tongue	C1 by way of the hypoglossal nerve

- Contains the
  — Internal jugular vein
  — Common carotid artery (distal part)
  — Internal and external carotid arteries (proximal portions)
  — Superior thyroid, lingual, and facial arteries (proximal portions)
  — Vagus and hypoglossal nerves

Table 8.2 *Deep Muscles of the Anterior Neck*

NAME	ORIGIN	INSERTION	ACTION	INNERVATION
Scalenus anterior	Anterior tubercles of transverse processes of third through sixth cervical vertebrae	Scalene tubercle of first rib	Laterally flexes neck; elevates first rib	Branches of ventral rami of fourth through sixth cervical spinal nerves
Scalenus medius	Transverse processes of all cervical vertebrae (on the posterior tubercles of three through seven)	First rib posterior to the groove for the subclavian artery	Laterally flexes neck; elevates first rib	Branches of ventral rami of third through eighth cervical spinal nerves
Scalenus posterior	Posterior tubercles of transverse processes of fourth through sixth cervical vertebrae	Outside of second rib	Laterally flexes neck; elevates second rib	Branches of ventral rami of sixth through eighth cervical spinal nerves
Scalenus minimus (frequently absent)	Anterior tubercle of transverse process of sixth or seventh cervical vertebra	First rib posterior to the groove for the subclavian artery or the suprapleural membrane	Laterally flexes neck; elevates first rib	Branch of ventral ramus of seventh cervical spinal nerve
Longus capitis	Anterior tubercles of transverse processes of third through sixth cervical vertebrae	Basilar part of occipital bone	Flexes head	Branches of ventral rami of first through third cervical spinal nerves
Longus colli	Vertical part: bodies of C5-T3 vertebrae	Vertical part: bodies of second through fourth cervical vertebrae	Flexes and rotates neck and head	Branches of ventral rami of second through seventh cervical spinal nerves
	Inferior oblique part: bodies of first through third thoracic vertebrae	Inferior oblique part: anterior tubercles of sixth and seventh cervical vertebrae		
	Superior oblique part: anterior tubercles of third through fifth cervical vertebrae	Superior oblique part: anterior arch of atlas		
Rectus capitis anterior	Lateral mass of atlas	Basilar part of occipital bone	Flexes head	Branches of ventral rami of first and second cervical spinal nerves
Rectus capitis lateralis	Transverse process of atlas	Jugular process of occipital bone	Laterally flexes head	Branches of ventral rami of first and second cervical spinal nerves

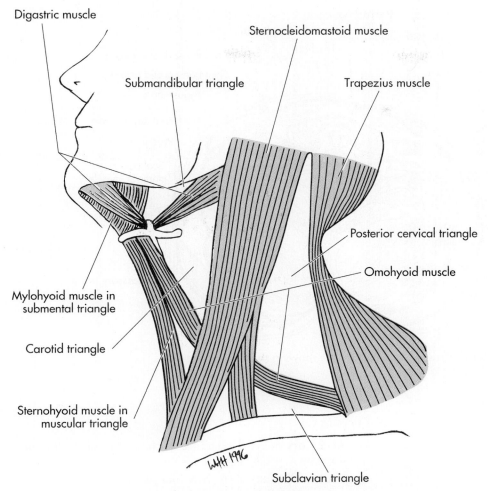

Fig. 8.1 Triangles of the neck.

Muscular triangle

- Is bounded by the anterior border of the **sternocleidomastoid,** the superior belly of the **omohyoid,** and the **anterior midline** of the neck
    - Has a **floor** formed by **sternohyoid** and **sternothyroid** muscles
    - Contains the anterior jugular vein

— *Posterior triangle*

- Is bounded by the anterior border of the **trapezius,** the posterior border of the **sternocleidomastoid,** and the superior border of the **clavicle**
- May be subdivided by the inferior belly of the omohyoid muscle into **occipital** and **subclavian** triangles
- Has a **roof** formed by the **superficial layer of deep cervical fascia** (investing layer)
- Has a **floor** formed **superiorly to inferiorly** by the splenius capitis, levator scapulae, scalenus posterior, and scalenus medius, all covered by the **prevertebral fascia**

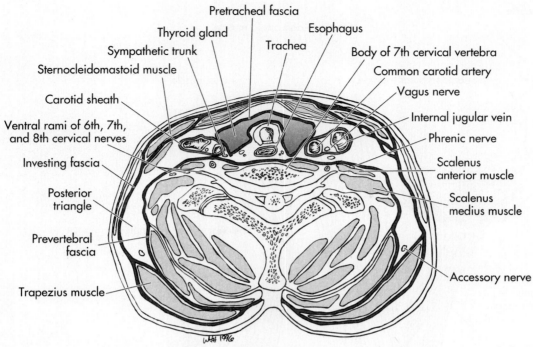

Fig. 8.2 Cross section of the neck showing the cervical fasciae.

- Contains the

    — **Accessory nerve** descending on the surface of the levator scapulae
    — Roots and trunks of the **brachial plexus**
    — **Subclavian artery** crossing the first rib
    — **Supraclavicular nerve**
    — **Suprascapular nerve**
    — **Dorsal scapular** and **long thoracic nerves** emerging through the scalenus medius muscle
    — **Nerves to the levator scapulae** from the ventral rami of C3 and C4
    — **Transverse cervical** and **suprascapular arteries**

- **Cervical fasciae (Fig. 8.2)**

    - Allows for the **free movement** of the different components of the neck
    - Generally serves as a barrier to the spread of infection and may direct the spread of infection from one region to another
    - Consists of the **superficial tela subcutanea** and the **deep cervical fascia,** which includes the superficial (investing) layer, the pretracheal layer, and the prevertebral layer

    — *Superficial cervical fascia*

        - Is the **tela subcutanea** lying immediately deep to the skin of the neck

- Contains the platysma muscle, superficial veins, cutaneous nerves, and variable amounts of fat
- Is continuous with the tela subcutanea over the head and thorax

— *Superficial layer of deep cervical fascia*

- Is also called the **investing fascia** because it surrounds or invests all of the structures of the neck deep to the superficial fascia
- Arises posteriorly from the cervical spinous processes and ligamentum nuchae
- Splits to enclose the **trapezius** and **sternocleidomastoid** muscles
- Is continuous across the midline anteriorly
- Is attached inferiorly to the spine of the scapula, the acromion, the clavicle, and the manubrium
- Is attached superiorly in a ringlike fashion to the external occipital protuberance, the superior nuchal line, the mastoid process, and the lower border of the mandible
- Splits superiorly to enclose the parotid and submandibular salivary glands

— *Pretracheal fascia*

- Lies deep to the infrahyoid muscles and over the front of the **larynx, thyroid,** and **trachea**
- Splits to **enclose** the **thyroid gland**
- Fuses on each side with the **carotid sheath**
- Attaches **superiorly** to the **thyroid cartilage** and **hyoid bone**
- Extends **inferiorly** into the thorax to blend with the **fibrous pericardium** around the great vessels thus providing a route for the **spread of infection** from the neck into the thorax
- Is **limited** to the **anterior part** of the neck as its name implies and **does not** completely ensheath the visceral structures of the neck
- Has a highly variable textbook description

— *Carotid sheath*

- Is a condensation of fascia around the **great vessels** of the neck
- Surrounds the **common and internal carotid arteries, internal jugular vein,** and **vagus nerve**
- Fuses with the **superficial layer of deep cervical fascia,** the **pretracheal fascia,** and the **prevertebral fascia**
- Extends from the base of the skull to the root of the neck

— *Buccopharyngeal fascia*

- Covers the outer surface of the pharyngeal constrictor muscles and the buccinator muscle

— *Pharyngeobasilar fascia*

- Lies between the mucosa of the pharynx and the pharyngeal constrictor muscles

— *Prevertebral fascia*

- Lies **deep** to the **superficial layer** of the deep cervical fascia

- Ensheaths the **vertebral column** and its related muscles
- Covers the **prevertebral muscles,** the **scalene muscles,** and the **intrinsic muscles** of the back
- Attaches posteriorly to the base of the skull and the **cervical spinous processes** and **ligamentum nuchae**
- Attaches anteriorly to the base of the skull and the **transverse processes** of the cervical vertebrae and then becomes **continuous across the midline** with the prevertebral fascia of the opposite side
- Divides over the front of the cervical vertebrae into the **interior lamina,** or **alar fascia,** that extends into the thorax to fuse with the fascia of the esophagus at the level of the body of the **third thoracic vertebrae,** and the **posterior laminae** that continues into the thorax over the front of the vertebral bodies
- Forms a "**danger space**" between the two layers on the front of the vertebral column that may facilitate the **spread of infection** from the deep neck into the thorax

- **Arteries of the neck**
  - *Subclavian artery (Fig. 8.3)*
    - On the **right** arises from the **brachiocephalic trunk** behind the right sternoclavicular joint
    - On the **left** arises from the **arch of the aorta** in the superior mediastinum
    - Arches laterally over the **cervical pleura** and **apex of the lung**
    - Grooves the **first rib** as it passes between the **scalenus anterior** and **scalenus medius** muscles
    - Is continuous with the **axillary artery** at the lateral border of the first rib
    - Is divided into **three parts** by the **scalenus anterior** muscle
    - Gives rise to the

      - Vertebral artery
      - Internal thoracic artery
      - Thyrocervical trunk
      - Costocervical trunk
      - Dorsal scapular artery (variable)

    Vertebral artery (see Fig. 8.3)

    - Arises from the **first part** of the subclavian artery
    - Ascends to the angle between the **longus colli** and **scalenus anterior** muscles and enters the **transverse foramen** of the **sixth cervical vertebra**
    - Is accompanied by the **vertebral vein** and a periarterial **sympathetic plexus**
    - Traverses the **transverse foramina** of the **upper six** cervical vertebrae
    - Passes medially on the posterior arch of the **atlas** and pierces the **posterior atlantooccipital membrane** to enter the cranial cavity through the **foramen magnum**
    - In the neck gives rise to

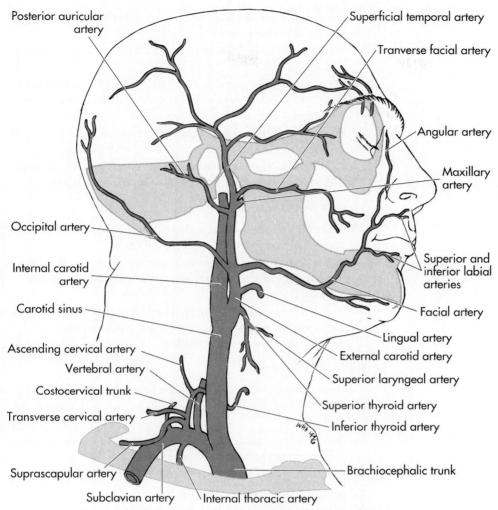

Fig. 8.3 The carotid arteries in the neck and the branches of the external carotid artery.

— **Radicular arteries,** which arise segmentally to supply the roots of the spinal nerves and reinforce the spinal arteries

— **Muscular branches,** as it lies on the posterior arch of the atlas, which anastomose with the deep arteries of the neck

Thyrocervical trunk (see Fig. 8.3)

- Arises from the **first part** of the subclavian artery at the medial border of the scalenus anterior muscle
- Is a short trunk that gives rise to the

— Inferior thyroid artery

— Transverse cervical artery

— Suprascapular artery

- **Inferior thyroid artery**

— Ascends anterior to the medial border of the scalenus anterior muscle

— Passes medially behind the **carotid sheath** and in front of the **vertebral artery**

— Reaches the lower pole of **thyroid gland** on its posterior surface

— Near the thyroid gland is intimately related to the **recurrent laryngeal nerve,** which is **vulnerable** in surgery on the thyroid gland

— Gives rise to the **ascending cervical artery,** which ascends on the scalenus anterior medial to the phrenic nerve

— Gives rise to the **inferior laryngeal artery,** which accompanies the inferior laryngeal nerve to supply the larynx

- **Transverse cervical artery**

  — Runs laterally across the scalenus anterior muscle and passes across the **posterior triangle** of the neck

  — Gives rise to a **superficial branch,** which descends on the deep surface of the **trapezius** muscle with the **accessory nerve**

  — Gives rise to a **deep branch,** which descends with the **dorsal scapular nerve** along the medial border of the scapula deep to the **rhomboid muscles**

- **Suprascapular artery**

  — Runs laterally across the scalenus anterior muscle

  — Passes across the **posterior triangle** of the neck behind the clavicle

  — Joins the **suprascapular nerve** to enter the supraspinous fossa deep to the **supraspinatus muscle**

Internal thoracic artery (see Fig. 8.3)

- Arises from the **first part** of the subclavian artery
- Descends on the anterior thoracic wall deep to the **costal cartilages**
- Terminates in the sixth intercostal space by dividing into the

  — Superior epigastric artery

  — Musculophrenic artery

Costocervical trunk (see Fig. 8.3)

- Arises from the posterior aspect of the **second part** of the subclavian artery
- Runs posteriorly over the **cervical pleura** to reach the neck of the first rib
- Terminates by dividing into the

  — **Deep cervical artery,** which ascends between the semispinalis capitis and semispinalis cervicis muscles to **anastomose** with the **occipital artery**

  — **Superior intercostal artery,** which gives rise to the first two **posterior intercostal arteries**

Dorsal scapular artery

- When present, **replaces** the deep branch of the transverse cervical artery (the superficial branch of which is then called the **superficial cervical artery**)

- Arises from the **third part** of the subclavian artery
- Accompanies the **dorsal scapular nerve** on the deep surface of the rhomboids

— *Common carotid artery (see Fig. 8.3)*

- On the **right** arises from the **brachiocephalic trunk** behind the right sternoclavicular joint
- On the **left** arises from the **arch of the aorta** in the superior mediastinum
- In the neck extends from the sternoclavicular joint to the **upper border of the thyroid cartilage** where it divides into the **internal** and **external** carotid arteries
- Lies deep to the anterior border of the **sternocleidomastoid muscle**
- Lies within the **carotid sheath** medial to the **internal jugular vein** with the **vagus nerve** lying posteriorly between the artery and vein

  - Carotid sinus

    — Is the dilated terminal portion of the **common carotid artery**
    — Functions as a **baroreceptor** sensing and relaying information on changes in arterial **blood pressure**
    — Is supplied by the carotid sinus branch of the **glossopharyngeal nerve**

  - Carotid body

    — Is a small rounded structure lying on the posterior side of the carotid bifurcation
    — Functions as a **chemoreceptor** sensing and relaying information on **oxygen** and **carbon dioxide** concentrations in arterial blood
    — Is supplied by the carotid sinus branch of the **glossopharyngeal nerve**

— *Internal carotid artery (see Fig. 8.3)*

- Has no branches in the neck

— *External carotid artery (see Fig. 8.3)*

- Begins at the **upper border of the thyroid cartilage** as a terminal branch of the **common carotid artery**
- Ends within the substance of the **parotid gland** deep to the **neck of the mandible** by dividing into the **maxillary** and **superficial temporal** arteries
- Lies at first anterior and then lateral to the internal carotid artery
- Gives rise to the

  — Superior thyroid artery
  — Lingual artery
  — Facial artery
  — Occipital artery
  — Posterior auricular artery

— Ascending pharyngeal artery
— Maxillary artery
— Superficial temporal artery

Superior thyroid artery

- Is usually the **first branch** of the **external carotid artery**
- Descends anteriorly and medially through the carotid triangle to reach the upper pole of the **thyroid gland**
- Accompanies the **external laryngeal nerve,** which supplies the cricothyroid muscle
- Gives rise to the **superior laryngeal artery,** which pierces the **thyrohyoid membrane** with the superior laryngeal nerve

Lingual artery

- Arises from the **external carotid artery** at the level of the **greater horn of the hyoid** bone
- Passes deep to the **hyoglossus** muscle to reach the tongue
- Is accompanied by the **deep lingual vein**
- Is divided into **three parts** by the hyoglossus muscle
- Near its origin is crossed superficially by the **hypoglossal nerve**
- Gives rise to the

  — **Suprahyoid branch,** which passes across the upper margin of the hyoid bone to the midline
  — **Dorsal lingual arteries,** which supply the dorsum of the tongue and the palatine tonsil
  — **Deep lingual artery,** which is the terminal branch of the lingual artery passing to the tip of the tongue
  — **Sublingual artery,** which supplies the sublingual gland and the floor of the mouth

Facial artery

- Typically arises from the external carotid just distal to the lingual artery but may arise in common as a **linguofacial trunk**
- As it loops deep to and over the **posterior digastric** and the **stylohyoid** muscles is related medially to the **pharyngeal constrictor** muscles
- Is related to the **submandibular salivary gland** deep to the mandible
- Winds around the lower border of the mandible to **enter the face** at the anterior margin of the masseter muscle
- Passes upward and medially to end at the **medial angle** of the eye
- In the **neck** gives rise to the

  — **Ascending palatine artery,** which passes deep to the styloglossus muscle and ascends over the upper border of the superior pharyngeal constrictor muscle to supply the soft palate
  — **Tonsillar artery,** which passes superficial to the styloglossus muscle to pierce the superior pharyngeal constrictor muscle and supply the palatine tonsil

— **Glandular branches** to the submandibular salivary gland

— **Submental artery,** which runs forward on the mylohyoid muscle in the submental triangle

- In the **face** gives rise to the

  — **Inferior labial artery**
  — **Superior labial artery**
  — **Lateral nasal artery**
  — **Angular artery**

Occipital artery

- Arises posteriorly from the **external carotid artery** at the level of the facial artery
- Passes posteriorly and superiorly along the lower border of the posterior belly of the **digastric muscle**
- Crosses lateral to the internal carotid artery, the internal jugular vein, and cranial nerves X, XI, and XII
- Grooves the **temporal bone** medial to the mastoid process
- Emerges onto the **scalp** at the apex of the posterior triangle
- Gives rise to the

  — **Sternomastoid branch,** which loops over the **hypoglossal nerve** before descending to supply the sternocleidomastoid muscle

  — **Meningeal branch,** which ascends through the jugular foramen to supply the dura of the posterior cranial fossa

  — **Descending branch,** which provides important collateral circulation by anastomosing with the **deep cervical artery** (from the costocervical trunk) and the **superficial branch of the transverse cervical artery** (from the thyrocervical trunk)

  — **Occipital branches** to the muscles and scalp of the occipital region

Posterior auricular artery

- Arises posteriorly from the **external carotid artery** above the posterior belly of the digastric muscle
- Passes posteriorly and superiorly deep to the **parotid gland** and lateral to the **styloid process**
- Ends posterior to the **external acoustic meatus** on the superficial surface of the **mastoid process**
- Gives rise to

  — **Auricular branches**
  — **Occipital branches**
  — **Stylomastoid branch,** which enters the stylomastoid foramen to supply the facial nerve and stapedius muscle

Ascending pharyngeal artery

- Is a small branch arising from the medial surface of the **external carotid artery** near its origin
- Ascends between the pharynx and the internal carotid artery

- Gives rise to the

  — **Pharyngeal branches**
  — **Meningeal branch,** which ascends through the jugular fo-
    ramen to supply the meninges of the posterior cranial fossa
  — **Palatine branch,** which supplies the soft palate and pal-
    atine tonsil
  — **Inferior tympanic artery** to the tympanic cavity

Maxillary artery

- Arises as a **terminal branch** of the **external carotid artery**
  deep to the neck of the mandible and within the substance of the parotid gland
- Traverses the **infratemporal fossa** and enters the **pterygopalatine fossa** through the **pterygomaxillary fissure**
- Supplies the muscles of mastication, the upper and lower jaws,
  the nasal cavity, the palate, and the dura
- Gives rise to the

  — Deep auricular artery
  — Anterior tympanic artery
  — Middle meningeal artery
  — Inferior alveolar artery
  — Branches to the muscles of mastication
  — Posterior superior alveolar artery
  — Infraorbital artery
  — Sphenopalatine artery
  — Descending palatine artery
  — Pharyngeal artery
  — Artery of the pterygoid canal

Superficial temporal artery

- Is the smaller of the two terminal branches of the **external carotid artery**
- Arises deep to the **neck of the mandible** in the substance of
  the **parotid gland**
- Ascends behind the **temporomandibular joint** and over the
  root of the **zygomatic arch** anterior to the auricle
- Supplies the **face** in front of the ear and the **scalp** of the temporal region
- Is accompanied by the **auriculotemporal nerve** and the
  superficial temporal vein
- Gives rise to the **transverse facial artery,** which passes across
  the face between the zygomatic arch and the parotid duct

- **Veins of the head, face, and neck (Fig. 8.4)**

  — *Facial vein*

    - The facial vein begins at the medial angle of the eye as the **an-
      gular vein.**
      - It descends in the face parallel and posterior to the **facial artery.**
      - It passes lateral to the angle of the mouth.

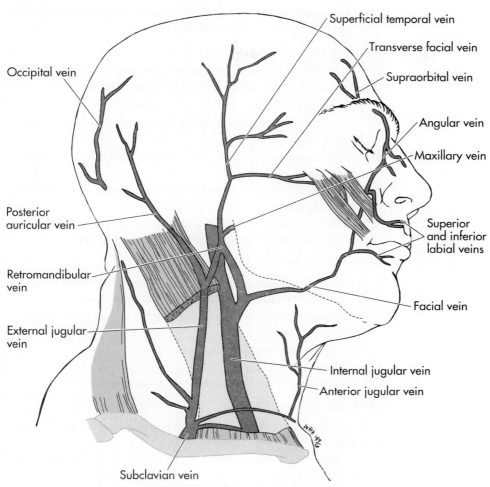

Fig. 8.4 Superficial veins of the head and neck.

- Below the mandible, the facial vein joins the **anterior division of the retromandibular vein** to form the **common facial vein,** which ends in the **internal jugular vein.**

- The facial vein communicates with the **cavernous sinus** via anastomoses with the **superior ophthalmic vein** at the angle of the eye and via anastomoses of the **deep facial vein** with the **pterygoid venous plexus.**

- Note that the distribution of the facial vein from the corner of the mouth to the angle of the eye is known as the **danger area** of the face because of the potential for the **spread of infection** through venous anastomoses to the dural venous sinuses.

— *Retromandibular vein*

- Is formed in the substance of the parotid gland by union of the maxillary vein and the **superficial temporal vein**

- Divides into

  — An **anterior division,** which joins the **facial vein** to form the common facial vein

— A posterior division, which joins the **posterior auricular vein** to form the **external jugular vein**

— *External jugular vein*

- Is formed by the union of the **posterior auricular vein** and the **posterior division of the retromandibular vein**
- Is a superficial vein but lies deep to the **platysma muscle**
- Crosses the **sternocleidomastoid muscle** obliquely to end in the **subclavian vein**
- Is usually inversely proportional in size to that of the internal jugular vein
- Lies on a line joining the **angle of the mandible** to the **middle of the clavicle**
- Usually receives the **suprascapular, transverse cervical, anterior jugular,** and **posterior external jugular** veins

— *Anterior jugular vein*

- Begins in the **submandibular region** above the hyoid bone and descends in the anterior neck just lateral to midline
- Above the sternum turns laterally to pass deep to the sternocleidomastoid
- Ends in the **external jugular vein**
- Just above the jugular notch of the sternum may be connected to the opposite vein by a **jugular venous arch**

— *Internal jugular vein*

- Begins in the **jugular foramen** as a continuation of the **sigmoid venous sinus**
- Descends within the **carotid sheath** lateral to the internal and common carotid arteries
- Ends behind the medial end of the clavicle by joining the **subclavian vein** to form the **brachiocephalic vein**
- Is dilated at its origin as the **superior bulb** and at its termination as the **inferior bulb**
- Usually has a single **valve** located just above the inferior bulb
- Receives blood from the sigmoid and inferior petrosal sinuses and from the superior thyroid, middle thyroid, pharyngeal, occipital, lingual, and common facial veins

— *Subclavian vein*

- Begins at the **lateral border of the first rib** as a continuation of the **axillary vein**
- Passes **anterior** to the **scalenus anterior** muscle; the **subclavian artery** passes **posterior** to the muscle
- Ends behind the medial end of the clavicle by joining the **internal jugular vein** to form the **brachiocephalic vein**
- Receives the **external jugular vein** as its only constant tributary (Note that the veins **corresponding** to the branches of the **subclavian artery** drain to the **brachiocephalic vein**, except for the suprascapular and transverse cervical veins, which end in the **external jugular vein**.)

- Lymphatic drainage of the head and neck
    - Drains directly or indirectly to the **deep cervical group of nodes**
    - May drain first to one of several **regional groups** of nodes, some of which form a **circular collar** at the junction of the head and neck
    - Is collected by the **jugular lymph trunk,** which on the **left side** usually joins the **thoracic duct** and on **the right side** either joins the **right lymphatic duct** or empties independently at the junction of the internal jugular and subclavian veins

    — *Regional groups of lymph nodes*
    Occipital nodes
    - Lie over the occipital bone at the attachment of the trapezius muscle
    - Drain the back of the scalp

    Mastoid (posterior auricular) nodes
    - Lie over the mastoid process behind the ear
    - Drain the back of the scalp, the auricle of the ear, and the external auditory meatus

    Parotid nodes
    - Lie on or within the parotid salivary gland
    - Drain the anterior scalp, the external and middle ear, and the parotid gland

    Buccal (facial) nodes
    - Lie on the buccinator muscle along the facial vein
    - Drain the eyelids, conjunctiva, nose, and cheek

    Submandibular nodes
    - Lie around or within the submandibular salivary gland
    - Drain the nose, lips, gums, cheeks, and tongue

    Submental nodes
    - Lie on the mylohyoid muscle in the submental triangle
    - Drain the tip of the tongue, floor of the mouth, lower lip, and chin

    Superficial cervical nodes
    - Lie along the external jugular vein
    - Drain the lower parotid region, the angle of the jaw, and the auricle of the ear

    Anterior cervical nodes
    - Lie along the anterior jugular vein
    - Drain the skin and subcutaneous tissue on the anterior neck below the hyoid bone

    Retropharyngeal nodes
    - Lie between the pharynx and the prevertebral fascia covering the vertebral column
    - Drain the nasopharynx and the auditory tube

    Tracheal nodes
    - Lie along the trachea
    - Receive lymph from the trachea and thyroid gland

— *Deep cervical lymph nodes*

- Lie along the **internal jugular vein** deep to the sternocleido-mastoid muscle
- Receive efferent vessels from the **regional lymph nodes**
- Are drained by the **jugular lymph trunk**
- Are often divided for descriptive purposes into **superior** and **inferior** groups of deep cervical nodes

Jugulodigastric node

- Is a large and fairly constant member of the **superior group** of deep cervical nodes
- Lies at the point where the posterior belly of the **digastric muscle** crosses the **internal jugular vein**
- Drains the **posterior third of the tongue** and the **palatine tonsil**

Juguloomohyoid node

- Is a large and fairly constant member of the **inferior group** of deep cervical nodes
- Lies above the intermediate tendon of the **omohyoid muscle** as it crosses the **internal jugular vein**
- Drains the anterior two thirds of the tongue

● **Nerves of the neck**

— *Cervical plexus (Fig. 8.5)*

- Is derived from the ventral rami of the first four cervical spinal nerves
- Gives rise to **cutaneous branches,** which supply the skin of the head and neck, including the

    — Lesser occipital nerve
    — Great auricular nerve
    — Transverse cervical nerve
    — Supraclavicular nerve

- Gives rise to **motor branches** to the muscles of the neck consisting of the

    — **Prevertebral muscles** (C1, C2, C3, C4), including the rectus capitis anterior and lateralis and the longus capitis and cervicis
    — **Levator scapulae muscle** (C3, C4)
    — **Scalenus anterior, medius, and posterior muscles** (C3, C4)
    — **Infrahyoid and geniohyoid muscles** (C1, C2, C3)

- Gives rise to the **phrenic nerve** (C3, C4, C5)
- Gives rise to branches to the **sternocleidomastoid muscle** (C2, C3) and the **trapezius muscle** (C3, C4), which contain afferent and sympathetic fibers but not GSE fibers (remember that these muscles receive their motor innervation [GSE] from the accessory nerve)

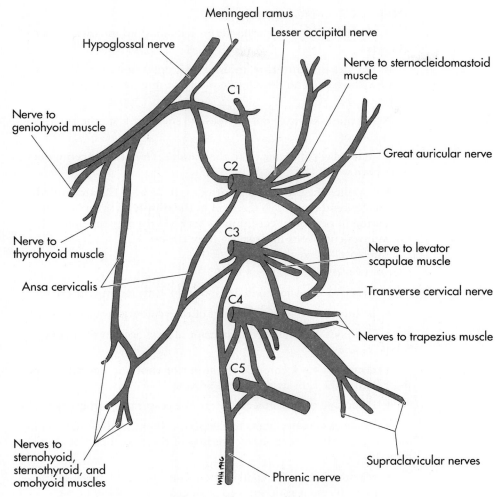

Fig. 8.5 The cervical plexus.

Lesser occipital nerve (C2)

- Is derived from the **ventral ramus** of C2; the **greater occipital** nerve is the **dorsal ramus** of C2
- Ascends along the posterior border of the sternocleidomastoid muscle
- Supplies the skin of the neck and scalp behind the ear

Great auricular nerve (C2, C3)

- Ascends vertically on the sternocleidomastoid toward the auricle
- Parallels the **external jugular vein**
- Supplies the skin over the auricle, parotid gland, and angle of the jaw

Transverse cervical nerve (C2, C3)

- Passes anteriorly across the sternocleidomastoid muscle toward the midline
- Supplies the skin of the anterior neck

Supraclavicular nerve (C3, C4)

• Emerges posterior to the sternocleidomastoid muscles as a single nerve

• Divides into **anterior, middle,** and **posterior** supraclavicular nerves, which descend deep to the platysma muscle to cross the clavicle

• Supplies skin over the clavicle and shoulder from the midline to the acromion

• May relay pain referred to the shoulder from the **phrenic nerve** distribution

• Supplies the skin of the **thorax** to the level of the **second rib** and may extend distally to the level of the **nipple** (Remember when evaluating upper spinal cord injury that the skin over the upper thorax receives cutaneous innervation from the cervical plexus as well as the intercostal nerves.)

Phrenic nerve (C3, C4, C5)

• Receives its major contribution from ventral ramus of **C4**

• Is formed at the lateral border of the **scalenus anterior** muscle

• Descends on the scalenus anterior muscle deep to the **prevertebral fascia**

• Leaves the neck through the **superior thoracic aperture** passing between the subclavian artery and vein

• Is the sole **motor** innervation to the **respiratory diaphragm**

• Provides **sensory** fibers to the pericardium, mediastinal pleura, and the pleural and peritoneal coverings of the central part of the diaphragm

• May receive the C5 contribution from the nerve to the subclavius in which case it is designated an **accessory phrenic nerve**

Ansa cervicalis (C1, C2, C3)

• Is a nerve loop derived from the **cervical plexus**

• Consists of a **superior root** and an **inferior root,** which form a loop anterior to the common carotid artery

• Supplies the **infrahyoid muscles** (strap muscles) **except** for the **thyrohyoid,** which is supplied by C1 and C2 fibers leaving the hypoglossal nerve more distally

• **Superior root**

— Is derived from fibers from C2, or C1 and C2, which loop upward to join and travel with the **hypoglossal nerve**

— Appears to arise from the hypoglossal nerve

— Is also known as the **descendens hypoglossi**

• **Inferior root**

— Is derived from C2 and C3

— Descends within the carotid sheath

— Often passes between the internal jugular vein and the common carotid artery

— *Brachial plexus in the neck (see Fig. 2.7)*

- Is formed in the neck from the **ventral rami** of spinal nerves **C5 to T1** and extends into the axilla
- Gives rise to the nerves supplying the upper extremity
- Emerges in the neck between the scalenus anterior and scalenus medius muscles
- Consists of roots, trunks, divisions, cords, and branches with only the **roots and trunks** (and their branches) lying in the **neck**

Dorsal scapular nerve (C5)

- Is a branch of the **C5 root** of the brachial plexus
- Passes posteriorly through the **scalenus medius** and deep to the levator scapulae muscle
- Runs on the deep surface of the rhomboid muscles with the **deep branch of the transverse cervical artery** (or the dorsal scapular artery)
- Supplies the **rhomboid major** and **rhomboid minor** muscles

Long thoracic nerve (C5, C6, C7)

- Arises in the neck from the **roots of C5, C6, and C7**
- Descends behind the brachial plexus and the first part of the axillary artery
- Passes inferiorly on the surface of the **serratus anterior** muscle, which it supplies

Suprascapular nerve (C5, C6)

- Arises in the neck from the **upper trunk** of the brachial plexus
- Passes across the neck deep to the trapezius
- Passes through the **scapular notch** deep to the **superior transverse scapular ligament**
- Runs with the **suprascapular artery** through the spinoglenoid notch to the infraspinous fossa
- Supplies the **supraspinatus and infraspinatus muscles** and the glenohumeral and acromioclavicular joints

Nerve to the subclavius (C5, C6)

- Arises in the neck from the **upper trunk** of the brachial plexus
- Descends anterior to the brachial plexus
- Supplies the subclavius muscle

— *Cranial nerves in the neck*

Hypoglossal nerve

- Exits the skull through the hypoglossal canal
- Descends anteriorly in the neck between the **internal carotid artery** and the **internal jugular vein**
- Appears below the posterior belly of the digastric muscle
- Hooks around the **sternocleidomastoid branch** of the **occipital artery**
- Passes anteriorly deep to the posterior belly of the digastric and between the hyoglossus and mylohyoid muscles
- In the neck gives rise to the

— Superior root of the ansa cervicalis

— Nerve to the thyrohyoid muscle

Accessory nerve

- Has two components, a **spinal root** and a **cranial root**
- Exits the skull through the **jugular foramen**
- **Cranial portion**

    — Arises as rootlets from the side of the **medulla** in a series with those of the glossopharyngeal and vagus nerves

    — **Joins** the **spinal root** before leaving the skull through the jugular foramen

    — Outside the skull separates from the spinal root to **join** the **vagus nerve** below the inferior vagal ganglion

    — Is distributed primarily with the external and inferior laryngeal nerves

    — Contains only **special visceral efferent** (SVE) fibers from cell bodies in the **nucleus ambiguus**

    — Supplies the muscles of the **larynx**

- **Spinal portion**

    — Arises as rootlets from the upper four or five **cervical spinal cord segments** (laterally between the dorsal and ventral rootlets)

    — **Ascends** through the **foramen magnum** to join the cranial root before leaving the skull through the jugular foramen

    — Descends in the neck deep to the **sternocleidomastoid** often passing for some distance through the substance of the muscle

    — Passes posteriorly across the **posterior triangle** of the neck and descends on the deep surface of the **trapezius muscle**

    — Contains only **general somatic efferent** (GSE) fibers from cell bodies in the **accessory nucleus**

    — Supplies the **sternocleidomastoid** and **trapezius** muscles

Vagus nerve

- Exits the skull through the **jugular foramen**
- Is joined below the inferior ganglion by the cranial root of the accessory nerve
- Descends in the neck within the **carotid sheath**
- Lies posteriorly between the **internal jugular vein** and the **internal and common carotid arteries**
- Gives rise to the

    — **Meningeal branch,** which arises from the superior ganglion and enters the cranial cavity through the **jugular foramen** to supply the **dura** of the **posterior cranial fossa**

    — **Auricular branch,** which enters the **mastoid canaliculus** in the lateral wall of the jugular fossa to supply **general somatic afferent** innervation of the **external ear and tympanic membrane**

— Pharyngeal branches to the pharyngeal plexus

— **Superior laryngeal nerve**, which divides into **internal** and **external** laryngeal nerves

— **Cardiac branches**, which descend to the cardiac plexuses of the thorax

— Branches to the **carotid sinus** and **carotid body**

— **Recurrent laryngeal nerve**, which returns to the neck from the thorax and terminates as the **inferior laryngeal nerve**

— *Sympathetic nerves in the neck*

Cervical sympathetic trunk

- Consists of **three or four** cervical sympathetic ganglia connected by a slender cord

- Ascends on the anterior surface of the **longus colli** and **longus capitis** muscles

- Lies posterior to the common and internal carotid arteries as they lie within the carotid sheath

- Lies between the **carotid sheath** and the **prevertebral fascia**

- Contains ascending **preganglionic sympathetic fibers (GVE)** from cell bodies in the intermediolateral cell column of the upper thoracic spinal cord segments (mostly T1 and T2) and **visceral afferent fibers (GVA)** from cell bodies in the dorsal root ganglia at the same level

- Distributes **postganglionic sympathetic fibers** via the **gray rami communicantes** to each of the **cervical spinal nerves**

- Distributes **postganglionic sympathetic fibers** and **general visceral afferent fibers**

— Via the **cervical sympathetic cardiac branches** to the **cardiac plexuses** of the thorax

— Via **periarterial plexuses** to the structures of the head and neck (for example, the internal and external carotid plexuses and the vertebral plexus)

— Via **communicating branches** to **cranial nerves** in the region

Superior cervical ganglion

- Is an elongated and flattened structure lying on the **longus capitis** muscle

- Lies at the level of the **first and second** cervical vertebrae (sometimes the second and third)

- Contains the cell bodies of **postganglionic sympathetic neurons,** which supply virtually **all** of the sympathetic innervation to the **smooth muscle** and **glands** of the **head**

- Gives rise to

— **Rami communicantes** to the upper four cervical spinal nerves

— **Superior cervical sympathetic cardiac nerve**

— **Internal carotid nerve** to the internal carotid plexus

— **External carotid nerve** to the external carotid plexus
— Variable **communicating branches** to cranial nerves IX, X, XI, and XII but most consistently to the **vagus** and **hypoglossal** nerves
— Branches to the **carotid body** and **carotid sinus**
— Branches to the **pharyngeal plexus**

Middle cervical ganglion

- Lies at the level of the transverse process of the **sixth cervical vertebra**
- Is variable and may fuse with the **superior cervical ganglion** or the **vertebral ganglion**
- Gives rise to

  — **Gray rami communicantes** to the fifth and sixth cervical spinal nerves
  — **Middle cervical sympathetic cardiac nerve**
  — Branches to the **perivascular plexus** around the **inferior thyroid artery**

Vertebral ganglion

- Lies over the **vertebral artery** below its entrance into the transverse foramen of C6
- May be absent but often is present together with the **middle ganglion**
- May give rise to

  — A **gray ramus communicans** (usually the sixth cervical spinal nerve)
  — Branches to the periarterial plexus around the vertebral **artery**

Inferior cervical ganglion

- Often fuses with the first thoracic ganglion to form the **cervicothoracic (stellate) ganglion**
- Lies on the transverse process of the seventh cervical vertebra and the neck of the first rib
- Gives rise to

  — **Gray rami communicantes** to the seventh and eight cervical spinal nerves
  — **Inferior cervical sympathetic cardiac nerve**
  — Branches to the **periarterial plexus** around the **vertebral** and **subclavian** arteries

Ansa subclavia

- Is a loop of the sympathetic trunk that passes anterior to the **subclavian artery**
- Connects the **inferior cervical ganglion** with either the **vertebral ganglion** or the **middle cervical ganglion**
- Is of unknown significance except that it contributes fibers to the periarterial plexus around the subclavian artery

Horner's syndrome

- Results from **interruption** of the **preganglionic sympathetic** input to the **superior cervical ganglion**
    - Is characterized by
        - A **warm and flushed skin** on the face resulting from denervation, and hence dilation, of the **blood vessels** in the skin
        - An **absence of sweating** on the head and face resulting from denervation of the **sweat glands** of the skin
        - A **small pupil** resulting from denervation of the **dilator pupillae muscle**
        - **Drooping of the upper eyelid** (ptosis) resulting from denervation of the **superior tarsal muscle** (smooth muscle)
    - May result from a high thoracic **spinal cord injury** or from invasion of the trunk by a **tumor** (commonly a Pancost's tumor of the lung)

● Other important structures of the neck

— *Thyroid gland*

- Is an **endocrine gland that arises** as a midline diverticulum from the floor of the embryonic **pharynx**
- Secretes the **hormones** thyroxine and triiodothyronine, which regulate the metabolic rate of body tissues, and thyrocalcitonin, which is concerned with the regulation of calcium metabolism in the body tissues
- Consists of **right and left lobes,** which are joined across the midline by the **isthmus**
- Is surrounded by a fibrous **capsule** and by a **sheath** derived from the **pretracheal fascia**
- **Lobes**
    - Lie below and posterior to the **oblique line** of the **thyroid cartilage**
    - Extend inferiorly to the level of the **fifth (or sixth) tracheal ring**
    - Lie on the sides of the **larynx** and **trachea**
    - Are covered superficially by the **sternothyroid** and **sternohyoid** muscles
- **Isthmus**
    - Lies over the **second and third tracheal rings**
    - Is **vulnerable** to injury and resulting hemorrhage during surgical **tracheostomy**
- **Pyramidal lobe**
    - When present, extends upward from the **isthmus**
    - May be **attached** to the **hyoid bone** by a ligamentous strand, which is called the **levator glandulae thyroideae** when the strand contains muscle

— Represents (together with any associated strand) a remnant of the lower end of the embryonic thyroglossal duct

- Is drained by the

    — **Superior and middle thyroid veins,** which empty into the internal jugular vein

    — **Inferior thyroid vein,** which empties into the left brachio-cephalic vein

- Is supplied by the paired **superior and inferior thyroid arter-ies** and by an inconstant **thyroid ima artery**

Superior thyroid artery

- Is usually the **first branch** of the **external carotid artery**
- Arises at the level of the **superior border** of the **thyroid carti-lage**
- Descends anteriorly and medially through the carotid triangle accompanied by the **external laryngeal nerve**
- At the upper pole of the thyroid lobe divides into **anterior** and **posterior** glandular branches

Inferior thyroid artery

- Arises in the root of the neck from the **thyrocervical trunk,** a branch of the subclavian artery

- Ascends anterior to the medial border of the scalenus anterior muscle

- Passes medially behind the **carotid sheath** and in front of the **vertebral artery**

- Reaches the lower pole of **thyroid gland** on its posterior surface

- Near the thyroid gland is intimately related to the **recurrent laryngeal nerve,** which is **vulnerable** in surgery on the thyroid gland

Thyroid ima artery

- The thyroid ima artery is an inconstant branch of the brachioce-phalic trunk or the arch of the aorta.

- It ascends through the superior mediastinum into the neck to reach the thyroid gland.

- It lies anterior to the trachea and therefore is **vulnerable** to injury during **thyroid surgery** or **surgical tracheostomy.** (Cutting the thyroid ima is particularly dangerous because it may retract into the thorax, making it more difficult to stop the bleed-ing.)

— *Parathyroid glands*

- Are small **endocrine glands,** usually four in number, which lie on or embedded in the posterior aspect of the thyroid gland

- Secrete **parathyroid hormone,** which is **essential** for the regu-lation of calcium metabolism in the body tissues

- May be found in the **lower neck** or in the superior or anterior **mediastinum**

- Arise as diverticulae of the third and fourth branchial pouches

— *Trachea*

- **Begins** in the neck at the **lower border** of the **cricoid cartilage** as the inferior continuation of the larynx
- Descends into the thorax to **terminate** by bifurcating at the level of the **sternal angle**
- Is 10 to 12 cm long and 1.5 to 2.0 cm in diameter
- Is characterized by a series of horseshoe shaped **cartilage rings** completed posteriorly by the **trachealis muscle** (smooth muscle)

— *Esophagus*

- Begins in the neck at the level of the **cricoid cartilage** as a continuation of the pharynx
- In the neck

    — Is **skeletal muscle** derived from mesoderm of the caudal **branchial arches**
    — Is innervated by SVE fibers from the **recurrent laryngeal nerves**
    — Is supplied by branches of the **inferior thyroid arteries**

■ **Bones of the Skull**

- For descriptive purposes, the bones of the skull are divided into the bones of the cranium and the bones of the **face.**
- Note that the term *cranium* is sometimes used to refer to the skull without the mandible.

● **Bones of the cranium (Figs. 8.6, 8.7, and 8.8)**

- Enclose the brain and brain stem
- Include the paired **parietal** and **temporal** bones and the unpaired **frontal, occipital, ethmoid,** and **sphenoid** bones

— *Parietal bones*

- Are paired bones that articulate with each other at the midline sagittal suture
- Articulate with the **temporal, frontal, occipital,** and **sphenoid** bones
- Have a **parietal eminence** (tuber) located posteriorly (the highest point of the bone)
- Are marked externally by the **superior and inferior temporal lines** for the attachment of the **temporal fascia** and the **temporalis muscle,** respectively

— *Frontal bone*

- Is an unpaired bone that forms the forehead and the roof of the orbit
- Articulates with the parietal, nasal, lacrimal, sphenoid, ethmoid, zygomatic, and maxilla bones
- Contains the

    — **Supraorbital foramen** (or notch) for passage of the supraorbital artery and nerve
    — **Supratrochlear notch** (frontal notch) for passage of the supratrochlear artery and nerve

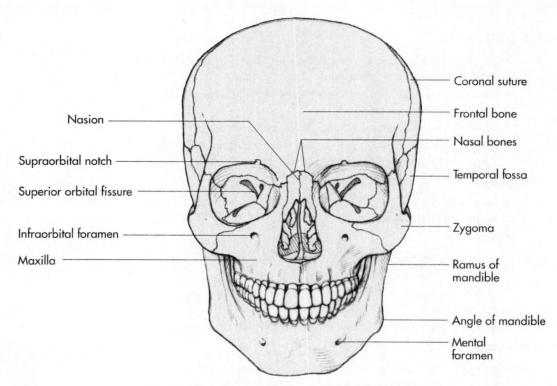

Coronal suture

Frontal bone

Nasal bones

Temporal fossa

Zygoma

Ramus of
mandible

Angle of mandible

Mental
foramen

Nasion

Supraorbital notch

Superior orbital fissure

Infraorbital foramen

Maxilla

Fig. 8.6 Anterior view of the skull (norma frontalis).

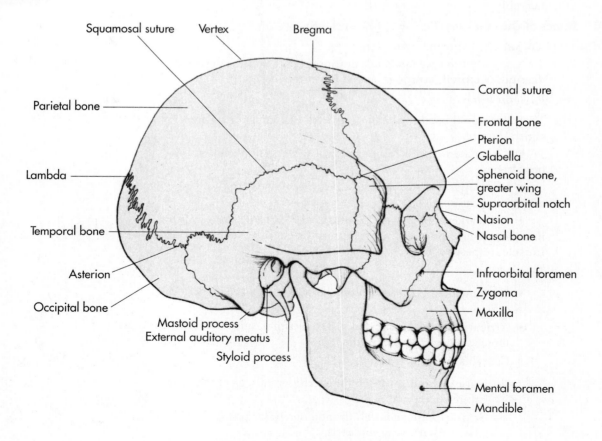

Squamosal suture   Vertex   Bregma

Parietal bone

Lambda

Temporal bone

Asterion

Occipital bone

Mastoid process
External auditory meatus

Styloid process

Coronal suture

Frontal bone

Pterion
Glabella

Sphenoid bone,
greater wing
Supraorbital notch
Nasion
Nasal bone

Infraorbital foramen

Zygoma

Maxilla

Mental foramen

Mandible

Fig. 8.7 Lateral view of the skull (norma lateralis).

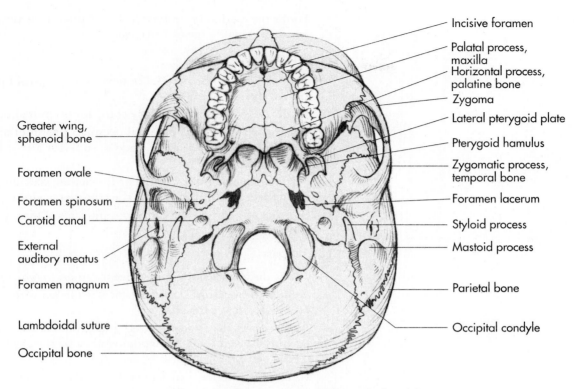

Fig. 8.8 Basal view of the skull (norma basalis).

- Is originally divided by a midline **frontal suture,** which may persist into adult life and is known as a **metopic suture**
- Has **squamous, orbital,** and **nasal** portions
- **Squamous portion**

    — Forms the convexity of the forehead
    — Contains the **frontal sinus**
    — Includes the **superciliary ridges** above the orbital margin

- **Nasal portion** articulates with the **nasal bones** and the **frontal processes** of the **maxillae**

— *Occipital bone*

- Is an unpaired bone that forms the base of the skull and the skull cap posteriorly
- Consists of **basilar, squamous,** and paired **lateral** (condylar) parts arranged around the **foramen magnum**
- The **basilar part** (basiocciput)

    — Articulates with the body of the sphenoid bone anteriorly and with the apex of the petrous temporal bone laterally
    — Is marked inferiorly by the **pharyngeal tubercle** for attachment of the **superior pharyngeal constrictor muscle** and the **pharyngeal raphe**
    — Forms the **anterior boundary** of the **foramen magnum**

— Forms the **medial boundary** of the **foramen lacerum**, which is closed in life by cartilage

- **Squamous part**

    — Articulates with the **parietal bones** and the **mastoid portion** of the **temporal bones**
    — Forms the **posterior boundary** of the **foramen magnum**
    — Externally includes the **external occipital protuberance**, the **external occipital crest**, and the **superior and inferior nuchal lines**
    — Internally includes the **cerebellar fossae**, the **cruciate eminence**, and the **groove for the transverse sinus**
    — Provides **attachment** for numerous **muscles** of the back and neck

- **Lateral part**

    — Forms the **lateral boundary** of the **foramen magnum**
    — Includes the **occipital condyles** for articulation with the **lateral masses of the atlas**
    — Also includes the **condylar fossa and canal** (for the condylar emissary vein) and the **hypoglossal canal** (for the hypoglossal nerve)
    — Forms the posterior boundary of the jugular foramen

— *Temporal bones*

- Are paired bones that articulate with the occipital, parietal, sphenoid, and zygomatic bones and with the head of the mandible
- Include **squamous, mastoid, petrous, tympanic,** and **styloid** parts
- **Squamous part**

    — Lies vertically on the side of the skull
    — Is related to the **temporal lobe** of the brain **medially** and to the **temporal fossa laterally**
    — Is grooved internally by the **middle meningeal artery**
    — Extends forward as the **zygomatic process** to articulate with the **temporal process of the zygomatic bone** and form the **zygomatic arch**
    — Includes the **mandibular fossa** and **articular tubercle**, which articulate with the **head of the mandible**

- **Tympanic part**

    — Is a curved plate that fuses with the mastoid and petrous parts
    — Forms a **sheath** around the **styloid process**
    — Forms the **floor** and **anterior wall** of the **external acoustic meatus**
    — Is separated from the squamous part in the mandibular fossa by the **tympanosquamous fissure**, which is partitioned medially by the tegmen tympani into a petrosquamous fissure anteriorly and a petrotympanic fissure poste-

riorly (the **chorda tympani** exits through the **petrotympanic fissure**)

- Styloid part

  — Includes the **styloid process**
  — Forms the anterior boundary of the **stylomastoid foramen**

- Mastoid part

  — Articulates with the **parietal** and **occipital** bones
  — Contains the **mastoid air cells,** which communicate with the **tympanic cavity** through the mastoid antrum
  — Includes a prominent **mastoid process,** which provides attachment for the sternocleidomastoid, splenius capitis, and longissimus capitis muscles
  — Includes the **mastoid notch** for attachment of the posterior belly of the digastric muscle
  — Is separated from the tympanic part by the **tympanomastoid fissure,** which transmits the **auricular branch of the vagus nerve**
  — Is grooved by the **occipital artery** as it passes posteriorly

- Petrous part

  — Articulates with the **occipital** and **sphenoid** bones
  — Contains the **inner ear** and parts of the **middle ear**
  — Contains the **carotid canal**
  — Forms the lateral boundary of the **jugular fossa** (the other being the lateral part of the occipital bone)
  — Includes the **mastoid canaliculus** in the lateral wall of the jugular fossa for passage of the **auricular branch of the vagus nerve**
  — Includes the **tympanic canaliculus** between the carotid canal and jugular fossa for the **tympanic branch of the glossopharyngeal nerve**
  — Has a **quadrate area** (between the carotid canal and the foramen lacerum) for attachment of the **levator veli palatini muscle**

— *Sphenoid bone*

  - Is an unpaired bone that articulates with the frontal, parietal, temporal, and zygomatic bones
  - Consists of a **body, greater and lesser wings,** and **pterygoid lamina**
  - Body

    — Lies in the **midline** at the junction of the anterior, middle, and posterior cranial fossae
    — Contributes to the **roof of the nasal cavity** anteriorly and the **roof of the nasopharynx** inferiorly
    — Forms the **hypophyseal fossa** for the pituitary gland superiorly
    — Contains the **sphenoid paranasal sinus**

— Is related to the **cavernous venous sinus** laterally

— Is grooved by the **optic chiasm** anteriorly and superiorly

— Articulates with and subsequently fuses with the basal part of the occipital bone posteriorly (the **sphenooccipital synchondrosis**)

- **Lesser wing**

    — Is a **paired** lateral extension from the anterior and superior part of the body

    — Arises by two roots, which form the **optic canal** for passage of the optic nerve and ophthalmic artery

    — Extends posteriorly as the **anterior clinoid process**

    — Forms the superior boundary of the **superior orbital fissure**

- **Greater wing**

    — Is a **paired** lateral extension from the inferior surface of the body

    — Articulates with the temporal, parietal, frontal, and zygomatic bones

    — Forms the roof of the **infratemporal fossa** and part of the **middle cranial fossa**

    — Forms the inferior margin of the **superior orbital fissure** and the posterolateral margin of the **inferior orbital fissure**

    — Includes the **foramen rotundum** (for the maxillary nerve), **foramen ovale** (for the mandibular nerve), and the **foramen spinosum** (for the middle meningeal artey)

    — Includes the **spine of the sphenoid,** which lies posterolateral to the foramen spinosum and provides attachment for the sphenomandibular ligament

- **Pterygoid process**

    — Is a paired process that extends inferiorly from the junction of the body and the greater wing

    — Consists of **medial and lateral pterygoid plates** (or laminae) with the **pterygoid fossa** between them

    — Separates the infratemporal fossa from the posterior nasal cavity (choanae)

    — Articulates with the maxilla, vomer, and palatine bones

    — Provides attachment on the **lateral plate** for the medial and lateral pterygoid muscles

    — Provides attachment on the **medial plate** for the cartilaginous auditory tube, the superior pharyngeal constrictor muscle, and the pharyngobasilar fascia

    — Includes the **pterygoid hamulus** from the posterior and inferior part of the **medial plate,** which serves as a pulley for the **tendon of the tensor veli palatini** muscle and provides attachment for the **pterygomandibular raphe**

— Includes the **scaphoid fossa** at the base of the medial plate for origin of the **tensor veli palatini** muscle

— *Ethmoid bone (see Figs. 8.35 and 8.36)*

- Is an unpaired cube-shaped bone
- Lies at the base of the cranium anterior to the sphenoid bone
- Forms part of the floor of the **anterior cranial fossa,** the medial wall of the orbit, and the medial and lateral walls of the **nasal cavity**
- Consists of **cribriform plate,** the **perpendicular plate,** and the **ethmoid labyrinth**
- **Cribriform plate**

    — Lies in the midline forming the **roof of the nasal cavity** and the central part of the **floor of the anterior cranial fossa**

    — Is perforated by the **olfactory foramina,** which transmit the **olfactory nerve** filaments

    — Projects superiorly as the **crista galli,** which provides attachment for the **falx cerebri**

- **Perpendicular plate**

    — Projects inferiorly from the middle of the cribriform plate

    — Forms the superior portion of the **bony nasal septum**

    — Articulates with the **vomer** bone

- **Ethmoid labyrinth**

    — Projects inferiorly from the lateral part of the cribriform plate

    — Forms the **lateral wall of the nasal cavity**

    — Includes the **superior nasal concha,** the **middle nasal concha,** and the **ethmoid air cells**

● **Sutures and landmarks of the cranium**

- *Coronal suture:* articulation between the frontal bone and the paired parietal bones
- *Sagittal suture:* articulation between the paired parietal bones
- *Lambdoid suture:* articulation between the paired parietal bones and the occipital bone
- *Squamous suture:* articulation between a parietal bone and the squamous part of the temporal bone
- *Parietomastoid suture:* articulation between a parietal bone and the mastoid portion of the temporal bone
- *Occipitomastoid suture:* articulation between the occipital bone and the mastoid portion of the temporal bone
- *Bregma:* the point at which the sagittal and coronal sutures meet
- *Lambda:* the point at which the sagittal and lambdoid sutures meet
- *Vertex:* the highest point of the skull near the midpoint of the sagittal suture
- *Nasion:* the point at which the frontal and nasal bones meet

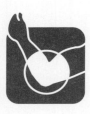

- *Pterion:* the area in the temporal region where the frontal and parietal bones meet the greater wing of the sphenoid bone and the squamous portion of the temporal bone
- *Inion:* the highest point of the external occipital protuberance
- *Glabella:* the region above the nasion between the paired superciliary arches

● **Bones of the face (see Figs. 8.6, 8.7, and 8.8)**

- Include the paired maxillae, zygomatic, lacrimal, nasal, palatine, and inferior nasal conchae bones and the unpaired vomer and mandible bones

— *Maxillae*

- Is a pair of bones that fuse to form the upper jaw
- Each consists of a **body,** a **zygomatic process,** a **frontal process,** a palatine process, and an **alveolar process**
- **Body**

    — Is pyramidal in shape
    — Contains the **maxillary paranasal sinus**
    — **Medially** contributes to the **inferior lateral nasal wall**
    — **Superiorly** forms most of the **floor of the orbit**
    — **Posteriorly** forms the anterior wall of the **infratemporal fossa**
    — **Anteriorly** is covered by **facial muscles**
    — Includes the **infraorbital canal and foramen,** which transmits the infraorbital nerve and artery

- **Frontal process**

    — Extends superiorly and medially to articulate with the nasal, frontal, and lacrimal bones
    — Forms part of the **medial margin of the orbit**

- **Zygomatic process**

    — Extends superiorly and laterally to articulate with the zygomatic bone

- **Palatine process**

    — Is a **horizontal extension** from the body
    — Fuses in midline with the opposite palatine process
    — Forms the bulk of the **bony palate**

- **Alveolar process**

    — Extends inferiorly from the body
    — Contains the sockets for eight teeth on each side

— *Zygomatic bone*

- Is a paired bone that forms the **prominence** of each **cheek**
- Articulates with the maxilla, sphenoid, frontal, and temporal bones
- Forms most of the **anterior boundary** of the **temporal fossa**

- Includes the **zygomaticofacial** and **zygomaticotemporal** foramina for the nerves of the same name
- Has a **frontal process,** which

  — Extends superiorly to articulate with the frontal bone
  — Forms most of the **lateral orbital margin**

- Has a **temporal process,** which

  — Extends posteriorly to articulate with the zygomatic process of the temporal bone
  — Forms the anterior part of the **zygomatic arch**

— *Nasal bones*

  - Are paired bones that fuse in the midline to form the central portion of the bony external nose
  - Articulate with the frontal bone, the frontal process of the maxilla, the perpendicular plate of the ethmoid bone (the bony nasal septum), and the nasal cartilage

— *Lacrimal bone*

  - Is a paired bone that contributes to the anterior part of the medial wall of the orbit
  - Articulates with the maxilla, ethmoid, and frontal bones
  - Includes the **lacrimal groove** and **posterior lacrimal crest,** which contain the **lacrimal sac**

— *Palatine bones*

  - Are **L-shaped** bones that consist of horizontal and perpendicular plates
  - **Horizontal plate**

    — Forms the posterior part of the bony palate
    — Fuses anteriorly with the palatine process of the maxilla

  - **Perpendicular plate**

    — Articulates with the maxilla, ethmoid, and sphenoid bones
    — Forms the posterior part of the **lateral wall of the nasal cavity**
    — Forms the medial wall of the **pterygopalatine fossa**
    — Contains the greater and lesser **palatine canals and foramina**
    — Contributes to the **sphenopalatine foramen**

— *Vomer (see Fig. 8.36)*

  - Is an unpaired midline bone that forms the posterior and inferior portion of the **nasal septum**
  - Separates the **choanae** posteriorly
  - Is grooved on each side by the **nasopalatine nerve**
  - Fuses anteriorly with the perpendicular process of the **ethmoid,** the palatine process of the **maxilla,** and the horizontal process of the **palatine** bones
  - Expands superiorly as the **alae of the vomer** to articulate with

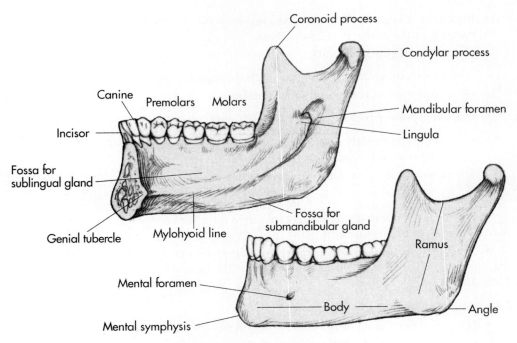

Fig. 8.9 Two views of the mandible.

the sphenoidal process of the **palatine bone** and the vaginal process from the medial pterygoid plate of the **sphenoid bone**

— *Inferior nasal concha (see Fig. 8.35)*

- Is a slender scroll of bone attached to the lateral wall of the nasal cavity
- Separates the middle meatus from the inferior meatus

— *Mandible (Fig. 8.9)*

- Is the bone of the lower jaw
- Articulates with the **temporal bones** of the skull at the **mandibular fossae**
- Consists of a **body** and paired **rami**
- **Body**

  — Is curved and horseshoe shaped
  — Joins the ramus at the **angle**
  — Is fused in the midline at the **symphysis menti**
  — Has a prominent **mental protuberance**, which expands laterally into paired **mental tubercles**
  — Has an **oblique line**, which extends upward and laterally from the mental tubercle to the anterior border of the ramus
  — Has a **mylohyoid line** on its inner surface for attachment of the mylohyoid muscle
  — Has a **mental spine** (and genial tubercles) on its inner sur-

face for attachment of the geniohyoid and genioglossus muscles

— Has **depressions** on its inner surface for the **submandibular** and **sublingual** salivary glands

— Has paired **digastric fossae** on the lower border near the midline for attachment of the **anterior belly of the digastric muscle**

— Includes the **mental foramen,** which transmits the **mental nerve and artery**

- Ramus

  — Has a roughened area on its outer surface marking the attachment of the **masseter muscle**

  — Has a roughened area on its inner surface marking the attachment of the **medial pterygoid muscle**

  — Includes the **mandibular foramen,** which opens into the **mandibular canal** and transmits the **inferior alveolar nerve and artery**

  — Includes the **lingula** above the mandibular foramen for attachment of the **sphenomandibular ligament**

  — Is grooved on its inner surface by the **mylohyoid nerve**

  — Expands superiorly as the **condylar process** and the **coronoid process** separated by the **mandibular notch**

- Coronoid process

  — Provides attachment for the **temporalis** muscle

- Condylar process

  — Includes the **head,** which articulates with the temporal bone at the mandibular fossa

  — Includes the **neck,** which receives the insertion of the lateral pterygoid muscle

● Major apertures of the skull (Table 8.3)

■ **Face and Scalp**

● Scalp

- Is the covering of the **cranial portion** of the head and is formed by a blending of the skin and fascia

- Consists of **five layers,** the first three of which are bound together and move as a unit

- Can be described so that the acronym **SCALP** is formed from the first letters of the descriptive terms (skin, connective tissue, aponeurosis, loose connective tissue, pericranium)

  - Skin

    — Is relatively thick compared with other areas of the body and usually has long, abundant hairs

  - Connective tissue

    — Is the fibrous superficial fascia between the skin and the galea aponeurotica

    — Contains the nerves and blood vessels

Table 8.3 *Major Apertures of the Skull*

APERTURE	BONE	COMMUNICATION BETWEEN	TRAVERSED BY
Cribriform plate	Ethmoid	Anterior cranial fossa and nasal cavity	Olfactory nerves (fila)
Optic canal	Sphenoid	Middle cranial fossa and orbit	Optic nerve, ophthalmic artery
Superior orbital fissure	Sphenoid	Middle cranial fossa and orbit	Oculomotor, trochlear, ophthalmic, and abducens nerves, ophthalmic vein
Foramen rotundum	Sphenoid	Middle cranial fossa and pterygopalatine fossa	Maxillary nerve
Foramen ovale	Sphenoid	Middle cranial fossa and infratemporal fossa	Mandibular nerve, accessory meningeal artery, lesser petrosal nerve (sometimes)
Foramen spinosum	Sphenoid	Middle cranial fossa and infratemporal fossa	Middle meningeal artery, meningeal branch of mandibular nerve
Innominate foramen (variable)	Sphenoid	Middle cranial fossa and infratemporal fossa	Lesser petrosal nerve
Foramen lacerum*	Between sphenoid and the apex of the petrous temporal bone	Middle cranial fossa and the base of the skull	Internal carotid artery, deep petrosal and greater petrosal nerves, origin of the nerve of the pterygoid canal
Lacrimal foramen	Sphenoid	Middle cranial fossa and orbit	Communicating branch between the middle meningeal and lacrimal arteries
Carotid canal	Temporal	Foramen lacerum and the base of the skull	Internal carotid artery, periarterial sympathetic plexus
Internal auditory meatus	Temporal	Posterior cranial fossa and the facial canal	Facial nerve, nervus intermedius, vestibulocochlear nerve, labyrinthine artery
Stylomastoid foramen	Temporal	Facial canal and the base of the skull	Facial nerve, stylomastoid artery
Jugular foramen	Between the occipital and temporal bones	Posterior cranial fossa and the base of the skull	Glossopharyngeal, vagus, and accessory nerves, internal jugular vein, inferior petrosal sinus, posterior meningeal arteries and nerves
Foramen magnum	Occipital	Posterior cranial fossa and the base of the skull	Brain stem, vertebral arteries and veins, spinal portion of the accessory nerve, spinal arteries
Hypoglossal canal	Occipital	Posterior cranial fossa and the base of the skull	Hypoglossal nerve, meningeal branches of cervical spinal nerves

*The foramen lacerum is an artifact found only in the dried skull. In life, this gap is filled by cartilage.

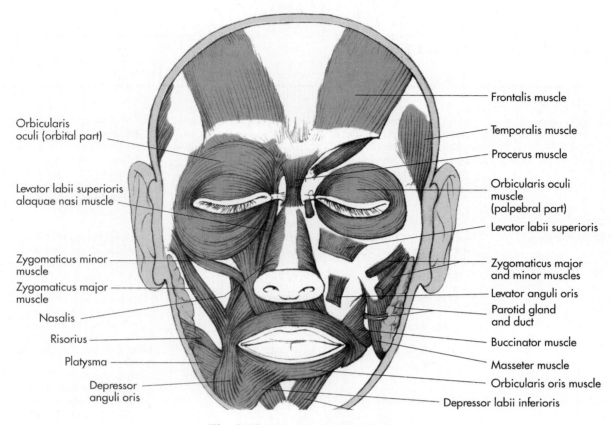

Fig. 8.10 Muscles of facial expression.

— Resists the contraction of blood vessels in lacerating wounds, resulting in profuse bleeding

- Aponeurosis

    — Is the membranous **galea aponeurotica,** which connects the frontalis and occipitalis components of the occipitofrontalis (epicranius) muscle

    — Functions as the deep fascia of the scalp

- Loose connective tissue

    — Allows movement of the first three layers on the skull

    — Is the plane of separation in scalping injuries

    — Readily allows the spread of infection deep to the galea aponeurotica with the potential for spread through the emissary veins to the intracranial dural venous sinuses

- Pericranium

    — Is the periosteum covering the outer surface of the skull

- **Muscles of the face and scalp (Fig. 8.10; Table 8.4)**

    - Are often called the muscles of facial expression

    - Are derived from the mesoderm of the **second branchial arch**

Table 8.4	*Muscles of the Face and Scalp**		
NAME	ORIGIN	INSERTION	ACTION
Muscles Around the Eye			
Orbicularis oculi	Orbital part: frontal and maxillary bones, medial palpebral ligament Palpebral part: medial palpebral ligament Lacrimal part: lacrimal crest behind to lacrimal sac	Orbital part: same as origin after making a complete loop around the orbit Palpebral part: lateral palpebral ligament and raphe Lacrimal part: lateral palpebral raphe	Orbital part: tightly closes the eye Palpebral part: closes eyelids as in blinking Lacrimal part: aspirates tears from the conjunctival sac by "pumping" the lacrimal sac
Corrugator supercilii	Medial part of superciliary arch of frontal bone	Skin of medial eyebrow	Pulls eyebrows medially wrinkling the skin over the bridge of the nose
Muscles Around the Nose			
Procerus	Nasal bone and cartilage	Skin between eyebrows	Depresses skin between eyebrows transversely wrinkling the skin over the bridge of the nose
Nasalis	Maxilla lateral to the incisive fossa	Alar part: ala of nose Transverse part: continuous across midline to the opposite side	Alar part: widens the nostril Transverse part: compresses the nostril
Depressor septi	Incisive fossa of maxilla	Nasal septum	Depresses nasal septum and constricts nostrils
Muscles Around the Mouth			
Orbicularis oris	Maxilla above the incisor and from other muscles of the mouth	Skin and mucous membrane of lips	Closes lips
Depressor anguli oris	Anterior part of oblique line of the mandible	Angle of the mouth	Pulls the corner of the mouth inferiorly and laterally
Depressor labii inferioris	Anterior part of oblique line of mandible	Orbicularis oris and skin of the lower lip	Pulls the lower lip inferiorly
Levator anguli oris	Canine fossa of maxilla	Angle of the mouth	Elevates the corner of the mouth
Levator labii superioris	Maxilla above the infraorbital foramen	Orbicularis oris and skin of the upper lip	Pulls the upper lip superiorly
Levator labii superioris alequae nasi	Frontal process of maxilla	Orbicularis oris and skin of the upper lip; ala of the nose	Pulls the upper lip superiorly and dilates the nostril
Mentalis	Incisive fossa of the mandible	Skin of the chin	Elevates and protrudes the lower lip
Risorius	Fascia over the parotid gland	Angle of the mouth	Pulls the angle of the mouth laterally
Zygomaticus major	Zygomatic bone	Angle of the mouth	Pulls the angle of the mouth superiorly and laterally
Zygomaticus minor	Zygomatic bone and orbicularis oculi below orbit	Orbicularis oris and skin of the upper lip	Pulls the upper lip superiorly

Table 8.4 *Muscles of the Face and Scalp—cont'd*

Name	Origin	Insertion	Action
Buccinator	Mandible, maxilla, and pterygomandibular raphe	Upper and lower lips at the angle of the mouth	Compression of the cheek
Auricularis anterior, superior, and posterior	Temporal fascia, galea aponeurotica, and mastoid bone	Anterior, superior, and posterior parts of the auricle	Movement of the auricle
Occipitofrontalis	Lateral part of the superior nuchal line, frontal bone above the orbit	Galea aponeurotica	Movement of the scalp, elevation of the eyebrows with wrinkling of the scalp
Platysma	Superficial fascia and skin over the pectoralis major	Inferior border of the mandible, skin and muscles of the lower lip, and angle of the mouth	Elevates the skin of the neck and upper thorax; pulls the lower lip and angle of the mouth inferiorly; opens mouth

Innervation: all of the muscles of the face and scalp are supplied by the **facial nerve**.

- Are innervated by the **facial nerve,** the nerve of the second branchial arch
- Generally lie between the skin and the underlying tissue and **attach to or affect the skin of the face and scalp**
- Some have a bony attachment and others do not

- Nerves of the face and scalp

    - The **motor nerve** to the muscles of the face is the **facial nerve (CN VII).**

    - Cutaneous innervation to the skin of the face and scalp is supplied by the ophthalmic, maxillary, and mandibular divisions of the **trigeminal nerve (CN V)** and by branches of the **cervical spinal nerves.**

    — *Facial nerve*

        - Exits the skull through the **stylomastoid foramen** deep to the parotid gland
        - Divides into **five groups** of terminal branches within the parotid gland

            — **Temporal** branches, which supply the orbicularis oculi, the corrugator supercilii, the frontalis, and the auricularis superior and anterior muscles
            — **Zygomatic** branches, which supply the orbicularis oculi
            — **Buccal** branches, which supply the muscles above the upper lip and angle of the mouth, including the muscles of the nose
            — **Marginal mandibular** branch, which supplies the muscles below the lower lip and angle of the mouth
            — **Cervical** branch, which supplies the platysma muscle

- Also gives rise to the

  — **Posterior auricular nerve,** which supplies the occipitalis and auricularis posterior muscles and is sensory to the posterior auricle
  — Nerve to the **stylohyoid** and **posterior digastric** muscles

Bell's palsy

- Is an idiopathic **unilateral paralysis** of the muscles of the face resulting from a lesion of the facial nerve
- Is **sudden in onset** (usually within 24 hours) and **transient** with recovery beginning in a few months
- Is characterized by

  — A drooping corner of the mouth
  — An inability to smile, whistle, or blow
  — A drooping upper eyelid and an everted lower eyelid
  — An inability to blink or close the eye

— *Trigeminal nerve*

- Provides sensory innervation to the face by way of cutaneous branches of the ophthalmic, maxillary, and mandibular nerves

Cutaneous branches of the ophthalmic nerve (Fig. 8.11)

- **Supraorbital nerve**

  — Arises from the **frontal nerve** in the orbit
  — Leaves the orbit through the **supraorbital notch** or foramen
  — Supplies the upper **eyelid** and the **forehead and scalp** as far as the vertex

- **Supratrochlear nerve**

  — Arises from the **frontal nerve** in the orbit
  — Leaves the orbit medial to the supraorbital nerve
  — Supplies the **upper eyelid** and the **medial forehead**

- **Infratrochlear nerve**

  — Arises from the **nasociliary nerve** in the orbit
  — Leaves the orbit **below** the **trochlea**
  — Supplies the medial part of the **upper eyelid**

- **Lacrimal nerve**

  — Arises from the **ophthalmic nerve** in the wall of the cavernous sinus
  — Gives cutaneous branches, which leave the orbit at the **lateral** corner of the **eye**
  — Supplies the lateral part of the upper eyelid

- **External nasal nerve**

  — Is a continuation of the **anterior ethmoidal nerve,** which arises from the **nasociliary nerve** in the orbit
  — Runs downward on the deep surface of the nasal bone and

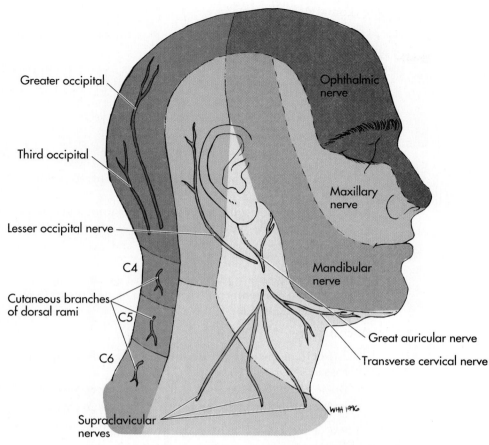

Greater occipital

Third occipital

Lesser occipital nerve

C4

Cutaneous branches of dorsal rami

C5

C6

Supraclavicular nerves

Ophthalmic nerve

Maxillary nerve

Mandibular nerve

Great auricular nerve

Transverse cervical nerve

Fig. 8.11 The cutaneous innervation of the head and neck.

leaves the nasal cavity by passing between the nasal bone and the lateral nasal cartilage

— Supplies the skin over the **dorsum of the nose**

Cutaneous branches of the maxillary nerve (see Fig. 8.11)

- **Infraorbital nerve**

    — Is a direct continuation of the **maxillary nerve**

    — Enters the orbit through the **inferior orbital fissure**

    — Traverses the floor of the orbit in the **infraorbital groove** and **canal**

    — Emerges onto the face through the **infraorbital foramen**

    — Supplies the **lower eyelid,** the side of the **nose,** the skin of the **upper lip,** and the mucosa of the **mouth**

- **Zygomaticofacial nerve**

    — Arises from the **zygomatic branch** of the **maxillary nerve** on the lateral wall of the orbit

    — Traverses the **zygomatic bone** and emerges onto the face at the lower lateral margin of the orbit

    — Supplies the skin of the face **lateral** to the orbit

- **Zygomaticotemporal nerve**

  — Arises from the **zygomatic branch** of the **maxillary nerve** on the lateral wall of the orbit

  — Traverses the **zygomatic bone** and exits its posterior surface into the temporal fossa

  — Penetrates the temporal fascia to supply the skin of the **temporal region** above and lateral to the eye

Cutaneous branches of the mandibular nerve (see Fig. 8.11)

- **Auriculotemporal nerve**

  — Arises from the **mandibular nerve** in the **infratemporal fossa**

  — Passes **behind** the **temporomandibular joint** and emerges from **deep** to the **parotid gland**

  — Crosses the root of the zygomatic arch and ascends **in front of the ear**

  — Supplies the parotid gland, the external ear and tympanic membrane, the temporomandibular joint, and the scalp of the temporal region

- **Buccal nerve**

  — Arises from the **mandibular nerve** in the **infratemporal fossa**

  — Branches on the outer surface of the buccinator muscle

  — Supplies the skin of the mucous membrane and cheek

- **Mental nerve**

  — Is the terminal branch of the **inferior alveolar branch** of the **mandibular nerve**

  — Emerges onto the face from the **mental foramen**

  — Supplies the skin of the **lower lip and chin**

— *Cutaneous branches of the cervical spinal nerves (see Figs. 8.5 and 8.11)*

- **Great auricular nerve**

  — Is derived from the ventral rami of **C2 and C3** via the **cervical plexus**

  — Ascends vertically on the sternocleidomastoid toward the auricle

  — Supplies the skin over the auricle, parotid gland, and angle of the jaw

- **Lesser occipital nerve**

  — Is derived from the **ventral ramus** of **C2** (the **greater occipital** nerve is the **dorsal ramus** of **C2**)

  — Ascends along the posterior border of the sternocleidomastoid muscle

  — Supplies the skin of the neck and scalp behind the ear

- **Greater occipital nerve**

  — Is the cutaneous branch of the **dorsal ramus** of **C2**

— Emerges onto the scalp after piercing the trapezius near its attachment to the occipital bone

— Supplies the posterior scalp anteriorly to the vertex

- **Blood vessels of the face and scalp (see Fig. 8.3)** The blood supply to the face and scalp is derived largely from branches of the **external carotid artery** but also from the **internal carotid artery** through branches of the ophthalmic artery.

   — *Superficial temporal artery*

   • Is the smaller of the two terminal branches of the **external carotid artery**

   • Arises deep to the **neck of the mandible** in the substance of the **parotid gland**

   • Ascends behind the **temporomandibular joint** and over the root of the **zygomatic arch** anterior to the auricle

   • Supplies the **face** in front of the ear and the **scalp** of the temporal region

   • Is accompanied by the **auriculotemporal nerve** and the **superficial temporal vein**

   • Gives rise to the **transverse facial artery**, which passes across the face between the zygomatic arch and the parotid duct

   — *Maxillary artery*

   • Arises as a **terminal branch** of the **external carotid artery** deep to the neck of the mandible and within the substance of the parotid gland

   • Passes medially through the infratemporal fossa and gives rise to branches that become cutaneous as the **mental, buccal,** and **infraorbital** arteries

      • **Mental artery**

         — Is a continuation of the **inferior alveolar artery** (from the maxillary artery)

         — Emerges onto the face through the **mental foramen**

         — Is distributed with the mental nerve to the chin and lower lip

      • **Buccal artery**

         — Arises from the **maxillary artery** in the infratemporal fossa

         — Is distributed with the **buccal nerve** (from the mandibular nerve)

         — Supplies the skin of the mucous membrane and cheek

      • **Infraorbital artery**

         — Arises from the **maxillary artery** in the pterygopalatine fossa

         — Courses through the infraorbital groove and canal to reach the face through the **infraorbital foramen**

         — Is distributed with the **infraorbital nerve** (from the maxillary nerve)

         — Supplies the **lower eyelid,** the side of the **nose,** the skin of the **upper lip,** and the mucosa of the **mouth**

— *Facial artery*

- Arises from the **external carotid artery** in the neck
- Is related to the **submandibular salivary gland** deep to the mandible
- Winds around the lower border of the mandible to **enter the face** at the anterior margin of the masseter muscle
- Passes upward and medially to end at the **medial angle** of the eye
- In the face gives rise to the

  — **Inferior labial artery,** which arises below the angle of the mouth and passes medially across the lower lip

  — **Superior labial artery,** which arises above the angle of the mouth and passes medially across the upper lip

  — **Lateral nasal artery,** which arises at the side of the nose to supply the ala and dorsum of the nose

  — **Angular artery,** which is its terminal branch

- Note that the **angular artery** anastomoses with the **dorsal nasal artery** (from the ophthalmic artery), forming an **anastomosis** between the **external and internal carotid arteries.**

— *Occipital artery*

- Arises posteriorly from the **external carotid artery** at the level of the facial artery
- Passes posteriorly and superiorly and grooves the **temporal bone** medial to the mastoid process
- Emerges onto the **scalp** at the apex of the posterior triangle
- Is distributed with the greater occipital nerve to the **posterior scalp**

— *Posterior auricular artery*

- Arises from the **external carotid artery** in the neck
- Passes posteriorly and superiorly deep to the **parotid gland** and lateral to the **styloid process**
- Ends behind the ear on the superficial surface of the mastoid process by dividing into

  — **Auricular branches,** which supply the back of the ear

  — **Occipital branches,** which supply the scalp above and behind the ear

— *Ophthalmic artery*

- Arises from the **internal carotid artery** in the cranial cavity
- Enters the orbit through the **optic canal**
- Gives rise to branches that become cutaneous **around the eye,** including the

  — **Supraorbital artery,** which is distributed with the supraorbital nerve to the upper **eyelid** and the **forehead and scalp**

  — **Supratrochlear artery,** which is distributed with the supratrochlear nerve to the upper **eyelid** and **medial forehead**

— **Lacrimal artery,** which gives **lateral palpebral arteries** to the upper eyelid

— **Dorsal nasal artery,** which leaves the orbit at the medial angle of the eye and is distributed to the root of the nose

• Remember that the internal and external carotid arteries anastomose by way of the **anastomosis** between the dorsal nasal branch of the **ophthalmic artery** and the angular branch of the **facial artery.**

Parotid, Temporal, and Infratemporal Regions

● Parotid gland

- Is the **largest** of the paired **salivary glands**
- Is an extensive gland that

— Lies below the **zygomatic arch** and below and inferior to the **external auditory meatus**

— Overlies the **masseter muscle** and **ramus of the mandible** anteriorly and the **sternocleidomastoid muscle** posteriorly

— Occupies the depression between the **ramus of the mandible** anteriorly and the **sternocleidomastoid muscle** and **mastoid process** posteriorly

— Inferiorly extends **deep** to the **ramus of the mandible**

— Is related on its deep surface to the posterior belly of the digastric muscle and the **styloid process**

- Is surrounded by the **parotid fascia,** which is a superior extension of the **superficial layer of deep cervical fascia**
- Is separated from the **submandibular salivary gland** by the **stylomandibular ligament**
- Is crossed superficially by the **platysma muscle** and the **great auricular nerve**
- Structures that lie partially **within the parotid gland** include the

— Facial nerve

— Retromandibular vein and its origin from the superficial temporal and maxillary veins

— External carotid artery and its posterior auricular, superficial temporal, and maxillary branches

— Parotid lymph nodes

- **Parotid duct**

— Is also called Stensen's duct

— Passes forward over the superficial surface of the **masseter muscle** about 1 cm below the **zygomatic arch**

— Turns medially at the anterior border of the masseter muscle to pierce the **buccal fat pad** and the **buccinator muscle**

— Opens into the oral cavity opposite the **upper second molar**

— *Innervation of the parotid gland*
Parasympathetic innervation

• Parasympathetic innervation is **secretomotor.**

- **Preganglionic parasympathetic** neuron cell bodies are located in the **inferior salivatory nucleus** of the brain stem.
- Preganglionic parasympathetic fibers traverse the glossopharyngeal nerve, its tympanic branch, the tympanic plexus, and the lesser petrosal nerve to synapse in the otic ganglion.
- **Postganglionic parasympathetic** neuron cell bodies are located in the **otic ganglion.**
- Postganglionic parasympathetic fibers join the mandibular nerve in the infratemporal fossa and are distributed to the parotid gland via the **auriculotemporal nerve.**

Sympathetic innervation

- Sympathetic innervation is **vasomotor.**
- **Preganglionic sympathetic** neuron cell bodies are located in the **intermediolateral cell column** of the upper thoracic spinal cord segments.
- **Postganglionic sympathetic** neuron cell bodies are located in the superior **cervical ganglion.**
- Postganglionic sympathetic fibers join the **external carotid nerve** and are distributed to the parotid gland via the periarterial **external carotid plexus.**

● Temporal and infratemporal fossae

— *Temporal fossa*

- Is bounded

    — Superiorly and posteriorly by the **inferior temporal line**
    — Anteriorly by the **frontal process of the zygomatic bone**
    — Inferiorly by the **zygomatic arch**

- Has a **floor** formed by parts of the

    — Greater wing of the sphenoid
    — Squamous temporal bone
    — Frontal bone
    — Parietal bone

- Contains

    — Most of the **temporalis muscle**
    — **Deep temporal nerves and artery** deep to the temporalis muscle
    — **Zygomaticotemporal nerve** on the anterior wall after it emerges from the zygomaticotemporal foramen

— *Infratemporal fossa*

- Is bounded

    — Anteriorly by the infratemporal surface of the maxilla
    — Superiorly by the infratemporal surface of the greater wing of the sphenoid
    — Medially by the lateral pterygoid plate of the sphenoid bone
    — Laterally by the coronoid process and ramus of mandible
    — Inferiorly is continuous into the neck

— Posteriorly by the temporomandibular joint and styloid process

- Is delineated from the temporal fossa superiorly by the **infratemporal crest** on the sphenoid and temporal bones
- Contains the

  — Mandibular nerve
  — Maxillary artery
  — Medial and lateral pterygoid muscles
  — Lower part of the temporalis muscle
  — Chorda tympani nerve
  — Otic ganglion

- Communicates with the

  — **Orbit** anteriorly through the **inferior orbital fissure**
  — **Pterygopalatine fossa** medially through the **pterygomaxillary fissure**

● Muscles of mastication (Fig. 8.12; Table 8.5)

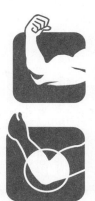

● Temporomandibular joint

- Is a **synovial joint** between the **head of the mandible** and the **mandibular fossa and articular tubercle** of the temporal bone
- Is surrounded by a loose **fibrous capsule,** which attaches to the margins of the articular surfaces (but encloses part of the neck of the mandible posteriorly)
- Has an **articular disc,** which

  — Is firmly **attached** at its margins to the **capsule**
  — Divides the joint into an **upper compartment** and a **lower compartment**
  — Anteriorly receives the insertion of fibers of the lateral pterygoid muscle
  — Moves with the head of the mandible in protraction and retraction

- Is reinforced **laterally by the lateral temporomandibular ligament,** which extends from the tubercle of the root of the zygoma (lateral to the articular tubercle) to the neck of the mandible
- Functions as both a **hinge joint** and a **gliding joint**
- Is innervated by the **auriculotemporal** and **masseteric** nerves (from the mandibular division of the trigeminal nerve)

— *Sphenomandibular ligament*

  - Is a thin fibrous band that extends from the **spine** of the sphenoid bone to the **lingula** of the mandible
  - Lies on the medial side of the temporomandibular joint and is not attached to the capsule
  - Has no established function relative to the temporomandibular joint
  - Is a **remnant** of the **cartilage** of the **second branchial arch** (Meckels's cartilage)

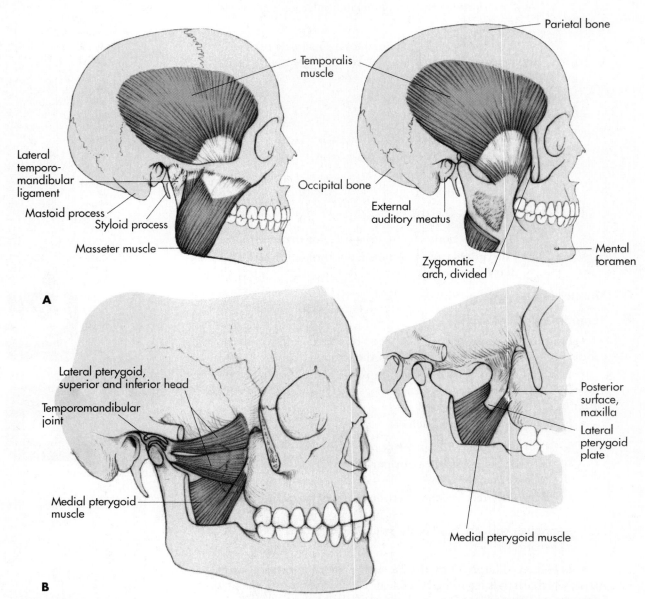

Fig. 8.12 Muscles of mastication. **A,** Superficial. On the right the zygomatic arch and masseter have been partially removed. **B,** Deep. On the left the coronoid process and part of the ramus have been removed.

— *Stylomandibular ligament*

- Extends from the **styloid process** of the temporal bone to the posterior border of the **ramus** of the mandible above the angle
- Separates the parotid gland from the submandibular gland
- Has no established function relative to the temporomandibular joint

- **Maxillary artery (Fig. 8.13)**

  - The maxillary artery arises as a **terminal branch** of the **external carotid artery** deep to the neck of the mandible and within the substance of the parotid gland.

Table 8.5   Muscles of Mastication

Name	Origin	Insertion	Action	Innervation*
Temporalis	Floor of the temporal fossa and the overlying temporal fascia	Coronoid process and anterior ramus of the mandible	Elevates and retracts the mandible	Anterior and posterior deep temporal nerves (from the mandibular nerve)
Masseter	Inferior and medial surface of the zygomatic arch	Lateral surface of the ramus and angle of the mandible	Elevates the mandible	Masseteric nerve (from the mandibular nerve)
Lateral pterygoid	Superior head: infra-temporal surface of the greater wing of the sphenoid. Inferior head: lateral surface of the lateral pterygoid plate	Pterygoid fovea on the neck of the mandible and the capsule and articular disc of the temporomandibular joint	Protracts and depresses the mandible; deviates the mandible to the opposite side	Nerve to the lateral pterygoid (from the mandibular nerve)
Medial pterygoid	Superficial head: tuber of the maxilla. Deep head: medial surface of the lateral pterygoid plate and the pyramidal process of the palatine bone	Medial surface of the ramus and angle of mandible	Protracts and elevates the mandible; deviates the mandible to the opposite side	Nerve to the medial pterygoid (from the mandibular nerve)

*All of the muscles of mastication are supplied by the **mandibular division** of the trigeminal nerve.

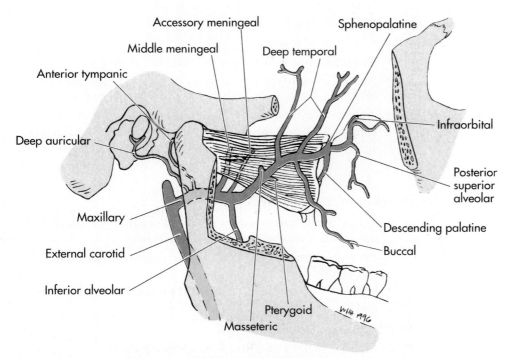

Fig. 8.13 The branches of the maxillary artery.

- It traverses the **infratemporal fossa,** where it may pass either superficial or **deep** to the **lateral pterygoid muscle.**
- It enters the **pterygopalatine fossa** through the **pterygomaxillary fissure.**
- The maxillary artery may be divided into three parts

    — The **first part** (mandibular part) extends from its origin to the lower margin of the lateral pterygoid muscle.

    — The **second part** (pterygoid part) lies either superficial or deep to the inferior head of the lateral pterygoid muscle.

    — The **third part** (pterygopalatine part) lies within the pterygopalatine fossa.

- The maxillary artery gives rise to branches that supply the muscles of mastication, the upper and lower jaws, the face, the nasal cavity, the nasopharynx, the palate, and the dura.

— *Deep auricular artery*

- Arises from the **first part** of the maxillary artery within the parotid gland
- Ascends posterior to the temporomandibular joint
- Supplies the temporomandibular joint, the external auditory meatus, and the outside of the tympanic membrane

— *Anterior tympanic artery*

- Arises from the **first part** of the maxillary artery or from the deep auricular artery within the parotid gland
- Ascends posterior to the temporomandibular joint and traverses the **petrotympanic fissure** to reach the tympanic cavity
- Supplies the tympanic cavity and the inner surface of the tympanic membrane

— *Middle meningeal artery*

- Arises from the **first part** of the maxillary artery
- Ascends **deep** to the **lateral pterygoid muscle** and passes between the two roots of the **auriculotemporal nerve**
- Traverses the **foramen spinosum** to enter the cranial cavity
- Supplies the skull and the dura mater as it passes between these structures
- Is often damaged in fractures of the temporal bone resulting in epidural hemorrhage

— *Accessory meningeal artery*

- Arises from the **first part** of the maxillary artery or as a common trunk with the middle meningeal artery
- Ascends anterior to the middle meningeal artery to pass through the **foramen ovale**
- Supplies the semilunar (trigeminal) ganglion and the dura mater

— *Inferior alveolar artery*

- Arises from the **first part** of the maxillary artery
- Passes between the **sphenomandibular ligament** and the **ramus** of the mandible with the **inferior alveolar nerve**

- Enters the **mandibular foramen** to traverse the **mandibular canal**
- Exits the mandibular canal through the **mental foramen** to terminate as the **mental artery**
- Gives rise to the **mylohyoid artery**, which accompanies the mylohyoid nerve
- Supplies the lower teeth and gums, the chin and lower lip, and the mucous membrane of the cheek

— *Branches to the muscles of mastication*

- Arise from the **second** (pterygoid) part of the maxillary artery
- Are **named** according to the **muscle supplied** and include the

   — **Masseteric artery,** which passes through the **mandibular notch** with the masseteric nerve to supply the **masseter muscle**

   — Anterior and posterior **deep temporal arteries,** which ascend in the **temporal fossa** with the deep temporal nerves to supply the **temporalis muscles**

   — **Pterygoid arteries,** which supply the **medial and lateral pterygoid muscles**

   — **Buccal artery,** which accompanies the buccal nerve to supply the skin and mucosa of the cheek

— *Posterior superior alveolar artery*

- Arises from the **third** (pterygopalatine) part of the maxillary artery as it passes through the pterygomaxillary fissure
- Descends on the posterior surface of the maxilla with the posterior superior alveolar nerve (from the maxillary nerve)
- Enters the maxilla to supply the upper molars and premolars

— *Infraorbital artery*

- Arises from the **third** (pterygopalatine) part of the maxillary artery
- Enters the orbit through the inferior orbital fissure
- Courses through the infraorbital groove and canal to reach the face through the **infraorbital foramen**
- Is distributed with the **infraorbital nerve** (from the maxillary nerve)
- Supplies the **lower eyelid,** the side of the **nose,** the skin of the **upper lip,** and the mucosa of the **mouth**
- While in the infraorbital canal gives rise to the **anterior** and **middle superior alveolar arteries,** which supply the molar and premolar teeth

— *Pharyngeal artery*

- Arises from the **third** (pterygopalatine) part of the maxillary artery
- Passes posteriorly with the **pharyngeal nerve** (from the maxillary nerve) through the **palatovaginal canal**
- Supplies the roof of the nasal cavity and nasopharynx and the sphenoid sinus

— *Artery of the pterygoid canal*

- Arises from the **third** (pterygopalatine) part of the maxillary artery
- Passes posteriorly through the **pterygoid canal** with the nerve of the same name
- Supplies the pharynx and the auditory tube

— *Sphenopalatine artery*

- Arises as a terminal branch from the **third** (pterygopalatine) part of the maxillary artery
- Passes medially to enter the **nasal cavity** through the **sphenopalatine foramen**
- Is the major supply to the nasal cavity and paranasal sinuses

— *Descending palatine artery*

- Arises as a terminal branch from the **third** (pterygopalatine) part of the maxillary artery
- Descends through the **pterygopalatine fossa** and the **palatine canal**
- In the palatine canal divides into **greater and lesser palatine arteries,** which exit through the greater and lesser palatine canals
- Supplies the **soft and hard palates**

● **Pterygoid venous plexus**

- Lies around the **maxillary artery** and the **lateral pterygoid muscle** within the infratemporal fossa
- Receives tributaries corresponding to the branches of the maxillary artery
- Coalesces to form the **maxillary vein,** which joins the **superficial temporal vein** deep to the neck of the mandible to form the **retromandibular vein**
- Communicates with the

  — **Facial vein** via the **deep facial vein**
  — **Cavernous dural venous sinus** through **emissary veins**

- Note that the latter two connections allow for the potential spread of infection from the face to the cranial cavity.

● **Mandibular nerve (Fig. 8.14)**

- Is the **third division** of the **trigeminal nerve**
- Arises from the **semilunar** (trigeminal) **ganglion** in the floor of the middle cranial fossa
- Exits the skull through the **foramen ovale**
- In the infratemporal fossa is joined by the **motor root**
- Is the only division of the trigeminal to innervate skeletal muscle
- Gives rise to branches that supply the muscles of mastication, the lower jaw, the temporomandibular joint, the face, the cheek and tongue, and the dura
- Supplies motor innervation (SVE) to eight paired muscles, including the

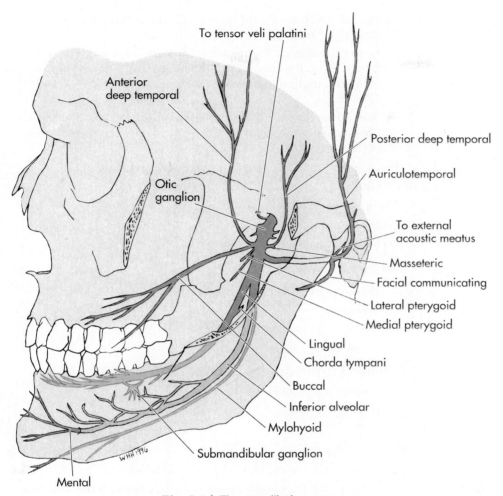

Fig. 8.14 The mandibular nerve.

— Temporalis muscle
— Masseter muscle
— Lateral pterygoid muscle
— Medial pterygoid muscle
— Mylohyoid muscle
— Anterior belly of the digastric muscle
— Tensor tympani muscle
— Tensor veli palatini muscle

• Contains

— **General visceral afferent** fibers from cell bodies in the **semilunar ganglion**

— **Special visceral efferent** fibers from cell bodies in the **trigeminal nucleus** (motor nucleus of V)

• Distributes

— **General visceral efferent** fibers (postganglionic parasympathetic) from the **otic ganglion** to the **parotid gland** (remember that these are accompanied by **GVA** fibers from the glosso-pharyngeal nerve)

— **General visceral efferent** fibers (preganglionic parasympathetic) from the **facial nerve** via the **chorda tympani** to the **submandibular ganglion** (remember that these are accompanied by GVA fibers)

— **Special visceral afferent** (taste) fibers from the **facial nerve** via the **chorda tympani** and lingual nerve to the anterior two thirds of the tongue

- Is described as having a **trunk,** which divides into **anterior** and **posterior divisions**

- **Trunk** gives rise to the

    — Meningeal branch
    — Nerve to the medial pterygoid

- **Anterior division** gives rise to the

    — Deep temporal nerves
    — Masseteric nerve
    — Nerve to the lateral pterygoid muscle
    — Buccal nerve

- **Posterior division** gives rise to the

    — Auriculotemporal nerve
    — Lingual nerve
    — Inferior alveolar nerve

— *Meningeal branch*

  - Arises from the **trunk** of the mandibular nerve
  - Passes with the middle meningeal artery through the **foramen spinosum**
  - Supplies the **dura** of the **middle cranial fossa**

— *Nerve to the medial pterygoid muscle*

  - Arises from the **trunk** of the mandibular nerve
  - Is closely associated with the **otic ganglion**
  - Supplies the medial pterygoid muscle
  - Gives rise to the

    — Nerve to the tensor tympani muscle
    — Nerve to the tensor veli palatini muscle

  - Note that the nerve to the tensor tympani muscle and the nerve to the tensor veli palatini muscle are often described as arising from the otic ganglion.

— *Deep temporal nerves*

  - Arise from the **anterior division** of the mandibular nerve
  - Are frequently described as **anterior** and **posterior** deep temporal nerves, which ascend in the temporal fossa along with the arteries of the same name
  - Supply the **temporalis muscle**

— *Masseteric nerve*

- Arises from the **anterior division** of the mandibular nerve
- Passes above the lateral pterygoid muscle and through the **mandibular notch**
- Supplies the masseter muscle

— *Nerve to the lateral pterygoid muscle*

- Arises from the **anterior division** of the mandibular nerve
- Supplies the lateral pterygoid muscle entering its deep surface

— *Buccal nerve*

- Arises from the **anterior division** of the mandibular nerve
- Passes between the two heads of the lateral pterygoid muscle
- Descends on the anterior border of the **temporalis muscle** and branches on the surface of the **buccinator muscle** (remember that the buccinator muscle receives its motor innervation from the **buccal branch of the facial nerve**)
- Supplies the skin and mucous membrane of the cheek and gums

— *Auriculotemporal nerve*

- Arises from the **posterior division** of the mandibular nerve by two roots, which embrace the **middle meningeal artery**
- Passes deep to the lateral pterygoid muscle and **posterior** to the **temporomandibular joint**
- Emerges from **deep** to the **parotid gland** and crosses the root of the zygomatic arch to ascend **in front of the ear**
- Supplies the parotid gland, the external ear and tympanic membrane, the temporomandibular joint, and the scalp of the temporal region
- Distributes **postganglionic parasympathetic fibers** to the **parotid gland** (from cell bodies in the **otic ganglion**)

— *Lingual nerve*

- Arises from the **posterior division** of the mandibular nerve
- Descends deep to the **lateral pterygoid muscle**
- Passes onto the lateral surface of the **medial pterygoid muscle** anterior to the **inferior alveolar nerve** and deep to the ramus of the mandible
- Deep to the lateral pterygoid muscle is joined on its posterior side by the **chorda tympani** nerve, which carries

  — **Parasympathetic preganglionic fibers** from the **facial nerve** to synapse in the **submandibular ganglion**
  — **Taste fibers (SVA)** from the **facial nerve** to be distributed to the **anterior two thirds of the tongue**

- Supplies **general somatic afferent** innervation to the **anterior two thirds of the tongue**
- Distributes **postganglionic parasympathetic fibers** from the **submandibular ganglion** to the **sublingual salivary gland**

— *Inferior alveolar nerve*

- Arises from the **posterior division** of the mandibular nerve

- Descends deep to the **lateral pterygoid muscle**
- Passes onto the lateral surface of the **medial pterygoid muscle** posterior to the **lingual nerve** and deep to the ramus of the mandible
  - Enters the mandibular canal through the mandibular foramen
  - Gives rise to the

    — Mylohoid nerve

    — **Inferior dental and gingival branches,** which arise in the mandibular canal to supply the lower teeth and gums

    — **Incisive branch,** which supplies the canine and incisor teeth

    — **Mental nerve,** which supplies the chin and the skin and mucosa of the lower lip

  - **Mylohyoid nerve**

    — Arises from the inferior alveolar nerve just before it enters the mandibular foramen

    — Lies at first in the **mylohyoid groove** on the medial surface of the ramus of the mandible and then on the lower border of the mylohyoid muscle

    — Innervates the **mylohyoid muscle** and the **anterior belly of the digastric muscle**

- **Otic ganglion**
  - Is one of the four parasympathetic ganglia of the head
  - Receives **preganglionic parasympathetic fibers** from the **glossopharyngeal nerve (CN IX)**, which traverse in sequence the tympanic nerve, the tympanic plexus, and the lesser petrosal nerve
  - Contains the cell bodies of postganglionic parasympathetic neurons with the postganglionic fibers distributed to the **parotid gland** via the **auriculotemporal nerve**
  - Lies in the roof of the infratemporal fossa **between** the **mandibular nerve** and the **tensor veli palatini** muscle
  - Is closely related to the **nerve to the medial pterygoid muscle** and is often described as giving rise to the nerves to the tensor tympani and the tensor veli palatini muscles

Cranial Cavity, Meninges, and Dural Venous Sinuses

- **Cranial cavity (Fig. 8.15)**
- **Meninges (Fig. 8.16)**
  - Consists of three sheaths, which surround and enclose the **brain** within the **cranial cavity**

  — *Pia mater*

    - Is a fine vascular layer that is **closely applied** to the surface of the **brain**
    - Dips into the **fissures** and **sulci** of the cerebral and cerebellar hemispheres
    - Forms a **sheath** around the **blood vessels** as they penetrate the surface of the brain

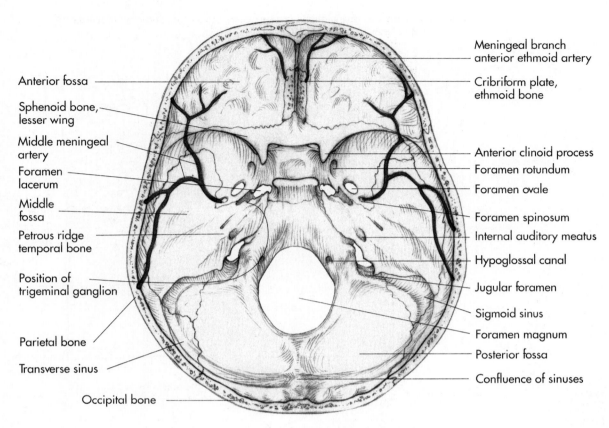

Anterior fossa

Sphenoid bone, lesser wing

Middle meningeal artery

Foramen lacerum

Middle fossa

Petrous ridge temporal bone

Position of trigeminal ganglion

Parietal bone

Transverse sinus

Occipital bone

Meningeal branch anterior ethmoid artery

Cribriform plate, ethmoid bone

Anterior clinoid process

Foramen rotundum

Foramen ovale

Foramen spinosum

Internal auditory meatus

Hypoglossal canal

Jugular foramen

Sigmoid sinus

Foramen magnum

Posterior fossa

Confluence of sinuses

Fig. 8.15 Floor of the cranial cavity.

— *Arachnoid mater*

- Is the delicate **intermediate** meningeal layer
- Is **attached** to the inner surface of the **dura mater**
- Is **attached** to the **pia mater** by fine strands that traverse the subarachnoid space
- Is separated from the pia mater by the **subarachnoid space,** which contains **cerebrospinal fluid**
- Exhibits numerous **arachnoid villi,** which

    — Are **microscopic** fingerlike **projections** through the meningeal layer of the dura into the **superior sagittal sinus** and **lateral lacunae**

    — Allow the **resorption** (leakage) of **cerebrospinal fluid** into the venous blood

    — May form **macroscopic** aggregations, **arachnoid granulations,** which often induce **pitting** of the adjacent bone (**fovea granulares**)

— *Dura mater*

- Is a tough connective tissue layer that forms a sac around the **brain** and is continuous at the foramen magnum with the dura matter surrounding the spinal cord

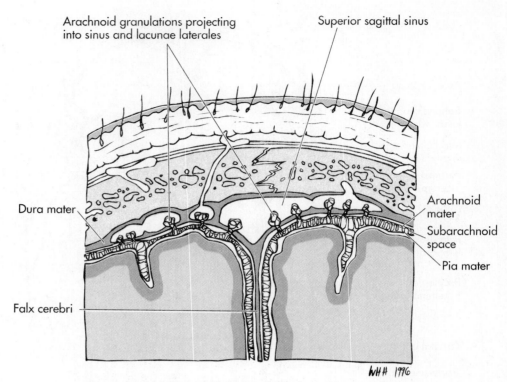

Fig. 8.16 Coronal section through the superior sagittal sinus.

- Has **no** associated **epidural space** because the dura fuses with the periosteum lining the inside of the skull
- Is often considered to consist of **two layers**, one being the true dura, or **meningeal layer**, and the other being the **periosteal layer** (note that so-called **epidural hemorrhages** occur into the potential space *between* the periosteal and meningeal **layers**
- Encloses the **dural venous sinuses**
- Gives rise to **projections** of the **meningeal layer** that partition the cranial cavity, including the falx cerebri and the falx and tentorium cerebelli

— *Other features related to the meninges*

Epidural space

- In the cranial cavity is only a **potential space** because the dura **fuses** with the **periosteum** lining the inside of the skull
- May collect leaking blood, which separates the **periosteal** and **meningeal** layers of the dura mater (an **epidural hemorrhage**)

Subdural space

- The subdural space is often referred to by clinicians as a real or potential space, but in reality it **does not exist.**
- Leaking blood may dissect the dura mater from the underlying arachnoid mater, allowing the blood to collect in the space created (a subdural hemorrhage).

Subarachnoid space

- Is the space between the **arachnoid mater** and the **pia mater**
- Contains **cerebrospinal fluid**
- Extends along the **optic nerve** to the back of the eyeball
- **Varies in width** because the pia follows the surface of the brain and the arachnoid is fused to the dura with the sites of greatest separation known as **cisterns**
  - **Cerebellomedullary cistern** (cisterna magna)
    — Lies posterior to the medulla and below the cerebellum
    — Is continuous inferiorly with the subarachnoid space around the spinal cord
  - **Pontine cistern**
    — Lies anterior to the pontomedullary junction
    — Contains the basilar artery at its midline
  - **Interpeduncular cistern**
    — Lies between the cerebral peduncles and extends forward to the optic chiasm
    — Contains the vessels of the arterial circle of Willis

— *Folds of the cranial dura mater*
  - Are formed by a double-layered infolding of the **meningeal layer** of the dura mater

Falx cerebri

- Is a sickle-shaped, midline fold that extends into the median fissure **between the cerebral hemispheres**
- Is attached
  — **Anteriorly** to the **crista galli** and the **frontal crest**
  — **Superiorly** to the inner surface of the **calvaria** at the margins of the sulcus for the **superior sagittal sinus** (on the frontal, parietal, and occipital bones)
  — **Posteriorly** to the **tentorium cerebelli**
- Encloses the **superior sagittal sinus** in its **superior border**
- Encloses the **inferior sagittal sinus** in its free lower border
- Arches over the **corpus callosum** inferiorly

Tentorium cerebelli

- Is a tentlike partition that **covers** the **posterior cranial fossa** and the **cerebellum** and **supports** the **occipital lobes** of the cerebral hemispheres
  - Is attached
    — **Posteriorly** to the inner surface of the **calvaria** at the margins of the sulcus for the **transverse sinus** (on the occipital and temporal bones)
    — **Anteriorly** to the anterior and posterior **clinoid processes** of the sphenoid bone

— **Anterolaterally** to the **petrous temporal bone** along the margins of the **superior petrosal sinus**

- Encloses the **transverse sinus** in its posterior border
- Has a free and concave anterior border, which together with the dorsum sellae forms the **tentorial notch** surrounding the midbrain
- Fuses on its superior surface in the midline with the **falx cerebri**

Falx cerebelli

- Is a small, sickle-shaped projection **between** the **cerebellar hemispheres**
- Encloses the **occipital sinus** in its posterior border
- Is attached superiorly to the lower border of the tentorium cerebelli and posteriorly to the internal occipital crest (of the occipital bone)

Diaphragma sellae

- Is a horizontal projection that forms the roof to the hypophyseal fossa
- Is open in the middle for the passage of the hypophyseal stalk

— ***Innervation of the cranial dura mater***

- Innervation of the cranial dura mater is supplied mainly by meningeal branches of the trigeminal nerve, the vagus nerve, and the upper cervical spinal nerves.
- The dura of the **anterior cranial fossa** is supplied by **meningeal branches** of the **anterior and posterior ethmoidal nerves** (from the nasociliary branch of the ophthalmic nerve).
- The dura of the **middle cranial fossa** is supplied by the

  — **Meningeal branch** of the **maxillary nerve,** which arises in the pterygopalatine fossa and enters the cranial cavity through the **foramen rotundum**

  — **Meningeal branch** of the **mandibular nerve,** which arises in the infratemporal fossa and enters the cranial cavity through the **foramen spinosum**

  — Note that both of these branches are further distributed along the course of the **middle meningeal artery** to the dura of the calvaria.

- The dura of the **posterior cranial fossa** is supplied by the

  — **Meningeal branch** of the **vagus nerve,** which enters the cranial cavity through the jugular foramen

  — **Meningeal branches** of the **upper cervical spinal nerves** (C1 and C2), which pass along the hypoglossal nerve to enter the cranial cavity through the hypoglossal canal

- The **tentorium cerebelli and the falx cerebri** are supplied by the **meningeal branch** of the **ophthalmic nerve,** which arises in the wall of the cavernous sinus and passes posteriorly onto the tentorium.

— ***Blood supply of the cranial dura mater***

- Anterior meningeal arteries

  — Arise from the anterior and posterior **ethmoidal arteries**

and from the **internal carotid artery** in the cavernous sinus

— Supply the floor of the **anterior cranial fossa**

- **Middle meningeal artery**

  — Arises from the **maxillary artery** in the infratemporal fossa

  — Enters the cranial cavity through the **foramen spinosum**

  — Supplies the floor of the **middle cranial fossa**

  — Divides into anterior and posterior branches, which supply the dura of the calvaria

  — Gives rise to a **communicating branch** to the **lacrimal artery** in the orbit

- **Accessory meningeal artery**

  — Arises from the **maxillary artery** or the **middle meningeal artery** in the infratemporal fossa

  — Enters the cranial cavity through the **foramen ovale**

  — Supplies the floor of the **middle cranial fossa**, including the **trigeminal ganglion**

- **Posterior meningeal arteries**

  — Arise as separate branches of the **ascending pharyngeal artery** and the **occipital artery**

  — Enters the orbit through the **jugular foramen**

  — Supply the floor of the **posterior cranial fossa**

● **Dura venous sinuses (Fig. 8.17)**

- Lie between the meningeal and periosteal layers of dura
- Drain the cerebral and meningeal veins
- Empty directly or indirectly into the internal jugular vein
- **Superior sagittal sinus**

  — Lies in the attached superior margin of the falx cerebri

  — Begins **anteriorly** at the **crista galli** and ends **posteriorly** in the **confluence of sinuses** (where the falx cerebri joins the tentorium cerebelli)

  — Presents several **lateral lacunae,** which are large expansions at the entrance of the smaller meningeal veins

  — Has accumulations of **arachnoid granulations** extending into the lateral lacunae

  — Drains the cerebral, meningeal, and diploic veins

- **Inferior sagittal sinus**

  — Lies in the free inferior margin of the falx cerebri

  — Posteriorly joins the great cerebral vein (of Galen) to form the straight sinus

- **Straight sinus**

  — Lies in the midline of the tentorium cerebelli along the attachment of the falx cerebri

  — Begins anteriorly at the union of the **inferior sagittal sinus** and the **great cerebral vein,** which drains the deeper parts of the brain

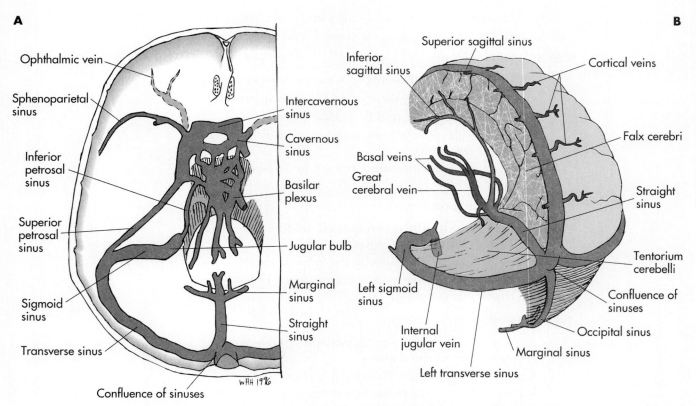

A

Ophthalmic vein

Sphenoparietal sinus

Inferior petrosal sinus

Superior petrosal sinus

Sigmoid sinus

Transverse sinus

Confluence of sinuses

Intercavernous sinus

Cavernous sinus

Basilar plexus

Jugular bulb

Marginal sinus

Straight sinus

WHH 1996

B

Superior sagittal sinus

Inferior sagittal sinus

Cortical veins

Falx cerebri

Basal veins

Great cerebral vein

Straight sinus

Left sigmoid sinus

Tentorium cerebelli

Internal jugular vein

Confluence of sinuses

Occipital sinus

Left transverse sinus

Marginal sinus

Fig. 8.17 Dural venous sinuses. **A,** Superior view. **B,** Superior oblique view.

— Ends posteriorly in the **confluence of sinuses**

- **Transverse sinus**

    — Begins at the **confluence of sinuses** and passes laterally
    — Lies along the attachment of the **tentorium cerebelli** to the occipital bone

- Note that the superior sagittal sinus typically drains to the right and the straight sinus to the left. Consequently, the transverse sinus, sigmoid sinus, and internal jugular vein are usually **larger on the right** than on the left.

- **Sigmoid sinus**

    — Is a continuation of the **transverse sinus**
    — Occupies an S-shaped groove on the petrous part of the temporal bone and the occipital bone
    — Ends at the **jugular foramen,** where it is continuous with the **internal jugular vein**

- **Occipital sinus**

    — Lies along the attachment of the **falx cerebelli** to the internal occipital crest
    — Begins with the union of the paired **marginal sinuses**
    — Ends above in the **confluence of sinuses**

- Superior petrosal sinus

  — Lies in the attachment of the **tentorium cerebelli** to the upper posterior border of the petrous temporal bone

  — Begins at the **cavernous sinus** and drains posteriorly to the junction of the transverse and sigmoid sinuses

- Inferior petrosal sinus

  — Begins at the **cavernous sinus** and drains inferiorly in the groove between the petrous temporal bone and the basilar part of the occipital bone

  — Exits the skull through the **jugular foramen** to end in the **internal jugular vein**

- Sphenoparietal sinus

  — Passes along the lesser wing of the sphenoid to end in the **cavernous sinus**

- Marginal sinus

  — Lies on each side of the **foramen magnum**

  — Ends in the **occipital sinus**

  — Communicates with the **basilar plexus** and the **internal vertebral venous plexus**

- Basilar plexus

  — Is a network of small venous channels on the basilar part of the occipital bone (the clivus)

  — Connects the **inferior petrosal sinuses** and communicates with the **internal vertebral venous plexus**

— *Cavernous sinus (see Figs. 8.17 and 8.18)*

  - Lies in the middle cranial fossa lateral to the body of the sphenoid bone

  - Extends from the **superior orbital fissure** anteriorly to the **apex of the petrous temporal bone** posteriorly

  - Is partitioned into numerous cavelike chambers

  - Forms the **lateral wall** of the **hypophyseal fossa**

  - Receives the terminations of the sphenoparietal sinus, the superior ophthalmic vein, and the superficial middle cerebral vein

  - Communicates with the

    — **Facial vein** via the **superior ophthalmic vein**

    — **Pterygoid venous plexus** via **emissary veins**

    — **Opposite cavernous sinus** via the **intercavernous sinuses**

    — **Sigmoid sinus** and **internal jugular vein** via the **superior and inferior petrosal sinuses**

Relationships of the cavernous sinus (Fig. 8.19)

  - The lateral wall contains (from superior to inferior) the oculomotor nerve, the trochlear nerve, and the ophthalmic nerve.

  - Structures passing through the sinus (separated from the blood

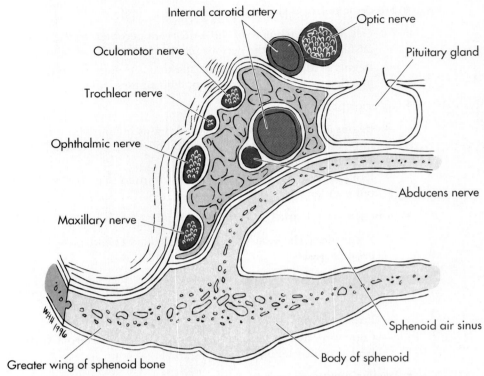

Fig. 8.18 Coronal section showing the relationships of the cavernous sinus.

only by vascular endothelium) include the internal carotid artery, the internal carotid perivascular plexus, and the abducens nerve.

- A tear of the internal carotid artery in the cavernous sinus may result in an **arteriovenous fistula** with pulsatile arterial blood filling the cavernous sinus and its tributaries.

- A **tumor** of the pituitary gland or an **aneurysm** of the internal carotid artery within the cavernous sinus may **impinge** on the **adjacent cranial nerves**, often affecting the **abducens nerve first** because of its proximity.

- Infectious material from the face may spread to the cavernous sinus (and subsequently to the cerebral veins) via emissary veins.

● **Emissary veins**

- Communicate between the dural venous sinuses and the veins outside the skull
- Allow blood to pass in either direction, although flow is normally away from the sinus
- May communicate with diploic veins
- Are always present, although not all are present within one individual
- Mastoid emissary vein

    — Is the largest and most constant emissary vein

    — Traverses the **mastoid foramen**

    — Connects the **sigmoid sinus** with the **occipital vein** or the **posterior auricular vein**

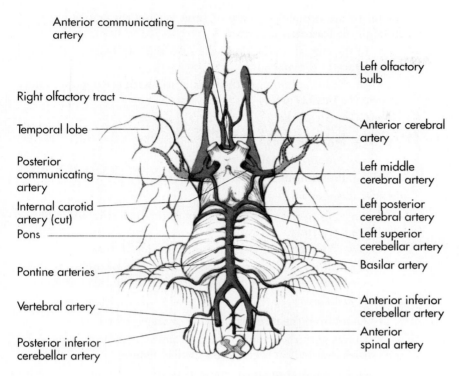

Anterior communicating artery

Right olfactory tract

Temporal lobe

Posterior communicating artery

Internal carotid artery (cut)

Pons

Pontine arteries

Vertebral artery

Posterior inferior cerebellar artery

Left olfactory bulb

Anterior cerebral artery

Left middle cerebral artery

Left posterior cerebral artery

Left superior cerebellar artery

Basilar artery

Anterior inferior cerebellar artery

Anterior spinal artery

Fig. 8.19 Arterial circle of Willis.

- **Parietal emissary vein**

  — Traverses the **parietal emissary foramen**
  — Connects the **superior sagittal sinus** with the veins of the **scalp**

- **Sphenoidal emissary vein**

  — Traverses the **sphenoidal emissary foramen** (of Vesalius)
  — Connects the **cavernous sinus** with the **pterygoid venous plexus**

- **Condylar emissary vein**

  — Traverses the **condylar canal**
  — Connects the **sigmoid sinus** with the **suboccipital venous plexus**

- **Emissary vein of the foramen cecum**

  — Traverses the **foramen cecum**
  — Connects the **superior sagittal sinus** with the veins of the **nasal cavity**

● **Blood supply of the brain** (see Fig. 8.19)

  — *Vertebral artery*

    • Arises from the **first part** of the subclavian artery
    • Traverses the **transverse foramina** of the **upper six** cervical vertebrae
    • Passes medially on the posterior arch of the **atlas** and pierces the

posterior atlantooccipital membrane to enter the cranial cavity through the **foramen magnum**

- In the cranial cavity lies in the subarachnoid space on the **ventral surface** of the **medulla**
- At the lower border of the pons unites with the opposite artery to form the **basilar artery**
- Gives rise to the

   — Posterior spinal artery
   — Anterior spinal artery
   — Posterior inferior cerebellar artery

Posterior spinal artery

- Arises from the **vertebral artery** or the **posterior inferior cerebellar artery**
- Descends along the attachment of the dorsal roots
- Is **reinforced** along its length by **radicular branches** of the vertebral, cervical, posterior intercostal, and lumbar arteries

Anterior spinal artery

- Arises from the terminal portion of the vertebral artery
- Unites with the artery of the opposite side to form a single artery, which descends in the anterior median fissure
- Like the posterior spinal artery is **reinforced** along its length by **radicular branches** of the vertebral, cervical, posterior intercostal, and lumbar arteries

Posterior inferior cerebellar artery

- Is the largest branch of the vertebral artery
- Supplies the medulla, the cerebellum, and the choroid plexus of the fourth ventricle

— **Basilar artery**

- Is formed at the lower border of the pons by the **union** of the **vertebral arteries**
- Ascends in the midline of the ventral pons
- Terminates at the upper border of the pons by **dividing** into the **posterior cerebral arteries**
- Gives rise to the

   — **Anterior inferior cerebellar arteries,** which supply the cerebellum and pons
   — **Labyrinthine arteries,** which enter the internal acoustic meatus with the facial and vestibulocochlear nerves to supply the inner ear
   — **Pontine arteries**
   — **Superior cerebellar arteries,** which supply the cerebellum and pons
   — **Posterior cerebral arteries**

— *Internal carotid artery*

- Gives rise to no branches in the neck
- Is invested by the **internal carotid plexus**

- Enters the skull through the **carotid canal** within the petrous part of the temporal bone
- Enters the middle cranial fossa through the foramen lacerum
- Runs forward through the **cavernous sinus** and leaves the sinus through the roof medial to the anterior clinoid process
- Terminates in the subarachnoid space by dividing into the **anterior cerebral artery** and the **middle cerebral artery**
- In its terminal part undergoes a characteristic U-shaped bend referred to as the **carotid siphon,** which is visible in lateral carotid arteriograms
- Within the **carotid canal** is related to the

  — Middle ear cavity
  — Cochlea of the inner ear
  — Auditory tube
  — Semilunar ganglion

- Within the **cavernous sinus** is related

  — Closely to the abducens nerve
  — Medially to the hypophyseal fossa and sphenoid sinus
  — Laterally to the oculomotor, trochlear, and ophthalmic nerves in the wall of the cavernous sinus

- Gives rise to the

  — **Caroticotympanic artery,** which passes through the caroticotympanic canaliculus (in the wall of the carotid canal) to supply the tympanic cavity
  — **Hypophyseal arteries** (superior and inferior), which supply the median eminence, the hypophyseal stalk, and the pituitary gland
  — **Ophthalmic artery,** which arises above the cavernous sinus and passes forward to enter the orbit through the optic canal
  — **Posterior communicating artery,** which connects the internal carotid artery and the posterior cerebral artery
  — **Anterior choroidal arteries,** which arise from the internal carotid artery near its termination to supply internal structures of the brain, including the choroid plexus
  — **Anterior cerebral artery**
  — **Middle cerebral artery**

— *Cerebral arteries (see Fig. 8.19)*
Anterior cerebral artery

- Is the smaller of the two **terminal branches** of the **internal carotid artery**
- Runs forward above the optic nerve and then upward and backward in the **longitudinal fissure** over the corpus callosum
- Supplies the orbital surface of the frontal lobe and the **medial surface** of the **cerebral hemisphere** posteriorly to the parietooccipital sulcus

Middle cerebral artery

- Is the larger of the two **terminal branches** of the **internal carotid artery**
- Runs upward and laterally in the **lateral sulcus**
- Supplies the adjacent parts of the frontal, parietal, and occipital lobes

Posterior cerebral artery

- Arises at the terminal bifurcation of the **basilar artery**
- Passes laterally around the midbrain and then passes posteriorly on the **medial surface** of the **cerebral hemisphere** below the parietooccipital sulcus
- Supplies the temporal lobe and the occipital lobe, including the visual area

— *Circle of Willis (arterial circle) (see Fig. 8.19)*

- Is a potentially important **anastomotic connection** between the **internal carotid artery**, the **vertebral artery**, and the same vessels of the opposite side
- Lies at the **base of the brain** in relation to the **optic chiasm** and the **hypophyseal stalk**
- Is formed by vessels on each side, including the

    — Anterior communicating artery
    — Anterior cerebral artery
    — Internal carotid artery
    — Posterior communicating artery
    — Posterior cerebral artery

■ **Orbit**

● Bony orbit (Fig. 8.20)

- Is the bony cavity that contains the eye and the associated muscles, nerves, and blood vessels
- Is said to be shaped like a **four-sided pyramid** with the **apex** pointed **posteriorly** and with the **base** formed by its anterior opening
- Is described as having a **roof, floor,** and **medial and lateral walls**
- Roof

    — Is formed mostly by the **orbital plate of the frontal bone** and only slightly by the **lesser wing of the sphenoid**
    — Is related to the **frontal lobe** of the cerebral hemisphere
    — **Laterally** includes the **fossa** for the **lacrimal gland**
    — **Medially** includes the **trochlear pit** and **trochlear spine**, which are related to the tendon of the **superior oblique muscle**

- Floor

    — Is formed by the **orbital plate of the maxilla**, the **zygomatic bone**, and to a small degree by the **orbital process of the palatine bone**
    — Is related to the **maxillary sinus**
    — Includes the **infraorbital groove and canal**, which contains the **infraorbital nerve and artery**

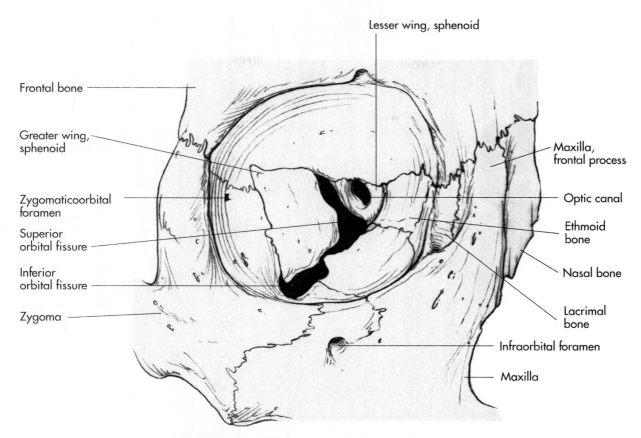

Fig. 8.20 Bony walls of the orbit.

- **Medial wall**

  — Is formed by the **orbital plate of the ethmoid**, the **lacrimal bone**, the **frontal bone**, and to a small degree by the **body of the sphenoid bone**

  — Is related to the **ethmoid air cells**, the **sphenoid sinus**, and the **nasal cavity**

  — Includes the **fossa for the lacrimal sac**, the **anterior and posterior lacrimal crests**, and the opening of the **nasolacrimal canal**

- **Lateral wall**

  — Is formed by the **zygomatic bone**, the **greater wing of the sphenoid bone**, and a small part of the **frontal bone**

  — Is related through the zygomatic and temporal bones to the **temporal fossa** containing the **temporalis muscle**

  — Is related through the greater wing of the sphenoid bone to the **middle cranial fossa**

● **Nerves of the orbit**

  — *Ophthalmic nerve (Fig. 8.21)*

      • The ophthalmic nerve arises from the **semilunar ganglion** in the **middle cranial fossa**.

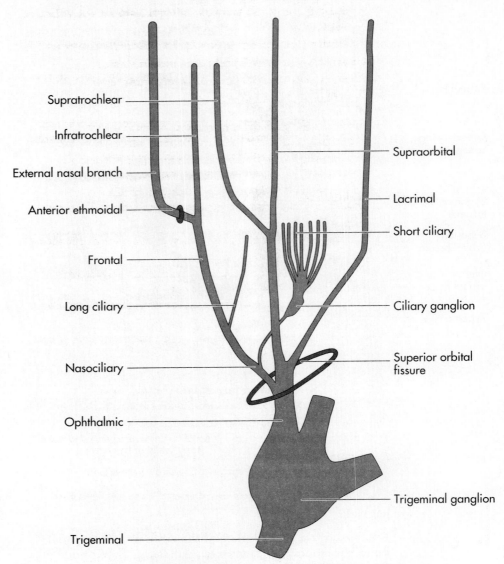

Fig. 8.21 Branches of the ophthalmic nerve.

Labels (top to bottom, left side):
Supratrochlear
Infratrochlear
External nasal branch
Anterior ethmoidal
Frontal
Long ciliary
Nasociliary
Ophthalmic
Trigeminal

Labels (right side):
Supraorbital
Lacrimal
Short ciliary
Ciliary ganglion
Superior orbital fissure
Trigeminal ganglion

- It is **entirely sensory**, containing only **general somatic afferent (GSA)** components. (Remember that the mandibular nerve is the only division of the trigeminal that supplies skeletal muscle.)
- The ophthalmic nerve passes forward in the **lateral wall** of the **cavernous sinus.**
- It divides into the lacrimal, frontal, and nasociliary nerves, which enter the orbit through the **superior orbital fissure.**

Frontal nerve

- Enters the orbit through the superior orbital fissure **superior** to the **common annular tendon**
- Passes forward on the superior surface of the **levator palpebrae superioris muscle**

- Divides into the

    — **Supraorbital nerve,** which exits the orbit through the supraorbital foramen or notch to supply the frontal sinus and the skin of the forehead, scalp, and upper eyelid

    — **Supratrochlear nerve,** which exits the orbit above the medial angle of the eye to supply the skin of the lower, medial forehead

Lacrimal nerve

- Enters the orbit through the superior orbital fissure **superior** to the **common annular tendon**
- Passes forward on the superior surface of the **lateral rectus muscle**
- Supplies the lacrimal gland, the conjunctiva, and the upper eyelid
- Receives a **communicating branch** from the **zygomaticotemporal nerve** (from the maxillary nerve), which carries **postganglionic parasympathetic fibers** originating in the **pterygopalatine ganglion** and destined for the **lacrimal gland**

Nasociliary nerve

- Enters the orbit through the superior orbital fissure **within** the **common annular tendon** and between the two divisions of the oculomotor nerve
- Passes medially **above** the **optic nerve** and **below** the **superior rectus muscle** accompanied by the ophthalmic artery
- Is the **sensory nerve** to the **eyeball**
- Also supplies the skin of the eyelid and nose and the mucosa of the nasal cavity and the ethmoid and sphenoid sinuses
- Gives rise to the

    — Communicating branch to the ciliary ganglion
    — Long ciliary nerves
    — Posterior ethmoidal nerve
    — Anterior ethmoidal nerve
    — Infratrochlear nerve

- **Communicating branch to the ciliary ganglion**

    — Often arises from the nasociliary nerve in the wall of the cavernous sinus and passes forward lateral to the optic nerve to reach the ciliary ganglion
    — Is also called the **sensory root** of the ciliary ganglion
    — Carries **general somatic afferent fibers,** which pass through the ciliary ganglion to be distributed through the **short ciliary nerves** to the eye

- **Long ciliary nerves**

    — Arise from the nasociliary nerve superior and medial to the optic nerve
    — Pass forward to pierce the sclera close to the optic nerve
    — Carry **postganglionic sympathetic fibers** and accompany-

ing **GVA fibers** (derived from the internal carotid plexus) to the **dilator pupillae muscle**

— Carry **GSA fibers** from the **iris and cornea**

- **Posterior ethmoidal nerve**

    — Is often absent
    — Is accompanied by the posterior ethmoidal artery
    — Leaves the orbit through the **posterior ethmoidal foramen** in the posterior **medial wall**
    — Supplies the sphenoidal and posterior ethmoidal sinuses

- **Anterior ethmoidal nerve**

    — Is accompanied by the anterior ethmoidal artery
    — Leaves the orbit through the **anterior ethmoidal foramen** in the anterior **medial wall**
    — Emerges into the **middle cranial fossa** above the **cribriform plate** of the ethmoid bone
    — Descends through the **nasal slit** into the roof of the **nasal cavity**
    — Divides into **internal and external nasal nerves**
    — Supplies the anterior and middle ethmoid sinuses, the mucosa of the upper nasal cavity, the skin over the dorsum of the nose, and the dura of the anterior cranial fossa

- **Infratrochlear nerve**

    — Is the terminal branch of the nasociliary nerve
    — Leaves the orbit below the trochlea
    — Supplies the skin and conjunctiva of the medial eyelids and the skin on the side of the nose

— *Trochlear nerve*

    • Is the smallest of the cranial nerves and is unusual in that it arises from the dorsal aspect of the brain stem
    • Curves around the midbrain to pierce the **roof of the cavernous sinus** near the attachment of the tentorium cerebelli to the **posterior clinoid process**
    • Passes forward in the lateral wall of the cavernous sinus below the oculomotor nerve
    • Enters the orbit through the superior orbital fissure **superior** to the **common annular tendon**
    • Passes medially across the levator palpebrae superioris muscle to enter the **superior oblique muscle**
    • Contains only GSE fibers (from cell bodies in the trochlear nucleus) and **supplies** only the **superior oblique muscle**

— *Abducens nerve*

    • Pierces the **posterior wall** of the **cavernous sinus** while in the **posterior cranial fossa**
    • Passes through the **cavernous sinus** adjacent to the **internal carotid artery**

- Enters the orbit through the superior orbital fissure **within** the **common annular tendon**
- Passes forward and laterally to enter the **lateral rectus muscle**
- Contains only GSE fibers (from cell bodies in the abducens nucleus) and **supplies** only the **lateral rectus muscle**

— *Oculomotor nerve*

- Pierces the roof of the cavernous sinus lateral to the posterior clinoid process
- Passes forward in the **lateral wall** of the **cavernous sinus** above the trochlear nerve
- Enters the orbit through the superior orbital fissure **within** the **common annular tendon** and lateral to the optic nerve
- Contains GSE fibers from cell bodies in the abducens nucleus, which supply the **extraocular muscles** except the lateral rectus and superior oblique muscles
  - Divides into the

    — **Superior division**, which supplies the **levator palpebrae superioris and superior rectus muscles**

    — **Inferior division**, which supplies the **inferior rectus, medial rectus,** and **inferior oblique** muscles

  - Gives rise to the **oculomotor root to the ciliary ganglion,** which

    — Is also called the **motor root** of the ciliary ganglion

    — Is a **branch** from the **inferior division** of the oculomotor nerve

    — Contains **preganglionic parasympathetic (GVE)** fibers from cell bodies in the Edinger-Westphal nucleus for synapse in the **ciliary ganglion** (postganglionic fibers reach the eye via the short ciliary nerves)

— *Optic nerve*

- The optic nerve is not a true peripheral nerve but a forward extension of the brain.
- It is surrounded by the meninges (and the subarachnoid space) to the back of the eyeball.
- It consists of the central **axons** of the **bipolar ganglion cells of the retina.**
- It passes posteromedially from the eyeball to leave the orbit through the **optic canal.**
- The optic nerve joins the opposite nerve at the **optic chiasm,** which is related

  — **Anteriorly** to the **anterior cerebral** and **anterior communicating arteries**

  — Laterally to the **internal carotid artery**

  — Posteriorly to the **hypophyseal fossa,** the **pituitary gland,** and the **hypophyseal stalk**

  — **Inferiorly** to the **sphenoid sinus**

  — Note that the optic chiasm may be impinged on by a tumor

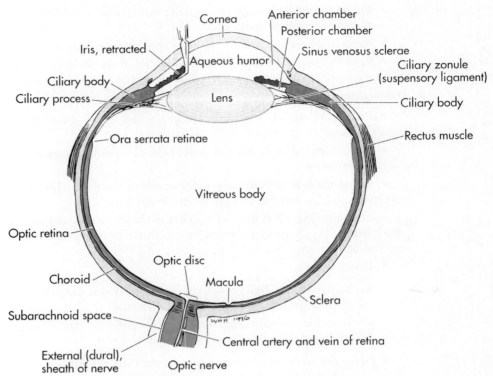

Fig. 8.22 Horizontal section of the eyeball.

of the pituitary or by an aneurysm of the internal carotid or anterior cerebral artery with resulting visual defects.

• The optic nerve contains the nerves of vision, which are classified functionally as special somatic **afferent** (SSA).

— *Ciliary ganglion (Fig. 8.22)*

• The ciliary ganglion is one of the four parasympathetic ganglia of the head and contains the cell bodies of **postganglionic parasympathetic neurons.**

• It is the only ganglion to distribute parasympathetic fibers to the **eye.**

• It lies **between** the **optic nerve** and the **lateral rectus muscle** in the posterior orbit.

• It receives the following:

— **Nasociliary (sensory) root** from the nasociliary nerve (a branch of the ophthalmic nerve) containing **general somatic afferent fibers**

— **Oculomotor (motor) root** from the oculomotor nerve containing **preganglionic parasympathetic fibers** for synapse in the ganglion

— **Sympathetic root** containing **postganglionic sympathetic** and accompanying **visceral afferent fibers** derived from the internal carotid plexus in the cavernous sinus

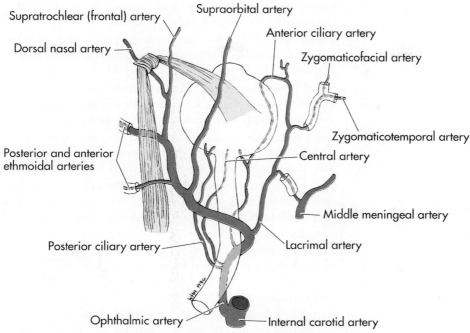

Fig. 8.23 Branches of the ophthalmic artery.

- **Short ciliary nerves** distribute fibers from the **ciliary ganglion** and contain the following:

  — **Parasympathetic postganglionic fibers,** which supply the **ciliary muscle** and the **sphincter pupillae muscle** (smooth muscles that constrict the pupil and focus the lens for accommodation to near vision)

  — **General somatic afferent fibers** from the cornea, ciliary body, and iris

  — **Postganglionic sympathetic** and accompanying **visceral afferent fibers** to the dilator pupillae muscle, the tarsal muscles of the eyelid, and the vascular smooth muscle of the eye

- Remember that only the parasympathetic fibers synapse in the ciliary ganglion. Sympathetic and afferent fibers pass through the ganglion without synapse.

● Blood vessels of the orbit

— *Ophthalmic artery (Fig. 8.23)*

  - The ophthalmic artery arises in the cranial cavity from the **internal carotid artery** medial to the anterior clinoid process.

  - It enters the orbit through the **optic canal** below the optic nerve and within the common annular tendon.

  - It passes with the nasociliary nerve from lateral to medial above the optic nerve.

  - It gives rise to the following:

    — **Central artery of the retina,** which enters the inferior surface of the optic nerve and passes forward in the center of the nerve to reach and supply the retina

— **Lacrimal artery,** which accompanies the lacrimal nerve to supply the lacrimal gland, the conjunctiva, and the upper eyelid

— **Short posterior ciliary arteries,** usually 6 to 10 in number, which enter the back of the eyeball close to the optic nerve and supply the choroid and the ciliary processes

— **Long posterior ciliary arteries,** usually two in number, which enter the eyeball to the outside of the short posterior ciliary arteries and supply the ciliary body and iris

— **Supraorbital artery,** which exits the orbit through the supraorbital foramen or notch with the supraorbital nerve to supply the frontal sinus and the skin of the forehead, scalp, and upper eyelid

— **Posterior ethmoidal artery,** which leaves the orbit through the posterior ethmoidal foramen with the nerve of the same name to supply the sphenoidal and posterior ethmoidal sinuses

— **Anterior ethmoidal artery,** which leaves the orbit through the anterior ethmoidal foramen with the nerve of the same name to supply the anterior and middle ethmoid sinuses, the mucosa of the upper nasal cavity, the skin over the dorsum of the nose, and the dura of the anterior cranial fossa

— **Medial palpebral arteries,** which arise distal to the anterior ethmoidal artery and supply the medial parts of the upper and lower eyelids

— **Supratrochlear artery,** which exits the orbit with the supratrochlear nerve above the medial angle of the eye to supply the skin of the lower, medial forehead

— **Dorsal nasal artery,** which accompanies the infratrochlear nerve to supply the skin and conjunctiva of the medial eyelids and the skin on the side of the nose

— Muscular branches

• **Obstruction** of the **central artery of the retina** or one of its branches will result in **partial or complete blindness** because there are no functional anastomoses with other vessels supplying the eyeball.

• The **dorsal nasal artery** anastomoses with the **angular artery** providing a potentially significant anastomosis **between the internal carotid and external carotid arteries.**

• The **anastomotic branch of the middle meningeal artery** communicates with the ophthalmic artery through the superior orbital fissure or the lacrimal foramen. It reinforces and may totally replace the ophthalmic artery.

— *Ophthalmic veins*
Superior ophthalmic vein

• Begins in the orbit with the union of branches from the **supraorbital vein** and the **angular vein**

- Passes posteriorly through the upper medial orbit
- Passes through the **superior orbital fissure** to open into the **cavernous sinus**
- Receives the terminations of the

    — Tributaries that correspond to branches of the ophthalmic artery

    — Two superior vorticose veins

    — Inferior ophthalmic vein

Inferior ophthalmic vein

- Arises from veins in the lower part of the orbit
- Receives the two inferior vorticose veins
- Ends in the superior ophthalmic vein
- Communicates through the inferior orbital fissure with the pterygoid plexus

— *Vorticose veins*

- Vorticose veins drain the **choroid layer** of the eyeball.
- They exit the sclera posteriorly, usually four in number, one for each quadrant.
- **Superior vorticose veins** end in the **superior ophthalmic vein.**
- **Inferior vorticose veins** end in the **inferior ophthalmic vein.**

● **Extraocular muscles (Fig. 8.24, Table 8.6)**

- Are derived from the pre-otic somites of the embryo
- Are innervated by GSE neurons in the oculomotor, trochlear, and abducens nerves

— *Testing the function of the extraocular muscles*

- The patient's head is held still and the patient is asked to follow the movement of an object (such as the examiner's finger) with the eyes.
- For each of the six muscles there is one position in which that muscle acts alone and at its maximum. These are the **six cardinal directions of gaze.**

    — To test the **lateral rectus** the patient is directed to look far **laterally.**

    — To test the **medial rectus** the patient is directed to look far **medially.**

    — To test the **superior rectus** the patient is directed to look far **laterally** and then **upward.**

    — To test the **inferior rectus** the patient is directed to look far **laterally** and then **downward.**

    — To test the **superior oblique** the patient is directed to look far **medially** and then **downward.**

    — To test the **inferior oblique** the patient is directed to look far **medially** and then **upward.**

- The medial rectus and lateral rectus adduct and abduct the pupil, respectively.

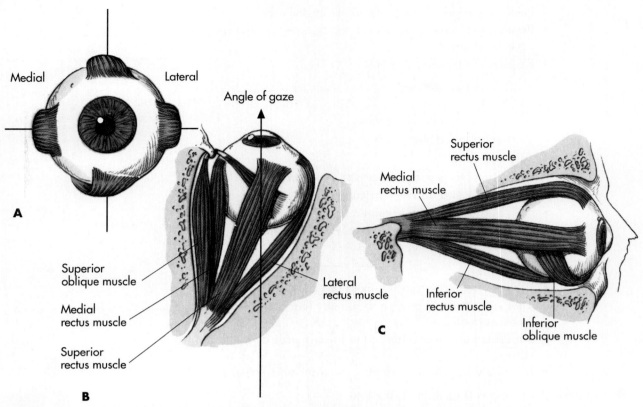

Fig. 8.24 The extraocular muscles. **A,** Anterior view. **B,** Superior view. **C,** Lateral view.

- • **When the pupil is abducted** the superior rectus and inferior rectus are, respectively, the only elevator and depressor of the pupil.
  - • **When the pupil is adducted** the inferior oblique and superior oblique are, respectively, the only elevator and depressor of the pupil.
- Features of the eyelids and lacrimal apparatus
  - — *Eyelids (palpebrae) (Fig. 8.25)*
    - • Consist of two folds of skin that lie anterior to the eye and are separated by the transverse **palpebral fissure**
    - • Are covered on their inner surface by the **conjunctiva,** which
      - — Reflects from the eyelid onto the sclera of the eyeball at the **conjunctival fornices**
      - — Is continuous over the front of the cornea with the **corneal epithelium**
      - — Forms a closed **conjunctival sac** when the eyelids are closed
    - • Contain the
      - — Palpebral part of the **orbicularis oculi** muscle
      - — Orbital septum
      - — Tarsal plates

Table 8.6	*Extraocular Muscles*			
NAME	**ORIGIN**	**INSERTION**	**ACTION***	**INNERVATION**
Superior rectus	Superior part of the common annular tendon	Sclera of the superior surface of the eye (anterior lateral quadrant)	Elevates and adducts the pupil	Oculomotor nerve (superior division)
Inferior rectus	Inferior part of the common annular tendon	Sclera of the inferior surface of the eye (anterior lateral quadrant)	Depresses and adducts the pupil	Oculomotor nerve (inferior division)
Medial rectus	Medial part of the common annular tendon	Sclera on the anteromedial surface of the eye	Adducts the pupil	Oculomotor nerve (inferior division)
Lateral rectus	Lateral part of the common annular tendon	Sclera on the anterolateral surface of the eye	Abducts the pupil	Abducens nerve
Superior oblique	Body of the sphenoid bone above and medial to the optic canal	Sclera on the superior surface of the eye (posterior lateral quadrant)	Depresses and abducts the pupil	Trochlear nerve
Inferior oblique	Orbital surface of the maxilla lateral to the nasolacrimal canal	Sclera on the inferior surface of the eye (posterior lateral quadrant)	Elevates and abducts the pupil	Oculomotor nerve (inferior division)
Levator palpebrae superioris	Lesser wing of the sphenoid above the common annular tendon	Skin and tarsal plate of the upper eyelid	Elevates the upper eyelid	Oculomotor nerve (superior division)

*The action relates to the eye moving from the primary position (the gaze is straight ahead).

— Levator palpebrae superioris muscle

— Tarsal muscles

- Are **closed** by action of the **orbicularis oculi muscle,** which is innervated by the **facial nerve** (note that denervation of the orbicularis oculi results in an inability to close the eye and in ptosis, or drooping of the lower eyelid)

- Are **opened** by the **levator palpebrae superioris** and **superior tarsal** muscles (note that ptosis of the upper eyelid can result from interruption of the oculomotor nerve to the levator palpebrae superioris or of the sympathetic innervation of the superior tarsal muscle)

Orbital septum

- Is continuous with the **periosteum** of the skull at the margin of the orbit

- Extends to the margin of the palpebral fissure attaching to the tarsal plates

- Anchors the tarsal plates to the medial and lateral walls of the orbit

Tarsal plates

- Are thin plates of **fibrous tissue in the upper and lower lid**

- Provide **support** for the lids, maintaining their shape

- Lie between the palpebral conjunctiva and the superficial fascia under the skin of the eyelid

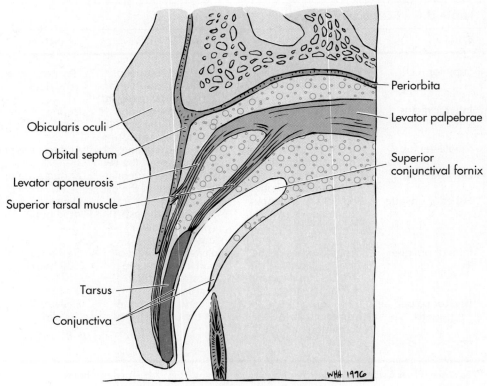

Fig. 8.25 The upper eyelid.

- Are attached to the margins of the orbit by the **orbital septum**, which is thickened **medially** to form the **medial palpebral ligament** and **laterally** to form the **lateral palpebral raphe**
- Contain numerous **tarsal glands** (modified sebaceous glands), which open at the margin of the lids

Superior tarsal muscle

- Is **smooth muscle** arising from the deep surface of the tendon of the levator palpebrae superioris
- Attaches into the upper margin of the **superior tarsal plate**
- Assists in holding the upper eyelid open

— *Lacrimal apparatus*

- **Lacrimal gland**

  — Lies in the **lacrimal fossa** of the frontal bone in the upper lateral portion of the orbit
  — Secretes **lacrimal fluid** (tears) by way of several ducts into the superior fornix of the **conjunctival sac**
  — Receives **parasympathetic innervation** from the **facial nerve** by way of (1) the greater petrosal nerve, (2) the nerve of the pterygoid canal, (3) the pterygopalatine ganglion, (4) the maxillary nerve, (5) the zygomatic nerve, (6) the zygomaticotemporal nerve, and (7) the communicating branch to the lacrimal nerve

- **Lacrimal fluid** (tears)

  — Nourishes the avascular cornea

  — Washes away irritants

  — Keeps the cornea moist

  — Contains the antibacterial enzyme lysozyme

  — Is swept across the eye by blinking to accumulate at the lacus lacrimalis, a triangular depression at the medial angle of the eye

  — Is aspirated through the **lacrimal puncta** and **lacrimal canaliculi** into the **lacrimal sac,** a membranous chamber occupying the **lacrimal fossa on the medial wall of the orbit**

- **Nasolacrimal duct**

  — Begins in the floor of the medial orbit as a continuation of the **lacrimal sac**

  — Descends in a bony canal to open on the lateral wall of the nasal cavity in the **inferior meatus**

● **Eyeball (see Fig. 8.2)**

  - Receives its blood supply from branches of the **ophthalmic artery**
  - Receives its innervation from the **nasociliary nerve** (from the ophthalmic nerve)

  — *Wall of the eyeball*

    - Consists of **three layers,** or tunics
    - **Fibrous tunic**

      — Is the outermost layer

      — Is differentiated anteriorly into the transparent **cornea**

      — Comprises the **sclera** over the remainder of the eye

    - **Vascular tunic**

      — Is the middle pigmented layer

      — Consists of the **iris, ciliary body,** and **choroid**

    - **Inner tunic**

      — Is formed by the **retina,** which is the **visual receptor organ**

  Chambers of the eyeball

    - **Anterior chamber**

      — Lies between the cornea and iris

      — Communicates with the posterior chamber through the pupil of the iris

      — Contains **aqueous humor** (fluid)

    - **Posterior chamber**

      — Lies between the iris and the lens and ciliary zonules

      — Communicates with the anterior chamber through the pupil of the iris

      — Contains **aqueous humor** (fluid)

- Vitreous chamber

    — Lies posterior to the lens and ciliary zonules
    — Comprises the bulk of the eyeball
    — Contains the gelatinous **vitreous body**

Other important features of the eyeball

- Optic disc

    — Is the point on the **posterior retina** where the ganglion cell **axons converge** to leave the eye through the **optic nerve**
    — Is referred to as the *blind spot* because it contains no visual receptors (rods or cones)
    — Is pierced by the **central artery of the retina,** which can be visualized as it ramifies over the retina

- Macula lutea (yellow spot)

    — Lies **lateral** to the **optic disc** around the optical axis of the eyeball
    — Has a **central depression,** the **fovea centralis**

- Fovea centralis

    — Is the central depression of the **macula lutea**
    — Is the area of **maximum visual acuity**
    — Contains **only cones** and **no rods**

- Pupil

    — Is a round defect in the **center** of the **iris**
    — Constantly **changes diameter** to adjust the amount of light that enters the eye
    — Is **constricted** by the **sphincter pupillae** muscle and **widened** by the **dilator pupillae** muscle

- Cornea

    — Is the **transparent** and **avascular** membrane comprising the anterior part of the fibrous tunic
    — Functions as a **lens** of fixed focal length that **refracts light** entering the eye

- Lens

    — Is a transparent biconvex disc
    — Lies **between** the **iris** anteriorly and the **vitreous body** posteriorly
    — Is suspended from the ciliary body by the ciliary zonules
    — Is maintained in a taut and slightly thinned state by tonic tension exerted by the **ciliary body** and **suspensory ligaments**
    — Rounds slightly when the tension is released by contraction of the **ciliary muscle**

Accommodation

- Is the reflex response that brings objects into focus for near vision (as in reading)

- Is characterized by

    — **Convergence** of the pupils to maintain binocular vision
    — **Constriction** of the **pupil** by action of the **sphincter pupillae** muscle
    — **Rounding** of the **lens** by action of the **ciliary muscle,** which reduces the tension exerted on the lens

- Is a parasympathetic response mediated by the oculomotor nerve via the ciliary ganglion

■ Pharynx

- Is a **fibromuscular tube**
- Is attached to the **base of the skull** superiorly
- Is continuous with the **esophagus** inferiorly
- Has a **wall** consisting of **four layers**

    — A **mucosa** lined by respiratory epithelium (ciliated pseudostratified columnar) in the nasopharynx and by stratified squamous epithelium elsewhere
    — The **pharyngobasilar fascia,** which is closely applied to and supports the mucosa (note that there is no submucosa in most of the pharynx so even slight edema will result in a painful "sore throat")
    — A **muscular coat** (skeletal muscle) consisting of the pharyngeal constrictor muscles externally and a group of longitudinal muscles internally
    — The **buccopharyngeal fascia,** which covers the outside of the **pharyngeal constrictor** and **buccinator** muscles and contains the **pharyngeal plexus** of nerves

- Is mostly **open anteriorly** where it **communicates** with the **nasal cavity,** the **oral cavity,** and the **larynx**
- Is described as having three parts, the **nasopharynx,** the **oropharynx,** and the **laryngopharynx**

● Nasopharynx (Fig. 8.26)

- Extends from the **base of the skull** to the **soft palate**
- **Communicates** anteriorly with the **nasal cavity** through the **choanae**
- Is functionally a part of the **respiratory system** and remains open at all times
- Is related within its wall to the **superior pharyngeal constrictor muscle**
- Is related superiorly to the **body of the sphenoid** and the **sphenoid sinus**
- Includes the **pharyngeal tonsils** and the pharyngeal opening of the **auditory tube**

    — *Pharyngeal tonsils*

    - Are embedded in the mucosa of the **posterior wall** of the nasopharynx
    - May impair breathing when enlarged and are then called **adenoids**

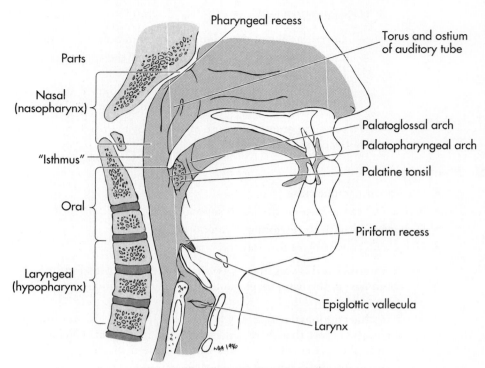

Fig. 8.26 The interior of the pharynx.

- May extend around the **pharyngeal ostium of the auditory tube** as **tubal tonsils**
- Are prominent in children but regress in adults

— *Auditory tube*

- Opens onto the **lateral wall** of the nasopharynx
- Pierces the **pharyngobasilar fascia** at the base of the skull above the upper border of the superior pharyngeal constrictor muscle
- Connects the **nasopharynx** to the **tympanic cavity**, allowing for equalization of pressure in the middle ear with the ambient pressure
- Is surrounded at its opening into the pharynx by a tubal elevation, the **torus tubarius**, which is formed by the mucosa overlying the projecting tubal cartilage
- Consists of **cartilaginous** and **bony** parts

  — The **cartilaginous part** is the **anterior two thirds**, which opens into the nasopharynx and lies at the **base of the skull** in the groove between the petrous temporal bone and the greater wing of the sphenoid. It is an invagination of the nasopharynx and is lined by **respiratory epithelium**. It is **normally closed** and opens only on **swallowing** or **yawning**.

  — The **bony part** is the **posterior one third**, which opens into the tympanic cavity and lies in the **lower part** of the **musculotubal canal** within the **petrous temporal bone**.

(The upper part is the semicanal containing the **tensor tympani muscle.**) It is an outgrowth of the tympanic cavity and remains **open** at all times.

- Provides a conduit for the spread of respiratory infections and infections of the pharyngeal tonsils to the tympanic cavity
- Is opened during swallowing and yawning by action of the tensor veli palatini and levator veli palatini muscles that attach to the cartilage of the auditory tube

- **Oropharynx** (see Fig. 8.26)

   - Extends from the **soft palate** above to the upper border of the **epiglottis** below
   - Lies at the level of the bodies of the **second** and **third** cervical vertebrae
   - Is functionally shared by the **respiratory system** and the **alimentary system,** conducting air during respiration and food and drink when swallowing
   - Has **lateral** and **posterior** walls related to the **pharyngeal constrictor** muscles
   - Is related anteriorly to the **oral cavity** through the **oropharyngeal isthmus** and to the **posterior one third of the tongue**
   - Contains the **palatine tonsils,** which lie between the **palatoglossal** and **palatopharyngeal** arches

   — *Palatine tonsil*

      - Is often simply called **the tonsil**
      - Is an accumulation of lymphoid tissue that lies in the **tonsillar fossa** between the **palatoglossal fold** anteriorly and the **palatopharyngeal fold** posteriorly
      - Lies in a **muscular bed** formed by the **superior pharyngeal constrictor** muscle
      - Has a "capsule" derived from the **pharyngobasilar fascia,** which facilitates its removal in a tonsillectomy
      - Is related at its lower pole to the **glossopharyngeal nerve** as it descends **between** the **superior** and **middle pharyngeal constrictor** muscles to reach the posterior one third of the tongue
      - Is prominent in children but regresses in adults
      - Receives **most** of its **blood supply** from the **tonsillar branch of the facial artery** but also from the ascending and descending palatine arteries, the ascending pharyngeal artery, and the lingual artery
      - Is innervated by the tonsillar branches of the glossopharyngeal nerve
      - Is drained by **lymph vessels,** which end primarily in the **jugulodigastric node** in the deep cervical group of nodes

- **Laryngopharynx** (see Fig. 8.26)

   - Extends from the upper border of the epiglottis to the lower border of the cricoid cartilage, where it is continuous with the esophagus
   - Lies at the level of the bodies of the **fourth, fifth,** and **sixth** cervical vertebrae

• Is functionally shared by the **respiratory system** and the **alimentary system,** conducting air during respiration and food and drink when swallowing

• Has **lateral** and **posterior** walls related to the **middle** and **inferior** pharyngeal constrictor muscles

• Is related anteriorly to the **aditus** of the **larynx** and to the **posterior surface** of the larynx

• Anteriorly extends lateral to the larynx as the **piriform recesses**

— *Piriform recess*

• The piriform recess is the part of the laryngopharynx lying lateral to the larynx.

• It lies between the thyrohyoid membrane and thyroid cartilage laterally and the aryepiglottic fold, arytenoid cartilage, and cricoid cartilage medially.

• **Food** or swallowed **foreign bodies** may become **lodged** in the recess.

• The **internal laryngeal nerve** (the sensory nerve to the larynx above the vocal fold) can be **anesthetized** where it lies deep to the mucosa of the piriform recess.

● **Deglutition**

• Deglutition is the act of **swallowing.** It includes several recognizable events:

— The bolus of food is pushed posteriorly through the oropharyngeal isthmus by the progressive contact of the dorsum of the tongue with the palate.

— The soft palate is elevated and the nasopharynx is closed off from the oropharynx by the action of the levator and tensor veli palatini muscles.

— The pharynx is elevated and shortened by the action of the longitudinal pharyngeal muscles.

— The bolus is pushed inferiorly by successive contractions of the superior, middle, and inferior pharyngeal constrictor muscles.

— The cricopharyngeal part of the inferior pharyngeal constrictor muscle relaxes, allowing the bolus to pass into the esophagus.

● **Muscles of the pharynx (Figs. 8.27 and 8.28; Table 8.7)**

• The muscles of the pharynx include three pairs of **circularly arranged** muscles (the pharyngeal constrictor muscles), which

— Have bony and cartilaginous attachments anteriorly and superiorly

— Are unattached posteriorly except at the **pharyngeal raphe,** where the paired constrictors meet

— Posteriorly overlap the constrictor above, forming a continuous muscular wall

— Diverge at their anterior attachments, leaving lateral gaps between adjacent constrictors

— Constrict the pharyngeal lumen to propel food and drink when swallowing

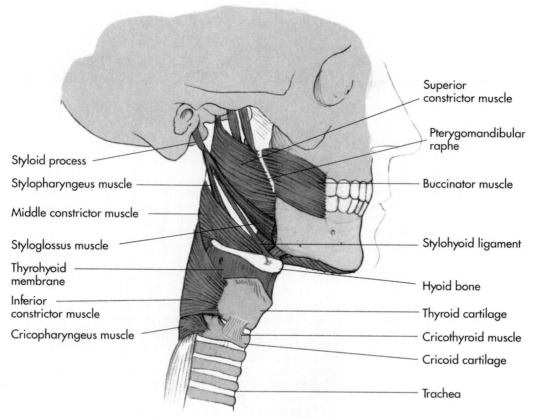

Superior
constrictor muscle

Pterygomandibular
raphe

Buccinator muscle

Styloid process

Stylopharyngeus muscle

Middle constrictor muscle

Styloglossus muscle

Stylohyoid ligament

Thyrohyoid
membrane

Hyoid bone

Inferior
constrictor muscle

Thyroid cartilage

Cricopharyngeus muscle

Cricothyroid muscle

Cricoid cartilage

Trachea

Fig. 8.27 Pharyngeal muscles and pterygomandibular raphe (lateral view).

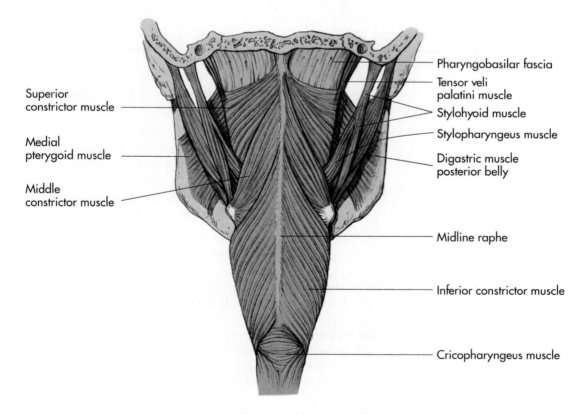

Pharyngobasilar fascia

Tensor veli
palatini muscle

Superior
constrictor muscle

Stylohyoid muscle

Stylopharyngeus muscle

Medial
pterygoid muscle

Digastric muscle
posterior belly

Middle
constrictor muscle

Midline raphe

Inferior constrictor muscle

Cricopharyngeus muscle

Fig. 8.28 Pharyngeal muscles from behind.

Table 8.7	***Muscles of the Pharynx***			
NAME	ORIGIN	INSERTION	ACTION	INNERVATION
Circular Muscles				
Superior pharyngeal constrictor	Medial pterygoid plate, pterygomandibular raphe, mylohyoid line of mandible, lateral side of tongue	Pharyngeal tubercle, median pharyngeal raphe	Constricts the pharynx	Vagus nerve by way of the pharyngeal plexus
Middle pharyngeal constrictor	Greater and lesser horns of hyoid bone, stylohyoid ligament	Median pharyngeal raphe	Constricts the pharynx	Vagus nerve by way of the pharyngeal plexus
Inferior pharyngeal constrictor	Arch of cricoid cartilage and oblique line of thyroid cartilage	Median pharyngeal raphe	Constricts the pharynx	Vagus nerve by way of the pharyngeal plexus. Lower part: external and recurrent larygneal nerves
Longitudinal Muscles				
Salpingopharyngeus	Cartilage of the auditory tube	Blends with the palatopharyngeus muscle in the lateral wall of pharynx	Elevates the pharynx in swallowing	Vagus nerve by way of the pharyngeal plexus
Palatopharyngeus	Posterior border of hard palate and the palatal aponeurosis	Pharyngobasilar fascia of lateral and posterior wall of pharynx, thyroid cartilage	Elevates the pharynx in swallowing	Vagus nerve by way of the pharyngeal plexus
Stylopharyngeus	Styloid process	Upper and posterior surface of thyroid cartilage (after blending with palatopharyngeus)	Elevates the pharynx in swallowing	Glossopharyngeal nerve

- The muscles of the pharynx include three pairs of **longitudinally arranged** muscles, which

  — Arise at the base of the skull and descend between the pharyngeal constrictor muscles and the pharyngobasilar fascia

  — Blend together in the pharyngeal wall and insert into the pharyngobasilar fascia and the thyroid cartilage

  — Together elevate and shorten the pharyngeal wall to assist in propelling food and drink when swallowing

- The **gap above** the **superior pharyngeal constrictor** muscle is closed by the **pharyngobasilar fascia** and is traversed by the auditory tube.

- The **gap between** the **superior constrictor** and the **middle constrictor** is traversed by the **stylopharyngeus muscle** and the **glossopharyngeal nerve.**

- The **lowest part** of the **inferior constrictor** arises from the **cricoid cartilage** and is often called the cricopharyngeus muscle. It is said to maintain a tonic contraction and function as a **sphincter** between the **pharynx** and **esophagus.** Innervation is from the **recurrent laryngeal nerve.**

- Innervation of the pharynx
  - *Pharyngeal plexus*
    - Provides most of the innervation to the pharynx
    - Lies in the **buccopharyngeal fascia** covering the **outer surface** of the **pharyngeal constrictor** muscles
    - Supplies the
      - **Muscles** of the **pharynx** except the **stylopharyngeus**
      - **Muscles** of the **palate** except the tensor veli palatini
      - **Mucosa** of the **pharynx** (except part of the roof, which is supplied by the pharyngeal branch of the maxillary nerve) and the cartilaginous portion of the **auditory tube**
    - Receives contributions from the pharyngeal branches of the
      - **Vagus nerve,** which provide SVE fibers to the muscles of the pharynx
      - **Glossopharyngeal nerve,** which carry **general visceral afferent (GVA)** fibers from the mucosa of the pharynx
      - **Superior cervical ganglion,** which **provide general visceral** efferent (GVE) and GVA fibers to the **blood vessels** and **glands** of the pharynx

- Blood supply of the pharynx
  - Is derived chiefly from the **ascending pharyngeal artery,** which
    - Is a small branch arising from the medial surface of the **external carotid artery** near its origin
    - Ascends between the pharynx and the internal carotid artery
  - Also is supplied regionally by the
    - Ascending palatine artery (from the facial artery)
    - Superior thyroid artery
    - Inferior thyroid artery

Pterygopalatine Fossa

- Is bounded
  - Anteriorly by the posterior surface of the maxilla
  - Posteriorly by the pterygoid process and greater wing of the sphenoid bone
  - Medially by the perpendicular plate of the palatine bone
  - Laterally is open through the pterygomaxillary fissure
  - Superiorly by the body of the sphenoid and the orbital process of the palatine bone
  - Inferiorly by the anterior and posterior walls, which meet to become continuous with the greater palatine canal.
- Communicates with the
  - **Orbit anteriorly through the inferior orbital fissure**
  - **Infratemporal fossa laterally through the pterygomaxillary fissure**
  - **Nasal cavity through the sphenopalatine foramen**

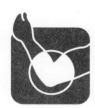

— **Middle cranial fossa** through the **foramen rotundum**
— **Oral cavity** (palate) through the **greater palatine canal**
— **Foramen lacerum** through the **pterygoid canal**
— **Nasopharynx** through the **palatovaginal canal**

- Contains the

— Third part of the maxillary artery
— Maxillary nerve
— Pterygopalatine ganglion

● **Pterygopalatine branches of the maxillary artery (see Fig. 8.13)**

— *Posterior superior alveolar artery*

- Arises as the maxillary artery passes through the pterygomaxillary fissure
- Descends on the posterior surface of the maxilla with the posterior superior alveolar nerve (from the maxillary nerve)
- Enters the maxilla to supply the **upper molars and premolars**

— *Infraorbital artery*

- Enters the orbit through the inferior orbital fissure
- Courses through the infraorbital groove and canal to reach the face through the **infraorbital foramen**
- Is distributed with the **infraorbital nerve** (from the maxillary nerve)
- Supplies the **lower eyelid,** the side of the **nose,** the skin of the **upper lip,** and the mucosa of the **mouth**
- While in the infraorbital canal gives rise to the **anterior** and **middle superior alveolar arteries,** which supply the molar and premolar teeth

— *Sphenopalatine artery*

- Passes medially to enter the **nasal cavity** through the **sphenopalatine foramen**
- Arises as a terminal branch of the maxillary artery (the other being the descending palatine artery)
- Enters the nasal cavity through the **sphenopalatine foramen** posterior to the middle concha
- Is the major supply to the nasal cavity and paranasal sinuses
- Is the most common source of serious bleeding in the posterior nasal cavity

— *Descending palatine artery*

- Arises as a terminal branch of the maxillary artery (the other being the sphenopalatine artery)
- Descends through the **pterygopalatine fossa** and the **palatine canal**
- In the palatine canal divides into **greater and lesser palatine arteries,** which exit through the greater and lesser palatine canals
- Supplies the **soft and hard palates**
- Note that the terminal branch of the **greater palatine artery**

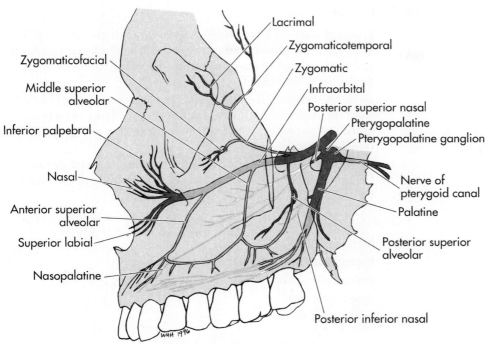

Fig. 8.29 The maxillary nerve.

ascends through the **incisive canal** to **anastomose** on the nasal septum with the septal branch of the **sphenopalatine artery.**

— *Pharyngeal artery*

- Passes posteriorly with the **pharyngeal nerve** (from the maxillary nerve) through the **palatovaginal canal**
- Supplies the roof of the nasal cavity and nasopharynx and the sphenoid sinus

— *Artery of the pterygoid canal*

- Passes posteriorly through the **pterygoid canal** with the nerve of the same name
- Supplies the pharynx and the auditory tube

● **Maxillary nerve (Fig. 8.29)**

- Is the **second division** of the **trigeminal nerve**
- Arises from the **semilunar** (trigeminal) **ganglion** in the floor of the middle cranial fossa
- Exits the skull through the **foramen rotundum** to enter the **pterygopalatine fossa**
- In the pterygopalatine fossa is joined to the **pterygopalatine ganglion** by communicating branches called **pterygopalatine nerves**
- Gives rise to branches that supply the nasal cavity and paranasal sinuses, the palate and upper jaw, the face and cheek, and the dura
- Contains **general visceral afferent** fibers from cell bodies in the **semilunar ganglion**

- Distributes

    — **General visceral efferent** fibers (parasympathetic postganglionic) from the **pterygopalatine ganglion** to the **lacrimal gland** and to the glands of the nasal cavity and palate (these are accompanied by **GVA** fibers from the facial nerve)

    — **General visceral efferent** fibers (sympathetic postganglionic) from the **superior cervical ganglion** to the **blood vessels** and **glands** of the nasal cavity and palate (these are accompanied by **GVA** fibers)

    — **Special visceral afferent** (taste) fibers from the **facial nerve** via the greater petrosal nerve and the nerve of the pterygoid canal to the **palate**

- **Trunk** gives rise to the

    — Meningeal branch
    — Pterygopalatine (communicating) nerves
    — Posterior superior alveolar nerves
    — Zygomatic nerve
    — Infraorbital nerve

- Pterygopalatine ganglion gives rise to the

    — Greater palatine nerve
    — Lesser palatine nerve
    — Posterior superior lateral nasal nerves
    — Posterior superior medial nasal nerves
    — Pharyngeal nerve
    — Orbital branches

— *Meningeal branch*

- Arises in the floor of the middle cranial fossa
- Supplies the dura of the middle cranial fossa and is distributed further along the course of the middle meningeal artery

— *Pterygopalatine (communicating) nerves*

- Leave the maxillary nerve in the pterygopalatine fossa to join the pterygopalatine ganglion
- Carry **GSA fibers** from the **maxillary nerve,** which pass through the ganglion **without synapse** to be distributed with the various branches arising from the ganglion
- Convey **postganglionic parasympathetic fibers** from the ganglion to the maxillary nerve for distribution to the **lacrimal gland** via the zygomatic and zygomaticotemporal nerves

— *Posterior superior alveolar nerves*

- Leave the pterygopalatine fossa through the pterygomaxillary fissure to enter the posterior surface of the maxilla
- Supply the upper molar teeth and gums, the maxillary sinus, and the cheek
- Contribute to the superior dental plexus

— *Zygomatic nerve*

- Enters the orbit through the inferior orbital fissure
- On the lateral wall of the orbit divides into **zygomaticotemporal** and **zygomaticofacial** branches
- **Zygomaticotemporal nerve**

    — Gives rise to a **communicating branch** to the **lacrimal nerve,** which conveys postganglionic parasympathetic fibers from the pterygopalatine ganglion to the **lacrimal gland**
    — Traverses the **zygomatic bone** and exits its posterior surface into the temporal fossa
    — Penetrates the temporal fascia to supply the skin of the **temporal region** above and lateral to the eye

- **Zygomaticofacial nerve**

    — Traverses the **zygomatic bone** and emerges onto the face at the lower lateral margin of the orbit
    — Supplies the skin of the face **lateral** to the orbit

— *Infraorbital nerve*

- Is a direct continuation of the **maxillary nerve**
- Enters the orbit through the **inferior orbital fissure**
- Traverses the floor of the orbit in the **infraorbital groove** and **canal**
- Emerges onto the face through the **infraorbital foramen**
- Supplies the **lower eyelid,** the side of the **nose,** the skin of the **upper lip,** and the mucosa of the **mouth**
- Gives rise to the

    — **Middle superior alveolar nerves,** which descend in the lateral wall of the maxillary sinus to supply the maxillary sinus and the upper premolar teeth and gums
    — **Anterior superior alveolar nerves** which descend in the anterior wall of the maxillary sinus to supply the maxillary sinus and the canine and incisor teeth and gums

— *Greater palatine nerve*

- Descends from the **pterygopalatine ganglion** to leave the pterygopalatine fossa through the **greater palatine canal**
- Emerges onto the palate through the **greater palatine foramen** to supply the mucosa of the **hard palate** and **gums**
- Gives rise to the **posterior inferior nasal nerves** while in the greater palatine canal

— *Lesser palatine nerve*

- Descends from the **pterygopalatine ganglion** to leave the pterygopalatine fossa through the **greater palatine canal**
- Emerges onto the palate through the **lesser palatine foramen** to supply the mucosa of the **soft palate**

— *Posterior superior nasal nerves*

- Pass medially from the pterygopalatine ganglion to enter the nasal cavity through the **sphenopalatine foramen**
- Include **lateral** and **medial** (septal) branches, which supply the mucosa of the nasal cavity
- The **nasopalatine nerve**

    — Is the largest of the medial posterior superior nasal nerves

    — Descends anteriorly on the nasal septum

    — Gives terminal branches, which pass through the **incisive canal** to supply the **hard palate** posterior to the incisors

— *Pharyngeal nerve*

- Passes posteriorly from the **pterygopalatine ganglion** to leave the pterygopalatine fossa through the **palatovaginal canal**
- Supplies the mucosa of the nasopharynx and sphenoid sinus

— *Orbital branches*

- Supply the periosteum of the orbit and the mucosa of the posterior ethmoid and sphenoid sinuses.

- **Pterygopalatine ganglion (see Fig. 8.29)**

    - Is one of the four parasympathetic ganglia of the head and contains the cell bodies of **postganglionic parasympathetic neurons**
    - Lies in the **pterygopalatine fossa** suspended from the maxillary nerve
    - Distributes parasympathetic fibers to the **lacrimal gland** and the **glands** of the **nasal cavity and palate**
    - Receives the

        — **Pterygopalatine nerves** (from the maxillary nerve) containing **general somatic afferent fibers,** which pass through the ganglion **without synapse** to be distributed with the various branches arising from the ganglion

        — **Nerve of the pterygoid canal** (the motor root) containing **preganglionic parasympathetic fibers** from the **facial nerve** for synapse in the ganglion

    - Is the site of synapse for the parasympathetic fibers but sympathetic and afferent fibers pass through without synapse

    — *Deep petrosal nerve*

    - The deep petrosal nerve arises in the **foramen lacerum** from the **internal carotid plexus.**
    - It joins the greater petrosal nerve in the foramen lacerum to form the nerve of the pterygoid canal.
    - It contains **postganglionic sympathetic** and accompanying **visceral afferent fibers** derived from the internal carotid plexus.
    - Remember that the cell bodies of the **postganglionic sympathetic neurons** are in the **superior cervical ganglion** and those of the associated **visceral afferent neurons** are in the **dorsal root ganglia** of the upper thoracic spinal nerves.

— *Greater petrosal nerve*

- Arises from the geniculate ganglion of the **facial nerve** within the facial canal
- Leaves the temporal bone through the **hiatus of the facial canal**
- Passes forward and medially in the floor of the **middle cranial fossa** and then descends into the foramen lacerum
- Joins the **deep petrosal nerve** to form the **nerve of the pterygoid canal**
- Contains

    — **Preganglionic parasympathetic fibers** from cell bodies in the **superior salivatory nucleus** for synapse in the **pterygopalatine ganglion**
    — Accompanying **general visceral afferent fibers** from cell bodies in the **geniculate ganglion**
    — **Special visceral afferent fibers** from cell bodies in the **geniculate ganglion** conveying **taste from the soft palate**

— *Nerve of the pterygoid canal*

- Arises in the foramen lacerum from the union of the **greater petrosal nerve** and the **deep petrosal nerve**
- Passes forward through the **pterygoid canal** to reach the **pterygopalatine ganglion**
- Contains the combined functional components of the **greater petrosal nerve** and the **deep petrosal nerve**

■ **Oral Cavity**

- Consists of the **vestibule** and the **oral cavity proper** (Fig. 8.30)
- **Vestibule**

    — Lies between the lips and cheeks externally and the teeth and gums internally
    — Is closed superiorly and inferiorly by the reflection of the mucosa from the inner to outer walls
    — **Opens** to the outside through the **oral fissure** between the lips
    — **Communicates** with the **oral cavity proper** behind the last molar tooth
    — Receives the opening of the **parotid duct** opposite the **upper second molar** tooth

- Oral cavity proper

    — Is bounded **anteriorly and laterally** by the **teeth and gums**
    — Is bounded **superiorly** by the **hard and soft palates**
    — Is bounded **inferiorly** by the **anterior two thirds of the tongue** and the surrounding **gutter** of the floor
    — **Communicates** posteriorly with the **pharynx** through the **oropharyngeal isthmus**

● Teeth

- Are of four types: incisors, canines, premolars, and molars

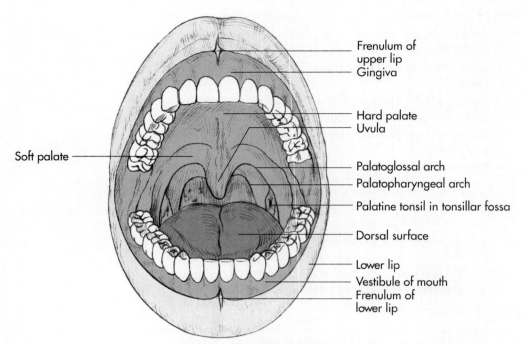

Fig. 8.30 Oral cavity and palatal arches.

- **Incisors**

  — Cut the food

  — Have a linear cutting edge, a chisel-shaped crown, and a single root

  — Are **eight** in number, four in the upper jaw and four in the lower jaw

  — Are referred to as **central incisors** (the medial two in each jaw) and **lateral** incisors (the two outer incisors in each jaw)

- **Canines**

  — Assist the incisors in cutting and tearing the food

  — Have a conical or cusplike crown and a single disproportionately large root

  — Are **four** in number, two in the upper jaw and two in the lower jaw

- **Premolars**

  — Assist in crushing the food

  — Are broad and have two cusps on the crown (thus they may be referred to as the bicuspids)

  — May have one or two roots

  — Are **eight** in number, four in the upper jaw and four in the lower jaw

— Are present only in the permanent dentition and not in the deciduous dentition

- Molars

    — Assist in chewing and grinding solid food
    — Increase in size from front to back
    — Have three to five cusps
    — Usually have three roots on the upper molars and two roots on the lower molars.
    — In the deciduous dentition are **eight** in number, four in the upper jaw and four in the lower jaw.
    — In the permanent dentition are **twelve** in number, six in the upper jaw and six in the lower jaw.
    — Note that the last molar is referred to as a "wisdom tooth" and its presence is variable.

— *Deciduous (primary) teeth*

    - Are also called milk teeth or baby teeth
    - Are 20 in number: **2 incisors, 1 canine,** and **2 molars** in each half jaw
    - Are smaller than permanent teeth
    - Erupt beginning with the **lower medial incisors** at about **6 months** of age and finishing with the **second molar** at about **2 years of age**
    - Are shed and replaced by the permanent teeth beginning at about 6 years and finishing at about 12 years of age

— *Permanent teeth*

    - There are typically 32 permanent teeth: **2 incisors, 1 canine, 2 premolars,** and **3 molars** in each **half jaw.**
    - Permanent teeth begin eruption at age 6, and all are present by age 12 except the last molar. ,
    - The last molar, the wisdom tooth, does not erupt until 18 to 20 years of age and may remain unerupted.

- Palate

    - Consists of the **bony palate** and the **soft palate**
    - Separates the **oral cavity** from the **nasal cavity**

    — *Bony palate (see Fig. 8.8)*

        - Is the **anterior two thirds** of the palate
        - Is formed by the

            — Palatine processes of the maxillae
            — Horizontal plates of the palatine bones

        - Contains the openings of the **incisive canal** anteriorly and the **greater and lesser palatine canals** posteriorly

    — *Soft palate*

        - Is a **fibromuscular fold** attached to the posterior border of the hard palate
        - Is the **posterior one third** of the palate

Table 8.8   *Muscles of the Palate*

Name	Origin	Insertion	Action	Innervation
Levator veli palatini	Apex of petrous temporal bone and the cartilaginous part of the auditory tube	Palatal aponeurosis	Elevates the soft palate	Vagus nerve by way of the pharyngeal plexus
Tensor veli palatini	Scaphoid fossa of the sphenoid bone and the cartilaginous part of the auditory tube	Palatal aponeurosis after hooking around the pterygoid hamulus	Tenses the soft palate	Nerve to the tensor veli palatini from the mandibular nerve
Musculus uvulae	Posterior nasal spine of the palatine bone and the palatal aponeurosis	Mucosa of the uvulae	Elevates the uvulae	Vagus nerve by way of the pharyngeal plexus
Palatoglossus	Palatal aponeurosis	Lateral surface of posterior tongue	Depresses the palate and narrows the oropharyngeal isthmus	Vagus nerve by way of the pharyngeal plexus
Palatopharyngeus	Posterior border of hard palate and the palatal aponeurosis	Pharyngobasilar fascia of lateral and posterior wall of pharynx, thyroid cartilage	Elevates the pharynx in swallowing	Vagus nerve by way of the pharyngeal plexus

- Projects posteriorly **between** the **nasopharynx** and the **oropharynx**
- Consists of the **palatal aponeurosis** and the **palatal muscles**
- Is continuous laterally with the **palatoglossal** and **palatopharyngeal** folds

— *Muscles of the palate (Table 8.8)*

— *Blood supply of the palate*

- Is derived from the **descending palatine artery** (from the maxillary artery) and the **ascending palatine artery** (from the facial artery)

Descending palatine artery

- Arises as a terminal branch from the **third** (pterygopalatine) part of the maxillary artery
- Descends through the **pterygopalatine fossa** and the **palatine canal**
- In the palatine canal divides into **greater and lesser palatine arteries** which exit through the greater and lesser palatine canals
- Supplies the **soft and hard palates**

Ascending palatine artery

- Arises from the **facial artery** deep to the posterior digastric muscle
- Ascends on the lateral wall of the upper pharynx
- Arches medially over the **upper border** of the **superior pharyngeal constrictor**

- Passes onto the palate **between** the **tensor veli palatini** and the **levator veli palatini**

— *Nerves of the palate*

  - Include the **greater palatine, lesser palatine,** and **nasopalatine** nerves
  - Contain

    — **Afferent (GSA)** fibers from the **maxillary nerve**
    — **Postganglionic parasympathetic (GVE)** fibers from the **pterygopalatine ganglion**
    — **Taste fibers (SVA)** from cell bodies in the **geniculate ganglion** of the **facial nerve** (by way of the greater petrosal nerve and the nerve of the pterygoid canal)

  Greater palatine nerve

  - Descends from the **pterygopalatine ganglion** to leave the pterygopalatine fossa through the **palatine canal**
  - Emerges onto the palate through the **greater palatine foramen** to supply the mucosa of the **hard palate** and **gums**

  Lesser palatine nerve

  - Descends from the **pterygopalatine ganglion** to leave the pterygopalatine fossa through the **palatine canal**
  - Emerges onto the palate through the **lesser palatine foramen** to supply the mucosa of the **soft palate**

  Nasopalatine nerve

  - Is the largest of the posterior superior medial nasal nerves
  - Descends anteriorly and inferiorly on the nasal septum
  - Passes through the **incisive canal** to emerge onto the **hard palate**

- **Tongue (Fig. 8.31)**

  - Is a mass of **skeletal muscle** covered by a **mucosa**
  - Lies partially in the **oral cavity proper** (the anterior two thirds) and partially in the **oropharynx** (the posterior one third)
  - Is attached by muscles to the mandible, hyoid bone, styloid process, palate, and pharynx
  - Functions in chewing, swallowing, speech, and taste
  - Four surfaces

    — **Tip and margin,** which rest against the lower teeth and gums
    — **Dorsum,** which faces the palate and is divided into **oral** and **pharyngeal** parts by the V-shaped **sulcus terminalis**
    — **Inferior surface,** which lies below the tip and margin entirely within the oral cavity
    — **Root,** which is the attachment to the floor of the mouth

  - **Oral part of the dorsal surface**

    — Is the two thirds lying **anterior** to the **sulcus terminalis**
    — Is **derived** from the **first branchial arch** and is innervated by its nerve, the **trigeminal nerve,** via the mandibular division

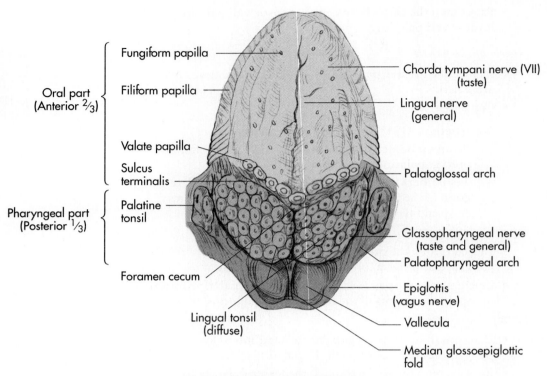

Oral part
(Anterior ⅔)

Fungiform papilla

Filiform papilla

Valate papilla

Sulcus
terminalis

Pharyngeal part
(Posterior ⅓)

Palatine
tonsil

Foramen cecum

Lingual tonsil
(diffuse)

Chorda tympani nerve (VII)
(taste)

Lingual nerve
(general)

Palatoglossal arch

Glossopharyngeal nerve
(taste and general)

Palatopharyngeal arch

Epiglottis
(vagus nerve)

Vallecula

Median glossoepiglottic
fold

Fig. 8.31 Dorsal view of the tongue.

— Is covered by numerous **filiform papillae** and fewer **fungiform papillae,** which bear **taste buds**

— Has a **row** of large, round **vallate papillae** with taste buds, which lies **anterior and parallel** to the **sulcus terminalis**

• **Pharyngeal part of the dorsal surface**

— Is the one third lying **posterior** to the **sulcus terminalis**

— Is **derived** from the **third branchial arch** and is innervated by its nerve, the **glossopharyngeal nerve**

— Is devoid of papillae

— Is covered by aggregations of lymphoid tissue forming the **lingual tonsil**

— Reflects onto the epiglottis as the median and lateral **glossoepiglottic folds**

• **Foramen cecum**

— Is a blind pouch lying at the **apex** of the **sulcus terminalis**

— Marks the site of **origin** of the **thyroid diverticulum** (the thyroglossal duct)

• **Frenulum**

— Is the midline **mucosal fold,** which connects the inferior surface of the tongue to the floor of the mouth

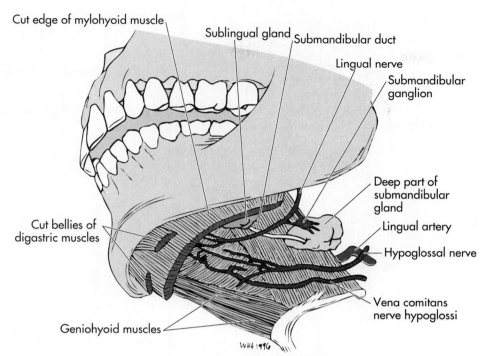

Fig. 8.32 The submandibular region.

— *Sublingual gland (Fig. 8.32)*

- Lies below the tongue on the upper surface of the **mylohyoid muscle** beneath the mucosa of the floor of the mouth
- Is related laterally to the **sublingual fossa** of the mandible
- Has numerous small **ducts,** which **open** onto the floor of the mouth over the **sublingual fold**
- Receives **postganglionic parasympathetic** innervation from **submandibular ganglion**
- Is supplied by the **sublingual artery** (from the lingual artery)

— *Muscles of the tongue (Fig. 8.33, Table 8.9)*

- Consist of **intrinsic** and **extrinsic** muscles
- Intrinsic muscles

  — Lie in the longitudinal, transverse, and vertical planes within the body of the tongue

- Extrinsic muscles

  — Have origins from the mandible, hyoid bone, and styloid process
  — Are described in Table 8.9

- Are derived from **occipital somites,** which migrate to their definitive position carrying the somitic nerves (the hypoglossal nerve) with them

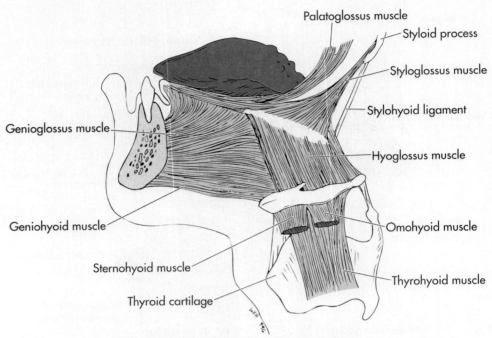

Fig. 8.33 Extrinsic muscles of the tongue.

Table 8.9 *Extrinsic Muscles of the Tongue*

Name	Origin	Insertion	Action	Innervation
Genioglossus	Superior part of the mental spine of the mandible	Fan out to blend with the intrinsic muscles from the root to the tip; body of hyoid bone	Depresses and protrudes the tongue; acting unilaterally deviates the protruded tongue to the opposite side	Hypoglossal nerve
Hyoglossus	Body and greater horn of the hyoid bone	Side of the tongue posteriorly	Depresses the tongue	Hypoglossal nerve
Styloglossus	Styloid process and stylohyoid ligament	Blends with the hyoglossus on the side of the tongue	Elevates and retracts the tongue	Hypoglossal nerve
Palatoglossus	Palatal aponeurosis	Lateral surface of posterior tongue	Depresses the palate, elevates the tongue, and narrows the oropharyngeal isthmus	Vagus nerve by way of the pharyngeal plexus

— *Innervation of the tongue*
Nerve supply of the muscles

• All of the intrinsic and extrinsic muscles of the tongue (except the palatoglossus) are innervated by the **hypoglossal nerve.**

• Note that the division of the tongue into an anterior two thirds and a posterior one third applies only to the mucosal covering and not to the musculature.

Mucosa of the anterior two thirds

- Receives **general somatic afferent fibers** from the **lingual nerve** (from the mandibular nerve)
- Receives **taste fibers** (SVA) from the **facial nerve** by way of the chorda tympani and lingual nerves

Mucosa of the posterior one third

- Receives **general visceral afferent fibers** from the **glossopharyngeal nerve**
- Receives **taste fibers** (SVA) from the **glossopharyngeal nerve**

Lingual nerve

- Arises from the posterior division of the **mandibular nerve** in the infratemporal fossa
- Descends anteriorly on the lateral surface of the **medial pterygoid** and **hyoglossus** muscles deep to the ramus of the mandible
- On the hyoglossus muscle **loops** laterally, inferiorly, and then medially **around** the **submandibular duct**
- Divides into **terminal branches** to supply the **mucosa** of the **anterior two thirds** of the tongue
- Is **joined** by communicating branches to the **submandibular ganglion**
- Is joined by the **chorda tympani,** which carries

  — **Preganglionic parasympathetic fibers** from the **facial nerve** to synapse in the **submandibular ganglion**
  — **Taste fibers** (SVA) from the **facial nerve** (with cell bodies in the geniculate ganglion) to be distributed to the **anterior two thirds of the tongue**

- Supplies **general somatic afferent** innervation to the **anterior two thirds** of the tongue
- Distributes **postganglionic parasympathetic fibers** from the **submandibular ganglion** to the **sublingual salivary gland** and the scattered small glands of the anterior two thirds of the tongue

Submandibular ganglion (see Fig. 8.32)

- Is one of the four parasympathetic ganglia of the head and contains the cell bodies of **postganglionic parasympathetic neurons**
- Lies in the **floor of the mouth** lateral to the hyoglossus muscle **suspended** from the **lingual nerve**
- Gives rise to **postganglionic parasympathetic** fibers to the **submandibular** and **sublingual** salivary glands and to small glands scattered on the anterior two thirds of the tongue
- Receives **preganglionic parasympathetic fibers** from the **facial nerve** via the **chorda tympani** and **lingual nerve** for synapse in the ganglion
- Remember that only the parasympathetic fibers synapse in the submandibular ganglion. Sympathetic and afferent fibers pass through the ganglion without synapse.

Glossopharyngeal nerve

- Exits the skull through the **jugular foramen**

- Descends on the wall of the pharynx between the internal and external carotid arteries
- Passes **between** the **superior** and **middle** pharyngeal constrictor muscles
- Passes through the **tonsillar bed** to reach the **posterior tongue**
- Gives rise to

    — Pharyngeal branches to the pharyngeal plexus
    — Motor branch to the stylopharyngeus muscle
    — Lingual branches to the posterior one third of the tongue

- Contains

    — **General visceral afferent** fibers to the middle ear, auditory tube, pharynx, palatine tonsils, and the posterior one third of the tongue
    — **Special visceral efferent** fibers to the stylopharyngeus muscle
    — Taste fibers (SVA) to the posterior one third of the tongue

Hypoglossal nerve (see Fig. 8.32)

- Exits the skull through the hypoglossal canal
- Descends anteriorly in the neck between the **internal carotid artery** and the **internal jugular vein**
- Passes anteriorly deep to the posterior belly of the digastric and then **between** the **hyoglossus** and **mylohyoid** muscles
- On the **lateral surface** of the **hyoglossus** muscle lies **inferior** to the deep part of the **submandibular gland,** the **submandibular duct,** and the **lingual nerve**
- Divides into its **terminal branches** over the **genioglossus muscle** anterior to the hyoglossus
- Contains GSE fibers only
- Supplies all of the **intrinsic and extrinsic muscles** of the tongue **except** the **palatoglossus** (supplied by the vagus via the pharyngeal plexus)

— ***Blood supply of the tongue***
Lingual artery (Fig. 8.34)

- Arises from the **external carotid artery** at the level of the **greater horn of the hyoid** bone
- Passes deep to the **hyoglossus** muscle to reach the tongue
- Is accompanied by the **deep lingual vein**
- Is divided into **three parts** by the hyoglossus muscle
- Near its origin is crossed superficially by the **hypoglossal nerve**
- Gives rise to the

    — **Suprahyoid branch,** which passes across the upper margin of the hyoid bone to the midline
    — **Dorsal lingual arteries,** which supply the dorsum of the tongue and the palatine tonsil
    — **Deep lingual artery,** which is the terminal branch of the lingual artery passing to the tip of the tongue

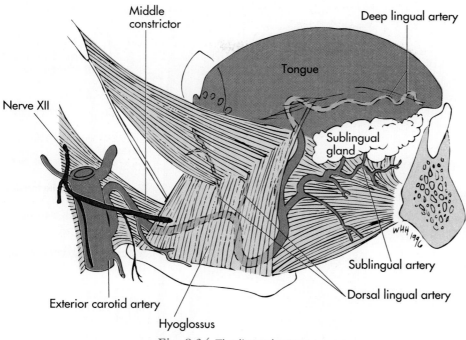

Fig. 8.34 The lingual artery.

— **Sublingual artery,** which supplies the sublingual gland and the floor of the mouth

■ Nasal Cavity and Paranasal Sinuses

● **External nose**

• Consists of the

— **Alae,** which are the flared parts lateral to the nares
— **Dorsum,** which is the ridge passing from the tip of the nose to the forehead
— **Bridge,** which is the root of the nose where it meets the forehead

• Has **bony skeleton** formed by the

— Nasal bones
— Frontal processes of the maxillae
— Nasal part of the frontal bone

• Has a **cartilaginous skeleton** consisting of the

— Septal cartilage
— Lateral nasal cartilages
— Alar cartilages

● **Nasal cavity (Fig. 8.35)**

• Is divided into **two cavities** by the **nasal septum**
• Extends from the **naris** (nostril) anteriorly to the **choana** posteriorly
• Is part of the **respiratory system** communicating posteriorly with the **nasopharynx**

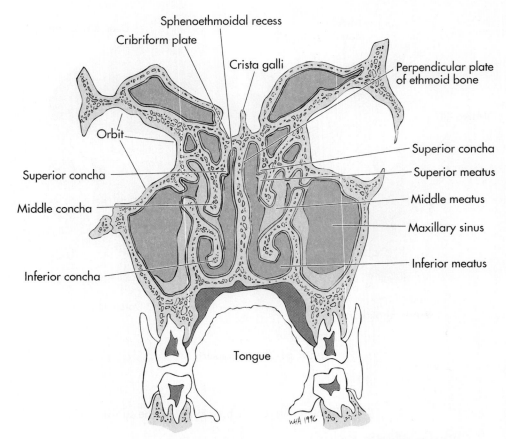

Fig. 8.35 Coronal section through the nasal cavity and paranasal sinuses.

- Consists of a **vestibule**, an **olfactory region**, and a **respiratory region**
- Extends posterior to the **superior nasal concha** as the **sphenoethmoidal recess**
- **Vestibule**

    — Is the dilation adjacent to the nostril
    — Is lined by **skin** provided with **hairs** and **sebaceous glands**
    — Functions to **filter** the incoming air

- **Olfactory region**

    — Lies in the **upper nasal cavity** below the **cribriform plate** of the ethmoid bone
    — Extends onto the **superior nasal concha** laterally and onto the **nasal septum** medially
    — Is covered by **olfactory mucosa** containing the receptor organs and neurons that convey the sense of smell (olfaction)

- **Respiratory region**

    — Includes most of the nasal cavity
    — Is covered by **respiratory mucosa,** which is highly vascular and glandular

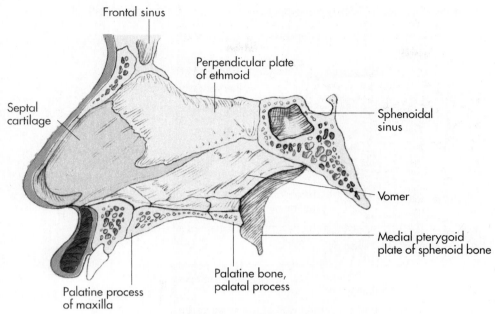

Fig. 8.36 The nasal septum.

— Is lined by **respiratory epithelium** (ciliated pseudostratified columnar epithelium)
— Functions to **warm and humidify** the incoming air

• Has a **roof**, a **floor**, a **medial wall**, and a **lateral wall**

• **Roof**

  — Is formed from anterior to posterior by the nasal, frontal, ethmoid, and sphenoid bones
  — Is related anteriorly to the **anterior cranial fossa** and the **olfactory nerves and bulb** and posteriorly to the **body of the sphenoid** and the **sphenoid sinus**

• **Floor**

  — Separates the nasal cavity from the oral cavity
  — Is formed by the hard palate
  — Consists of the **palatine process of the maxilla** anteriorly and the **horizontal plate of the palatine bone** posteriorly

• **Medial wall** (Fig. 8.36)

  — Is formed by the **nasal septum,** which separates the two nasal cavities
  — Consists of the **septal cartilage,** the **perpendicular plate of the ethmoid bone,** and the **vomer**

• **Lateral wall**

  — Is a complicated structure consisting of parts of the lacrimal, ethmoid, maxillary, palatine, sphenoid, and inferior conchal bones

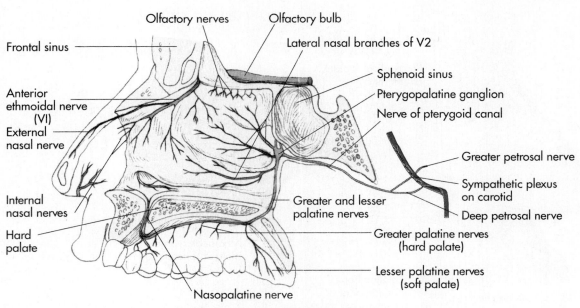

Fig. 8.37 Innervation of the lateral wall of the nasal cavity.

— Includes the superior, middle, and inferior **nasal cochae and meatuses**

— *Nasal conchae (see Fig. 8.35)*

  • The nasal conchae lie on the **lateral wall** of the nasal cavity.

  • They are thin, curved **bony processes** covered by **respiratory mucosa.**

  • They function to **increase the surface area** of the respiratory epithelium to facilitate **warming** and **humidifying** of the **inhaled air.**

  • There are usually three: a **superior, middle,** and **inferior.**

  • The superior and **middle** nasal conchae are processes of the **ethmoid bone.**

  • The **inferior** nasal concha is a **separate bone.**

— *Nasal meatuses (see Fig. 8.35)*

  • The nasal meatuses lie below and lateral to each of the nasal conchae.

  • The **superior nasal meatus** receives the opening of the posterior ethmoidal air cells.

  • The **middle nasal meatus** receives the openings of the frontal and maxillary sinuses and the anterior and middle ethmoid air cells.

  • The **inferior nasal meatus** receives the opening of the nasolacrimal duct.

— *Innervation of the nasal cavity (Fig. 8.37)*

  • **General somatic afferent** innervation to the mucosa of the nasal cavity is supplied by branches of **ophthalmic** and **maxillary nerves.**

- **Parasympathetic innervation** (GVE) to the **glands** of the nasal cavity is derived from the **facial nerve** via the **pterygopalatine ganglion** and is distributed through the branches of the maxillary nerve and pterygopalatine ganglion.
- **Sympathetic innervation** (GVE) to the **blood vessels** of the nasal cavity is derived from the **superior cervical ganglion** and is distributed through the branches of the maxillary nerve and the pterygopalatine ganglion and also through the perivascular plexuses.
- The sense of smell (olfaction) is conveyed through the olfactory nerves.

Branches of the maxillary nerve

- **Posterior superior lateral nasal nerves**

    — Arise from the **pterygopalatine ganglion** in the pterygopalatine fossa
    — Enter the **nasal cavity** through the **sphenopalatine foramen**
    — Supply the posterior and superior portion of the lateral wall of the nasal cavity

- **Posterior inferior lateral nasal nerves**

    — Arise from the **greater palatine nerve** as it descends in the greater palatine canal
    — Supply the posterior and inferior portion of the lateral wall of the nasal cavity

- **Posterior superior medial nasal nerves**

    — Arise from the **pterygopalatine ganglion** in the pterygopalatine fossa
    — Enter the **nasal cavity** through the **sphenopalatine foramen**
    — Supply the posterior and superior portion of the nasal septum

- **Nasopalatine nerve**

    — Is the largest of the posterior superior medial nasal nerves
    — Descends anteriorly and inferiorly on the nasal septum
    — Passes through the **incisive canal** to emerge onto the **hard palate**
    — Supplies the **nasal septum** and the **hard palate** behind the upper incisors

Branches of the ophthalmic nerve

- **The internal nasal nerve** provides GSA innervation to the mucosa of both the septum and the lateral wall of the **anterior part** of the nasal cavity. It is a branch of the **anterior ethmoidal nerve** after it leaves the anterior cranial fossa and enters the nasal cavity through the nasal slit.
- The **external nasal nerve** is the other terminal branch of the anterior ethmoidal nerve. It exits the nasal cavity between the nasal bone and septal cartilage to supply the dorsum of the nose.

Olfactory nerves (see Fig. 8.37)

- Arise from neuron cell bodies in the **olfactory mucosa** of the nasal cavity
- Consist of collections of axons that pass through the cribriform plate to synapse in the olfactory bulb
- Convey the sense of **smell** (olfaction)
- Are classified functionally as **special visceral afferent** (SVA) neurons

— *Blood supply of the nasal cavity*

- The blood supply of the nasal cavity is derived mostly from the **sphenopalatine** and **anterior ethmoidal** arteries but also from the greater palatine artery, the superior labial artery, and the posterior ethmoidal artery.
- **Nosebleed** (epistaxis) most often occurs from the **anterior part** of the **nasal septum** anterior to the inferior concha. This is the area where the distribution of the septal branches of the **sphenopalatine** and **superior labial** arteries meet and is referred to as **Kiesselbach's area.**

Sphenopalatine artery

- Arises in the pterygopalatine fossa as a **terminal branch** of the **maxillary artery**
- Enters the nasal cavity through the **sphenopalatine foramen** posterior to the middle concha
- Terminates promptly by dividing into lateral and medial **posterior nasal arteries**
- Supplies the posterior part of the nasal septum and the lateral nasal wall
- Is the most common source of serious bleeding in the posterior nasal cavity

Anterior ethmoidal artery

- Arises from the **ophthalmic artery** in the **medial orbit**
- Traverses the **anterior ethmoidal canal** and the **anterior cranial fossa** before entering the **nasal cavity** through the **nasal slit**
- Divides into medial and lateral branches, which supply the **anterior part** of the nasal **septum** and the **lateral nasal wall**

— *Paranasal sinuses (see Fig. 8.35)*

- Are **outgrowths** of the **nasal cavity** and retain a communication for drainage into the nasal cavity
- Are lined by a **mucoperiosteum** covered by **respiratory epithelium** continuous with that of the nasal cavity
- Are innervated in general by the **maxillary** and **ophthalmic** nerves
- Function to
  - Reduce the weight of the skull
  - Serve as resonators for sound production
  - Warm and humidify the inspired air

Maxillary sinus

- Is the largest of the paranasal sinuses and is present at birth
- Lies within the **body of the maxilla**
- Drains into the **middle meatus** of the nasal cavity through the **semilunar hiatus**
- Is supplied by the **superior alveolar** and **infraorbital nerves** and arteries
- **Roof**
    — Is the **floor** of the **orbit**
    — Contains the **infraorbital groove** and **canal**
- **Floor**
    — Lies against the **alveolar process** of the maxilla
    — Contains **elevations** produced by the **roots** of a variable number of **teeth**
- **Posterior wall**
    — Forms the **infratemporal** surface of the maxilla
- **Anterior wall**
    — Lies below the infraorbital margin of the orbit
    — Contains the **roots** of the **premolar** and **canine** teeth
- **Medial wall**
    — Is the thin bone forming the **lateral wall** of the **nasal cavity**
    — Contains the opening of the sinus into the nasal cavity
- **Lateral wall**
    — Lies in the zygomatic process of the maxilla

- Note that **maxillary sinusitis** is frequently accompanied by a toothache because of the relationship of the roots of the upper teeth to the maxillary sinus.

Sphenoid sinus

- Lies within the **body of the sphenoid bone**
- Drains into the nasal cavity through the **sphenoethmoidal recess**
- Is divided into **left** and **right** sinuses by a deviated **bony septum**
- Is supplied by the **lateral posterior superior nasal nerves** (from the maxillary nerve), the **lateral posterior nasal arteries** (from the sphenopalatine artery), and the **posterior ethmoidal nerve and artery** (from the ophthalmic artery)
- Is related
    — **Superiorly** to the **hypophyseal fossa** and the **optic nerve** and **chiasm**
    — **Inferiorly** to the **nasal cavity** and **nasopharynx**
    — **Anteriorly** to the **nasal cavity**

      — **Posteriorly** to the **brain stem** (pons) in the posterior cranial fossa

      — **Laterally** to the **cavernous sinus** and **internal carotid artery**

Ethmoid sinus

- Lies within the ethmoid bone
- Consists of numerous ethmoid cells grouped together as **anterior, middle,** and **posterior** ethmoid cells
- Is related

      — **Medially** to the **nasal cavity**

      — **Laterally** to the **orbit**

      — **Superiorly** to the **anterior cranial fossa**

- **Anterior ethmoid cells**

      — Open into the infundibulum of the middle meatus

      — Are supplied by the anterior ethmoidal nerve and artery

- **Middle ethmoid cells**

      — Open onto or above the ethmoid bulla of the middle meatus

      — Form the ethmoid bulla of the middle meatus

      — Are supplied by the anterior ethmoidal nerve and artery

- **Posterior ethmoid cells**

      — Open into the superior meatus

      — Have the same nerve and blood supply as the sphenoid sinus

Frontal sinus

- Lies in the squamous and orbital parts of the **frontal bone**
- Is a paired sinus of highly variable size
- Is often considered to be a large anterior ethmoid cell that has invaded the frontal bone
- Is related

      — **Anteriorly** to the **forehead**

      — **Posteriorly** and **superiorly** to the **anterior cranial fossa**

      — **Inferiorly** to the roof of the **orbit**

- Opens by way of the **frontonasal duct** into the **ethmoidal infundibulum of the middle meatus**
- Is supplied by the **supratrochlear** and **supraorbital** nerves and arteries

■ Larynx

- Opens and closes the airway during

      — Swallowing

      — Coughing and sneezing

      — Fixation of the thoracic wall in powerful movements of the upper limb and trunk muscles

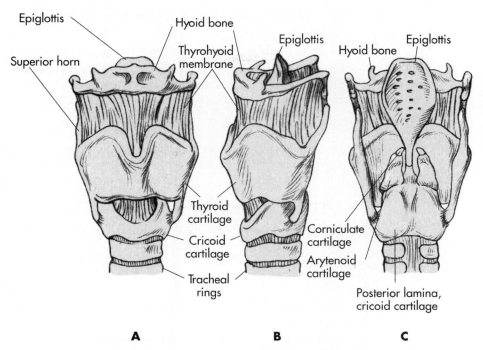

Fig. 8.38 Cartilages of the larynx. **A,** Anterior view. **B,** Lateral view. **C,** Posterior view.

- Regulates the passage of air during

  — Phonation (speech)
  — Normal variations in inspiration and expiration

● **Laryngeal skeleton (Fig. 8.38)**

  - Is a cartilaginous framework that is firmly anchored to the hyoid bone
  - Moves up or down with movement of the hyoid bone
  - Consists of the paired arytenoid, corniculate, and cuneiform cartilages and the unpaired thyroid, cricoid, and epiglottic cartilages

  — *Thyroid cartilage*

    - Is the largest of the laryngeal cartilages
    - Is connected

      — **Superiorly** to the **hyoid bone** by way of the **thyrohyoid membrane**
      — **Inferiorly** to the **cricoid cartilage** by way of the **cricothyroid joint** and the **cricothyroid membrane**

    - Consists of paired **laminae,** each of which has a **superior horn** and an **inferior horn**
    - **Laminae**

      — Meet in the midline anteriorly but diverge posteriorly forming the shape of an **open shield**
      — Meet anteriorly and superiorly to form the V-shaped **superior thyroid notch**

— Meet at a 90° angle in the **male** and a 120° angle in the **female**

— In the **male** form a midline **laryngeal prominence**

— On their outer surface have an **oblique line** for attachment of the inferior pharyngeal constrictor, sternothyroid, and thyrohyoid muscles

- The **superior horn** (cornua)

    — Is connected to the greater horn of the hyoid bone by the **thyrohyoid ligament,** a lateral thickening of the thyrohyoid membrane

- The **inferior horn** (cornua)

    — Articulates with the **cricoid cartilage** at the synovial cricothyroid joint

— *Cricoid cartilage*

- Is an unpaired hyaline cartilage
- Is **ring shaped** having a narrow **anterior arch** and a wide **posterior lamina**
- Lies at the level of the **sixth cervical vertebra**
- Is connected

    — **Superiorly** to the **thyroid cartilage** by way of the **cricothyroid joint** and the **cricothyroid membrane**

    — **Inferiorly** to the **first tracheal ring** by way of the **cricotracheal ligament**

- Articulates with the **inferior horn** of the **thyroid cartilage** at the **cricothyroid joint**
- Articulates on the **lamina** with the paired **arytenoid cartilages** at the **cricoarytenoid joints**

— *Arytenoid cartilage*

- Is a paired hyaline cartilage
- Is shaped like a three-sided pyramid
- Sits on the superior surface of the cricoid lamina
- Has an **apex,** which

    — Is directed superiorly

    — Supports the **corniculate cartilage** within the **aryepiglottic fold**

- Has a **base,** which

    — Is directed inferiorly

    — Forms a **synovial joint** with the lamina of the **cricoid cartilage**

- Has a **muscular process,** which

    — Extends **laterally** from the base

    — Provides attachment for the **lateral cricoarytenoid, posterior cricoarytenoid,** and **thyroarytenoid** muscles

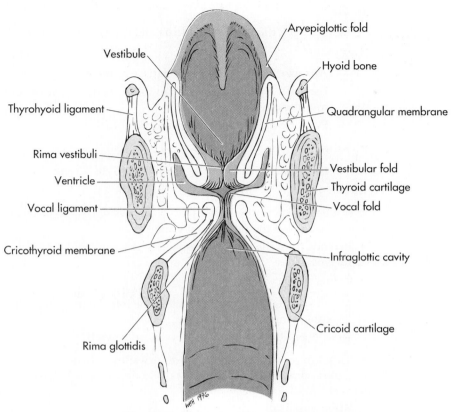

Fig. 8.39 Coronal section of the larynx.

- Has a **vocal process,** which

  — Extends **anteriorly** from the base
  — Provides attachment for the **vocal ligament**

— *Epiglottic cartilage*
  - Is a leaf-shaped cartilaginous plate
  - Lies posterior to the root of the tongue and anterior and superior to the laryngeal aditus
  - Is **attached** at its narrow **stalk** to the posterior surface of the **thyroid cartilage** at the union of the laminae

— *Corniculate cartilage*
  - Is a paired elastic cartilage that rests on the apex of the arytenoid cartilage
  - Lies within the aryepiglottic fold

— *Cuneiform cartilage*
  - Is a paired elastic cartilage that lies in the aryepiglottic fold superior to the corniculate cartilage

● **Laryngeal cavity and folds (Fig. 8.39)**

- The laryngeal cavity is divided into three distinct parts, the **vestibule,** the **ventricle,** and the **infraglottic cavity,** by the **vestibular folds** and **ventricular folds.**

— *Vestibule*

- Lies between the **laryngeal aditus** and the **vestibular** folds
- Is bounded

  — **Anteriorly** by the posterior surface of the **epiglottis**
  — **Laterally** by the **aryepiglottic folds** and the **quadrangular membrane**
  — **Posteriorly** by the **interarytenoid fold**

- **Aditus**

  — Is the **entrance** from the pharynx into the larynx

— *Vestibular fold*

- Is a paired transverse fold lying on the side of the larynx
- Is often called the **false vocal chord**
- Extends from the thyroid cartilage to the arytenoid cartilage above the vocal fold
- Contains the

  — **Vestibular ligament,** which is the inferior margin of the **quadrangular membrane**
  — Upper fibers of the **thyroarytenoid muscle**

- Closes to protect the airway during swallowing and during forced expiration against a closed airway (straining as in Valsalva's maneuver)
- **Rima vestibuli**

  — Is the space between the paired vestibular folds

— *Ventricle*

- Is a boat-shaped depression extending laterally **between** the **vestibular fold** and the **vocal fold**

- **Saccule**

  — Is an anterior and superior **evagination** of the **ventricle**
  — Is variable in size and may extend through the thyrohyoid membrane
  — Contains numerous glands, the secretions of which **lubricate** the **vocal fold**

— *Ventricular fold*

- Is also called the **vocal fold** or the **true vocal chord**
- Lies inferior to the vestibular fold
- Extends between the **thyroid cartilage** and the **vocal process** of the arytenoid cartilage
- Contains the

  — **Vocal ligament**
  — **Vocalis** portion of the thyroarytenoid muscle

- Functions to

  — Control the flow of air through the rima glottidis
  — Produce the sounds of **speech**

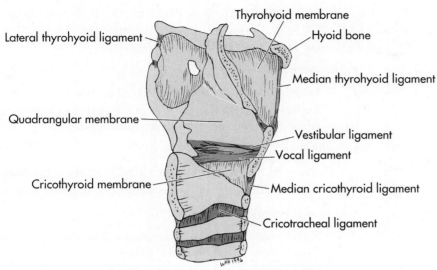

Lateral thyrohyoid ligament

Thyrohyoid membrane

Hyoid bone

Median thyrohyoid ligament

Quadrangular membrane

Vestibular ligament

Vocal ligament

Cricothyroid membrane

Median cricothyroid ligament

Cricotracheal ligament

Fig. 8.40 Membranes and ligaments of the larynx.

- **Rima glottidis**

    — Is the interval **between** the paired **vocal folds**
    — Is the narrowest part of the laryngeal cavity
    — Opens and closes to regulate the passage of air

- Note that **obstruction** of the laryngeal airway at the **rima glottidis** may result from **aspirated food** such as a piece of meat or from **edema** in the mucosa resulting from an **allergic response**.

— *Infraglottic cavity*

    - Lies between the **vocal fold** and the **lower border** of the **cricoid cartilage**
    - Is continuous inferiorly with the trachea
    - Is related **anteriorly** to the **cricothyroid membrane**
    - Note that an **emergency airway** made through the **cricothyroid membrane** will enter the airway **below the vocal folds** where obstruction of the airway most commonly occurs.

- Ligaments and membranes of the larynx (Fig. 8.40)

— *Thyrohyoid membrane*

    - Is a tough, fibrous membrane that **connects** the upper border of the **thyroid cartilage** to the lower border of the **hyoid bone**
    - Is pierced by the **internal laryngeal nerve** and **superior laryngeal artery** (from the superior thyroid artery)
    - Is thickened in midline to form the **median thyrohyoid ligament**
    - **Lateral thyrohyoid ligament**

        — Is the thickened posterior margin of the thyrohyoid membrane
        — Connects greater horn of the thyroid cartilage with the greater horn of the hyoid bone

—— May contain a small cartilaginous nodule, the **cartilago triticea**

— *Cricothyroid membrane*

- Is attached

    —— **Inferiorly** to the arch of the **cricoid cartilage**
    —— **Superiorly** to the deep surface of the **thyroid cartilage** and to the vocal process of the **arytenoid cartilage**

- Is thickened

    —— Along its **free upper border** to form the **vocal ligament**
    —— In the **midline** to form the **median cricothyroid ligament**

- **Conus elasticus**

    —— Is that part of the **cricothyroid membrane** which extends upward deep to the thyroid cartilage
    —— Lies **between** the **mucous membrane** and the **thyroarytenoid muscle**
    —— Has a free border, which forms the **vocal ligament**

— *Vocal ligament*

- Extends between the deep surface of the **thyroid cartilage** and the **vocal process** of the **arytenoid cartilage**
- Is the thickened free border of the **conus elasticus** portion of the cricothyroid membrane

— *Quadrangular membrane*

- Connects the **arytenoid cartilage** and the **epiglottic cartilage**
- Lies in the **lateral wall** of the **vestibule** separating it from the piriform recess
- **Vestibular ligament**

    —— Is the free **lower border** of the **quadrangular membrane**
    —— Lies in the **vestibular fold**

● **Intrinsic muscles of the larynx (Table 8.10)**

● **Innervation of the larynx**

— *Superior laryngeal nerve*

- Arises from the **vagus nerve** at the level of the **inferior vagal ganglion**
- Descends on the lateral wall of the pharynx to divide above the level of the hyoid bone into the **internal laryngeal nerve** and **external laryngeal nerve**

— *Internal laryngeal nerve*

- Arises from the **superior laryngeal nerve** above the level of the hyoid bone
- Pierces the thyrohyoid membrane along with the superior laryngeal artery (from the superior thyroid artery)
- Descends deep to the mucosa of the **piriform recess**
- Supplies the **laryngeal mucosa above the level of the vocal fold** and also the mucosa of the **piriform recess** and **valleculae**

Table 8.10 *Intrinsic Muscles of the Larynx*

NAME	ORIGIN	INSERTION	ACTION	INNERVATION
Cricothyroid	External surface of arch of the cricoid cartilage	Lower border of lamina and inferior horn of thyroid cartilage	Tenses and lengthens the vocal ligament by tilting the thyroid cartilage forward	Vagus nerve by way of the external laryngeal nerve
Posterior cricoarytenoid	Posterior surface of the cricoid lamina	Muscular process of the arytenoid cartilage	Abducts the vocal fold by laterally rotating the arytenoid cartilage	Vagus nerve by way of the inferior laryngeal nerve
Lateral cricoarytenoid	Upper border of the arch of the cricoid cartilage	Muscular process of the arytenoid cartilage	Adducts the vocal fold by medially rotating the arytenoid cartilage	Vagus nerve by way of the inferior laryngeal nerve
Transverse arytenoid	Posterior surface of the arytenoid cartilage	Posterior surface of the opposite arytenoid cartilage	Adducts the vocal folds by pulling the arytenoid cartilages together	Vagus nerve by way of the inferior laryngeal nerve
Oblique arytenoid	Muscular process of the arytenoid cartilage	Apex of the opposite arytenoid cartilage	Adducts the vocal folds by pulling the arytenoid cartilages together	Vagus nerve by way of the inferior laryngeal nerve
Thyroarytenoid	Posterior surface of the thyroid cartilage near the midline	Anterolateral surface of the arytenoid cartilage (between the vocal and muscular processes)	Decreases the tension and length of the vocal ligament by tilting the thyroid cartilage posteriorly	Vagus nerve by way of the inferior laryngeal nerve
Vocalis (portion of the thyroarytenoid lying within the vocal fold)	Posterior surface of the thyroid cartilage near the midline	Along the length of the vocal ligament to the vocal process	Varies the length, thickness, and tension of the vocal ligament	Vagus nerve by way of the inferior laryngeal nerve
Thyroepiglotticus	Posterior surface of the thyroid cartilage above the thyroarytenoid at the midline	Lateral margin of the epiglottic cartilage and the quadrangular membrane	Depresses the epiglottis and narrows the aditus in swallowing	Vagus nerve by way of the inferior laryngeal nerve
Aryepiglotticus (upward continuation of the oblique arytenoid)	Apex of the arytenoid cartilage	Lateral margin of the epiglottic cartilage	Depresses the epiglottis and narrows the aditus in swallowing	Vagus nerve by way of the inferior laryngeal nerve

- Can be **anesthetized** where it lies in the floor of the **piriform recess**

— *External laryngeal nerve*

- Arises from the **superior laryngeal nerve** above the level of the hyoid bone
- Descends with the **superior thyroid artery** below the **oblique line** of the thyroid cartilage
- Passes between the **inferior pharyngeal constrictor** and the **sternothyroid** muscles
- Supplies the **cricothyroid muscle** and the lowest part of the **inferior pharyngeal constrictor**

— *Inferior laryngeal nerve*

- Is the **terminal part** of the **recurrent laryngeal nerve**
- Enters the larynx posterior to the cricothyroid joint in the

gap between the inferior pharyngeal constrictor and the esophagus
- Is **motor (SVE)** to the **intrinsic muscles** of the larynx except the cricothyroid muscle
- Is **sensory (GVA)** to the **mucosa** of the larynx **below the level of the vocal fold**

● Blood supply of the larynx

— *Superior laryngeal artery*

- Is a branch of the superior thyroid artery (from the external carotid artery)
- Pierces the thyrohyoid membrane with the internal laryngeal nerve
- Supplies the upper part of the larynx
- Anastomoses with the inferior laryngeal artery

— *Inferior laryngeal artery*

- Is a branch of the inferior thyroid artery (from the thyrocervical trunk)
- Accompanies the inferior laryngeal nerve into the larynx
- Supplies the lower part of the larynx
- Anastomoses with the superior laryngeal artery

■ **Ear**

● **External Ear**

— *Auricle*

- Collects the **sound waves,** directing them into the external auditory meatus
- Consists of a **double layer of skin** supported by a framework of **elastic cartilage,** except for the lobule, which contains fibrous fatty tissue and no cartilage
- Is anchored to the skull by **anterior** and **posterior ligaments**
- Receives the insertions of the anterior, superior, and posterior **auricular muscles**
- Is supplied by the great auricular nerve, the auriculotemporal nerve, and lesser occipital nerve

— *External acoustic (auditory) meatus (Fig. 8.41)*

- Extends from the **auricle** to the **tympanic membrane** and is about 2.5 cm long
- Consists of a **cartilaginous portion** (the outer one third) and a **bony** portion (the inner two thirds)
- Is S shaped and narrows at the junction of the cartilaginous and bony parts
- Is lined by **skin** containing numerous **ceruminous glands,** which secrete **earwax**
- Is supplied by the **auriculotemporal nerve** and by the **auricular branch of the vagus** joined by branches of the facial and glossopharyngeal nerves
- Is supplied by the **superficial temporal, deep auricular,** and **posterior auricular** arteries

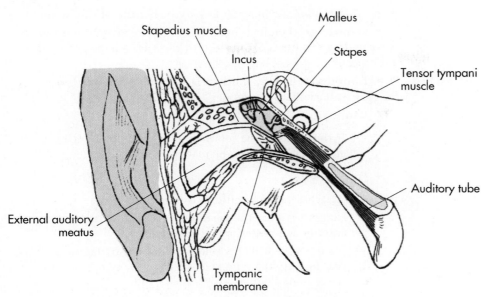

Fig. 8.41 The external, middle, and inner ear.

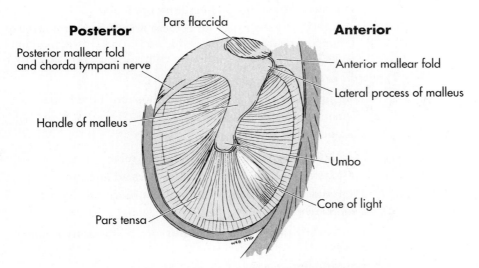

Fig. 8.42 Lateral surface of the tympanic membrane.

● **Middle ear (tympanic cavity)**

— *Tympanic membrane (Fig. 8.42)*

• Is a thin oval-shaped membrane that forms the lateral wall of the tympanic cavity

• Separates the **external acoustic meatus** from the **tympanic cavity**

• Conducts sound vibrations to the ossicles of the middle ear

• Consists of a dense **fibrous membrane** covered by **skin externally** and by **mucosa internally**

• Has a **concave lateral surface,** which is directed **forward** and **downward**

- Is attached on its inner surface to the **handle of the malleus**
- Is **innervated** on its **outer surface** by the **auriculotemporal nerve** and by the **auricular branch of the vagus** joined by branches of the facial and glossopharyngeal nerves
- Is **innervated** on its inner surface by the **tympanic branch of the glossopharyngeal nerve**

  - **Umbo**

    — Is the center of the concavity of the membrane lying at the end of the handle of the malleus

  - **Pars tensa**

    — Attaches to the **handle of the malleus**
    — Comprises all of the membrane except that between the anterior and posterior malleolar folds
    — Is supported at its periphery by a **fibrocartilaginous ring** that fits into the tympanic sulcus in the tympanic part of the temporal bone

  - **Pars flaccida**

    — Is the **anterosuperior part** of the membrane lying **between** the anterior and posterior **malleolar folds**
    — Is relatively loose (flaccid) because it has **no central layer** of supporting fibrous tissue and is **not** supported at its periphery by the **fibrocartilaginous ring**

  — *Tympanic cavity*

  - Is an air-filled **cavity** within the **petrous temporal bone**
  - Contains the **auditory ossicles**
  - Communicates with the

    — **Nasopharynx** through the auditory tube
    — **Mastoid air cells** through the **aditus ad antrum**
    — Is described as having **four walls**, a roof, and a floor

Lateral wall (Fig. 8.43)

- Is formed by the **tympanic membrane** and the **epitympanic recess**
- **Epitympanic recess**

  — Is the extension of the tympanic cavity **above the tympanic membrane** and is often referred to as the "attic"
  — Contains the **head of the malleus** and the body of the **incus**

Medial wall (Fig. 8.44)

- Separates the tympanic cavity from the inner ear
- **Promontory**

  — Is the rounded **bulge** in the central part of the wall formed by the **basal turn of the cochlea**
  — Is covered by the **tympanic plexus** of nerves derived from the **tympanic branch of the glossopharyngeal nerve** and

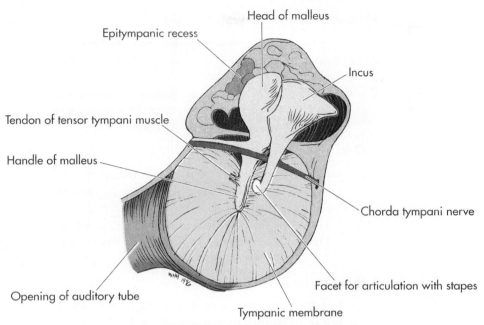

Fig. 8.43 Lateral wall of the tympanic cavity.

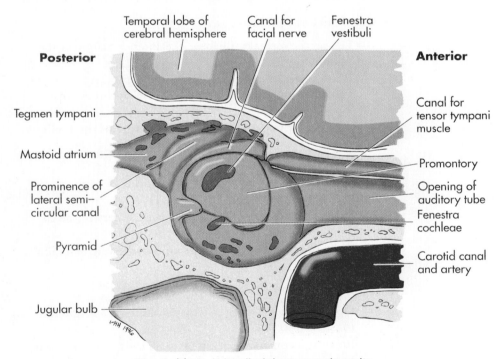

Fig. 8.44 Medial wall of the tympanic cavity.

the **caroticotympanic nerve** (from the internal carotid plexus)

- **Round window** (fenestra cochleae)

  — Lies **below** and **posterior** to the **promontory**
  — Is an opening between the **tympanic cavity** and the **bony cochlea** of the inner ear
  — Is **closed** by the **secondary tympanic membrane,** which undergoes compensatory excursions in response to the movement of the **stapes** in the oval window

- **Oval window** (fenestra vestibuli)

  — Lies **above** and **posterior** to the **promontory**
  — Is an opening between the **tympanic cavity** and the **vestibule** of the inner ear
  — Is **closed** by the **footplate of the stapes,** which undergoes compensatory excursions in response to the movement of the **tympanic membrane**

- **Prominence of the facial canal**

  — Lies **above** the **promontory** and the **oval window**
  — Is formed by the **facial nerve** in the facial canal as it passes posteriorly from the geniculate ganglion

- **Prominence of the lateral semicircular canal**

  — Overlies the ampullary end of the lateral semicircular canal

- **Cochleariform process**

  — Lies on the medial wall above the anterior margin of the promontory
  — Is the posterior end of the bony ridge separating the **semicanals** for the **tensor tympani** and the **auditory tube**
  — Serves as a **pulley** for the tendon of the **tensor tympani** muscle as it passes to attach to the **handle of the malleus** on the medial wall

Anterior wall (see Fig. 8.44)

- Superiorly receives the openings of the **auditory tube** and the **semicanal for the tensor tympani** muscle
- Inferiorly is related to the **internal carotid artery** in the **carotid canal**
- Is pierced by the opening of the **caroticotympanic canaliculus**

Posterior wall (see Fig. 8.44)

- **Aditus ad antrum**

  — Opens superiorly from the **epitympanic recess** into the **mastoid antrum**
  — Provides a **communication** between the **tympanic cavity** and the **mastoid air cells**
  — Can become infected (mastoiditis) by the spread of infection from the middle ear

- Pyramidal eminence

  — Is a tiny cone-shaped projection on the posterior wall at the level of the oval window

  — Houses the **stapedius muscle,** the tendon of which emerges at the apex to insert into the neck of the **stapes**

- **Facial canal**

  — Descends in the posterior wall to the stylomastoid foramen

Roof (Fig. 8.44)

- Is formed by the **tegmen tympani,** which is a thin plate of the petrous temporal bone
- Separates the **tympanic cavity** from the **middle cranial fossa** and the **temporal lobe** of the brain

Floor (see Fig. 8.44)

- Is formed by the **jugular fossa** of the temporal bone
- Separates the **tympanic cavity** from the **jugular bulb** (the beginning of the internal jugular vein)
- Is pierced by the **tympanic branch of the glossopharyngeal nerve,** which passes to the tympanic plexus over the promontory

Important relationships of the tympanic cavity

- Lateral wall: tympanic membrane, epitympanic recess
- Medial wall: inner ear, facial nerve
- Anterior wall: auditory canal, internal carotid artery
- Posterior wall: mastoid antrum, facial nerve
- Floor: bulb of internal jugular vein
- Roof: middle cranial fossa, temporal lobe

— *Auditory ossicles*

- Transmit the sound waves received at the tympanic membrane to the perilymph of the inner ear
- Are covered by the mucous membrane, which lines the tympanic cavity
- Are connected by synovial joints (note that arthritis may affect these joints and impair their function)

Malleus (hammer) (see Figs. 8.43 and 8.45)

- Consists of a head, neck, handle, and anterior and lateral processes
- Head

  — Is the rounded upper end that lies in the **epitympanic recess**

  — **Articulates** with the body of the **incus**

- Handle (manubrium)

  — Is attached to the medial surface of the **tympanic membrane**

  — Provides **attachment** for the tendon of the **tensor tympani muscle**

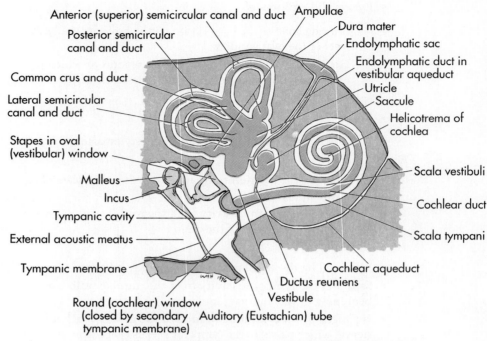

Anterior (superior) semicircular canal and duct
Ampullae
Posterior semicircular canal and duct
Dura mater
Endolymphatic sac
Common crus and duct
Endolymphatic duct in vestibular aqueduct
Lateral semicircular canal and duct
Utricle
Saccule
Helicotrema of cochlea
Stapes in oval (vestibular) window
Malleus
Incus
Scala vestibuli
Tympanic cavity
Cochlear duct
External acoustic meatus
Scala tympani
Tympanic membrane
Cochlear aqueduct
Ductus reuniens
Vestibule
Round (cochlear) window (closed by secondary tympanic membrane)
Auditory (Eustachian) tube

Fig. 8.45 Schematic illustration of the middle and inner ear.

Incus (anvil) (see Figs. 8.43 and 8.45)

- The incus (anvil) consists of a body and a short crus and long crus.
- The **body articulates** with the head of the **malleus.**
- The **long crus** descends vertically, lying medial and parallel to the handle of the malleus, and ends in a cartilaginous nodule, the **lenticular process,** which **articulates** with the **stapes.**
- The **short crus** is **attached** by a ligament to the **posterior wall** of the tympanic cavity.

Stapes (stirrup) (see Fig. 8.45)

- The stapes (stirrup) has a head and neck connected by two crura to the base.
- The **head articulates** with the lenticular process of the incus.
- The **neck** receives the attachment of the **stapedius tendon.**
- The **base** (footplate) is anchored into the **oval window** by the **annular ligament.**

— ***Muscles related to the middle ear***

Stapedius muscle

- Arises from the inner surface of the **pyramidal eminence** on the **posterior wall** of the **tympanic cavity**
- Has a **tendon** that emerges at the apex to insert into the neck of the **stapes**
- Contracts **reflexly** in response to **loud sounds** and limits the excursion of the stapes at the oval window

- Is innervated by the **facial nerve** as it descends in the posterior wall of the tympanic cavity

Tensor tympani muscle (see Fig. 8.41)

- Arises from the cartilaginous portion of the auditory tube and occupies the upper semicanal of the musculotubal canal
- Has a **tendon** that hooks around the **cochleariform process** (on the medial wall of the tympanic cavity) to insert into the **handle of the malleus**
- Contracts **reflexly** in response to **loud sounds** and limits the excursion of the tympanic membrane
- Is innervated by the **nerve to the tensor tympani** from the **nerve to the medial pterygoid** (a branch of the **mandibular nerve**)

— *Nerves related to the middle ear*

Tympanic nerve

- Arises from the inferior ganglion of the **glossopharyngeal nerve**
- Passes through the **tympanic canaliculus** to enter the **floor** of the **tympanic cavity**
- Contributes to the **tympanic plexus,** which ramifies over the **promontory**
- Supplies **afferent fibers (GSA)** to mucosa of the **tympanic cavity,** the **mastoid air cells,** and the **auditory tube**
- Also contains **preganglionic parasympathetic (GVE)** fibers for distribution to the **otic ganglion**

Lesser petrosal nerve

- Arises from the **tympanic plexus** from fibers of the **tympanic nerve**
- Leaves the tympanic cavity through the roof to enter the floor of the **middle cranial fossa**
- Descends through the **foramen ovale** (or the innominate foramen) to reach the **infratemporal fossa** and end in the **otic ganglion**
- Contains

    — **Preganglionic parasympathetic (GVE)** fibers for synapse in the otic **ganglion**
    — General visceral afferent fibers, which accompany the parasympathetic fibers.

- Remember that **parasympathetic fibers** from the **otic ganglion** are distributed to the **parotid gland** via the **auriculotemporal nerve.**

Caroticotympanic nerve

- Is derived from the **internal carotid plexus** in the carotid canal
- Reaches the **tympanic cavity** through the **caroticotympanic canaliculus** in the anterior wall
- Joins the **tympanic plexus** over the promontory
- Contains

— **Postganglionic sympathetic** fibers (from the superior cervical ganglion)

— Accompanying general visceral afferent fibers

Facial nerve

- Is the **seventh cranial nerve (CN VII)**
- Leaves the **posterior cranial fossa** through the **internal acoustic meatus**
- Traverses the **petrous temporal bone** within the **facial canal**
- Within the facial canal is related to the inner ear and the medial and posterior walls of the **tympanic cavity**
- Exits the skull through the **stylomastoid foramen**
- Gives rise to its **terminal branches** within the substance of the **parotid gland**
- Includes the **nervus intermedius,** which

  — Enters the internal acoustic meatus below the facial nerve

  — Joins the facial nerve in the proximal part of the facial canal

  — **Contains the preganglionic parasympathetic fibers** and the **taste fibers** of the facial nerve

- Within the facial canal gives rise to the

  — Greater petrosal nerve

  — Nerve to the stapedius

  — Chorda tympani

- Outside the skull gives rise to the

  — Nerves to the stylohyoid and posterior digastric muscles

  — Posterior auricular nerve

  — Communicating branch to the auricular branch of the vagus nerve

  — Terminal branches to the muscles of facial expression (temporal, zygomatic, buccal, marginal mandibular, and cervical branches)

- Contains

  — **Special visceral efferent** fibers from cell bodies in the **facial nucleus,** which are distributed to the muscles of **facial expression,** the **stapedius,** and the **stylohyoid** and **posterior digastric** muscles

  — **Special visceral afferent** (taste) fibers from cell bodies in the geniculate ganglion, which are distributed to the **palate** and the **anterior two thirds of the tongue**

  — **General visceral efferent** fibers (preganglionic parasympathetic) from the **superior salivatory nucleus,** which are distributed to the **submandibular ganglion** and the **pterygopalatine ganglion**

  — **General visceral afferent** fibers from cell bodies in the **geniculate ganglion,** which accompany the parasympathetic fibers

— **General somatic afferent fibers** from cell bodies in the **geniculate ganglion,** which are distributed to the external ear

Chorda tympani

- Arises from the **facial nerve** in the terminal part of the **facial canal**
- Enters the tympanic cavity on the posterior wall
- Passes across the lateral wall of the tympanic cavity **between the tympanic membrane** and the **handle of the malleus**
- Leaves the tympanic cavity and enters the **infratemporal fossa** through the **petrotympanic fissure**
- Ends by joining the **lingual nerve**
- Contains

  — **Preganglionic parasympathetic (GVE)** fibers for synapse in the **submandibular ganglion**
  — **General visceral afferent** fibers, which accompany the parasympathetic fibers
  — **Taste fibers (SVA),** which are distributed along the lingual nerve to the anterior two thirds of the tongue

- **Inner ear (see Fig. 8.45)**
  - Lies in the **petrous** part of the **temporal bone** medial to the middle ear
  - Consists of a **bony labyrinth** and a **membranous labyrinth**
  - Is supplied by the **labyrinthine artery,** which arises from the basilar artery and enters the inner ear through internal auditory meatus

  — *Bony labyrinth (see Fig. 8.45)*
    - Is a series of communicating bony chambers lined by periosteum
    - Includes the **cochlea,** the **vestibule,** and the **semicircular canals**
    - Contains the **membranous labyrinth** suspended in **perilymph**
    - **Cochlea**

      — Resembles a snail's shell
      — **Spirals** around a central bony core, the **modiolus,** making $2\frac{3}{4}$ **turns**
      — Contains the **cochlear duct** (part of the membranous labyrinth), which **divides** the bony cavity into the **scala vestibuli** and the **scala tympani,** except at the tip of the cochlea, where the two parts communicate
      — Receives the opening of the **round window** (fenestra cochleae)

    - **Vestibule**

      — Is the middle part of the bony labyrinth
      — Contains the **utricle** and **saccule** (parts of the membranous labyrinth)

Table 8.11 *Summary of Cranial Nerves*

Name	Functional Components	Cells of Origin	Chief Function
CN I—olfactory nerve	Special visceral afferent	Olfactory mucosa	Smell
CN II—optic nerve	Special somatic afferent	Ganglion cells of retina	Vision
CN III—oculomotor nerve	General somatic efferent	Oculomotor nucleus	Extraocular muscles: superior rectus, inferior rectus, medial rectus, inferior oblique, levator palpebrae superioris
	General visceral efferent	Edinger-Westphal nucleus	Accommodation to near vision: sphincter pupillae and ciliary muscles
CN IV—trochlear nerve	General somatic efferent	Trochlear nucleus	Extraocular muscle: superior oblique
CN V—trigeminal nerve	General somatic afferent	Semilunar ganglion	General sensation: scalp, face, upper and lower jaws, oral cavity, nasal cavity, eye
	Special visceral efferent	Motor nucleus of V (trigeminal nucleus)	Movements of the mandible: temporalis, masseter, medial pterygoid, lateral pterygoid, mylohyoid, anterior digastric; plus tensor tympani, tensor veli palatini
CN VI—abducens nerve	General somatic efferent	Abducens nucleus	Extraocular muscle: lateral rectus
CN VII—facial nerve	Special visceral efferent	Facial nucleus	Muscles of facial expression plus stylohyoid, posterior digastric, stapedius
	General visceral efferent	Superior salivatory nucleus	Secretomotor to lacrimal gland, submandibular and sublingual salivary glands, small glands of oral and nasal cavities
	Special visceral afferent	Geniculate ganglion	Taste from anterior two thirds of tongue
	General visceral afferent	Geniculate ganglion	Visceral sensation: distributed with general visceral efferent
	General somatic afferent	Geniculate ganglion	Somatic sensation: external ear and tympanic membrane

   — Receives the opening of the **oval window** (fenestra vestibuli)

- **Semicircular canals**

   — Are termed anterior, posterior, and lateral

   — Open into the vestibule

   — Are arranged in three planes, a horizontal plane and two vertical planes at right angles to each other

— *Membranous labyrinth (see Fig. 8.45)*

- Is a series of communicating membranous chambers
- Lies within the **bony labyrinth** and is **surrounded by perilymph**
- Contains the **endolymph**

| **Table 8.11** | *Summary of Cranial Nerves—cont'd* | | |

NAME	FUNCTIONAL COMPONENTS	CELLS OF ORIGIN	CHIEF FUNCTION
CN VIII—cochlear nerve	Special somatic afferent	Vestibular ganglion	Equilibrium (balance)
Vestibulocochlear nerve		Spiral ganglion	Hearing
CN IX—glosso-pharyngeal nerve	Special visceral efferent	Nucleus ambiguus	Stylopharyngeus muscle
	General visceral efferent	Inferior salivatory nucleus	Secretomotor to parotid salivary gland
	Special visceral afferent	Inferior ganglion (inferior petrosal)	Taste from posterior one third of tongue
	General visceral afferent	Inferior ganglion (inferior petrosal)	Visceral sensation: pharynx and posterior one third of tongue; visceral reflexes
	General somatic afferent	Superior ganglion (superior petrosal)	Somatic sensation: tympanic membrane and middle ear
CN X—vagus nerve	Special visceral efferent	Nucleus ambiguus	Muscles of pharynx, larynx, and soft palate excluding the stylopharyngeus but including the palatoglossus
	General visceral efferent	Dorsal motor nucleus	Cardiac muscle, smooth muscle, and glands of the thorax and abdomen
	Special visceral afferent	Inferior ganglion (nodose ganglion)	Taste over epiglottis
	General visceral afferent	Inferior ganglion (nodose ganglion)	Visceral sensation and reflexes: distributed with general visceral efferent
	General somatic afferent	Superior ganglion (jugular ganglion)	Somatic sensation: external ear and dura
CN XI—accessory nerve	Special visceral efferent	Nucleus ambiguus	Joins the vagus to distribute to the larynx (and possibly the pharynx)
Spinal portion	General somatic efferent	Accessory nucleus	Sternocleidomastoid and trapezius muscles
CN XII—hypoglossal nerve	General somatic efferent	Hypoglossal nucleus	Intrinsic and extrinsic muscle of the tongue except the palatoglossus

- Includes the **cochlear duct,** the **utricle** and **saccule,** and the semicircular ducts
- **Cochlear duct**

  — Ends blindly at the tip of the cochlea

  — Contains the spiral **organ of Corti,** the organ of hearing

- **Utricle and saccule**

  — Lie within the **vestibule** of the bony labyrinth

  — Are joined by the tiny **utriculosaccular duct**

  — Each **contain** a specialized epithelial organ, the **macula,** which senses **linear acceleration** and the pull of **gravity**

- **Semicircular ducts**

  — Lie within the **semicircular canals** of the bony labyrinth

  — Open into the utricle at five points (note that one limb

Table 8.12   *Parasympathetic Innervation of the Head*

Origin	Route of Preganglionic Fibers	Ganglion	Route of Postganglionic Fibers	Distribution
Oculomotor nerve/ Edinger-Westphal nucleus	Oculomotor nerve, inferior division, motor root to ciliary ganglion	Ciliary ganglion	Short ciliary nerves	Ciliary muscle, sphincter pupillae
Facial nerve/superior salivatory nucleus	Nervus intermedius, facial nerve, greater petrosal nerve, nerve of the pterygoid canal	Pterygopalatine ganglion	Pterygopalatine nerves, maxillary nerve, zygomatic nerve, zygomaticotemporal nerve, communicating branch to the lacrimal nerve	Lacrimal gland
			Greater and lesser palatine nerves, posterior nasal nerves	Glands of nasal cavity and palate
Facial nerve/superior salivatory nucleus	Nervus intermedius, facial nerve, chorda tympani, lingual nerve	Submandibular ganglion	Lingual nerve	Sublingual gland, small glands of the oral cavity
			Submandibular branches	Submandibular gland
Glossopharyngeal nerve/inferior salivatory nucleus	Tympanic nerve, tympanic plexus, lesser petrosal nerve	Otic ganglion	Communicating branch to the mandibular nerve, auriculotemporal nerve	Parotid gland

         of the anterior semicircular duct and one limb of the posterior semicircular duct unite before reaching the utricle)

— Are dilated at one end to form the **ampulla,** which **contains** a specialized epithelial organ, the **crista ampullaris,** which senses **rotational acceleration** in each of the three planes

Endolymphatic duct

* Extends posteriorly from the **utriculosaccular duct**
* Passes through the **vestibular aqueduct** in the temporal bone
* Ends blindly as the **endolymphatic sac,** which lies beneath the dura covering the posterior surface of the temporal bone above the termination of the sigmoid sinus
* May allow for **resorption** of the **endolymph** into the cerebrospinal fluid of the subarachnoid space

— *Vestibulocochlear nerve*

* Is the eighth cranial nerve (CN VIII)
* Is the nerve of the inner ear
* Leaves the **posterior cranial fossa** through the **internal auditory meatus** in the petrous temporal bone
* In the internal auditory meatus divides into the **vestibular nerve** and the **cochlear nerve**

Vestibular nerve

- At the end of the internal auditory meatus divides into numerous rootlets that pierce the medial wall of the vestibule
- Supplies the

    — Maculae of the utricle and saccule
    — Cristae ampullares of the semicircular ducts

- Contains SSA fibers, which have cell bodies located in the **vestibular ganglion**
- **Vestibular ganglion**

    — Lies on the vestibular nerve in the internal acoustic meatus
    — Contains **bipolar neurons** rather than the more common pseudounipolar neurons

Cochlear nerve

- At the end of the internal auditory meatus pierces the bony wall to reach the **modiolus** of the **cochlea**
- Supplies the spiral organ of Corti
- Contains SSA fibers, which have cell bodies located in the **spiral ganglion**
- **Spiral ganglion**

    — Lies in the core of the modiolus
    — Contains bipolar **neurons** rather than the more common pseudounipolar neurons

■ Cranial Nerves (Tables 8.11 and 8.12)

MULTIPLE CHOICE
REVIEW QUESTIONS

1. You are confident that you can create an artificial airway without damaging the thyroid gland because you know that the isthmus of the thyroid is located at which of the following levels?

   a. Cricothyroid membrane
   b. Laminae of the thyroid cartilage
   c. Second and third tracheal rings
   d. Cricoid cartilage
   e. Jugular notch

2. The superior thyroid artery is usually the first branch of which of the following?

   a. Costocervical trunk
   b. Thyrocervical trunk
   c. Common thyroid artery
   d. Internal carotid artery
   e. External carotid artery

3. Which of the following is the important muscle that opens the rima glottidis?

   a. Thyroarytenoid
   b. Vocalis
   c. Cricothyroid
   d. Lateral cricoarytenoid
   e. Posterior cricoarytenoid

4. Which of the following arteries lies between the anterior and middle scalene muscles?

   a. Internal thoracic
   b. Vertebral
   c. Thyrocervical trunk
   d. Common carotid
   e. Second part of the subclavian

5. Your patient has incurred a direct injury to the right orbit. He is unable to depress the fully adducted pupil on this side, but the left side is unaffected. Which muscle is affected?

   a. Superior rectus
   b. Inferior rectus
   c. Medial rectus
   d. Inferior oblique
   e. Superior oblique

6. The muscle that closes the eye is innervated by which of the following nerves?

   a. Buccal branch of the mandibular nerve
   b. Infraorbital nerve
   c. Ophthalmic nerve
   d. Oculomotor nerve
   e. Facial nerve

7. Preganglionic parasympathetic fibers destined for the submandibular ganglion arise from neuron cell bodies in which of the following areas?

   a. Geniculate ganglion
   b. Otic ganglion
   c. Superior cervical ganglion
   d. Superior salivatory nucleus
   e. Inferior salivatory nucleus

8. The sensory innervation to the scalp over the pterion is largely carried by which of the following?

   a. Auriculotemporal nerve
   b. Great auricular nerve
   c. Lesser occipital nerve
   d. Greater occipital nerve
   e. Supraorbital nerve

9. The infratemporal fossa communicates with the pterygopalatine fossa through which of the following?

   a. Superior orbital fissure
   b. Inferior orbital fissure
   c. Foramen spinosum
   d. Pterygomaxillary fissure
   e. Sphenopalatine foramen

10. Branches of the maxillary artery supply all *except* which of the following?

    a. Nasal cavity
    b. Meninges
    c. Upper eyelid
    d. Upper teeth
    e. Soft palate

11. A knife wound to the posterior triangle of the neck could reasonably be expected to produce all *except* which of the following?

    a. An inability to shrug the shoulder
    b. Paralysis of the rhomboid muscles
    c. Paralysis of the vocal fold
    d. Difficulty in abducting the shoulder
    e. Loss of sensation over the upper pectoral region

12. The dura of the cranial cavity is innervated by all *except* which of the following?

    a. Ophthalmic nerve
    b. Mandibular nerve

c. Glossopharyngeal nerve
d. Vagus nerve
e. Upper cervical spinal nerves

13. The facial nerve provides parasympathetic innervation to all *except* which of the following?

a. Parotid gland
b. Submandibular gland
c. Lacrimal gland
d. Sublingual gland
e. Glands of the nasal mucosa

14. The mandibular nerve innervates all *except* which of the following muscles?

a. Tensor veli palatini
b. Anterior belly of the digastric
c. Buccinator
d. Lateral pterygoid
e. Masseter

15. The inferior laryngeal nerve innervates all *except* which of the following muscles?

a. Cricothyroid
b. Thyroarytenoid
c. Lateral cricoarytenoid
d. Posterior cricoarytenoid
e. Transverse arytenoid

16. All *except* which of the following cranial nerves contain SVA fibers?

a. CN I
b. CN II
c. CN VII
d. CN IX
e. CN X

17. All *except* which of the following cutaneous nerves are derived from ventral rami?

a. Great auricular nerve
b. Greater occipital nerve
c. Lesser occipital nerve
d. Transverse cervical nerve
e. Supraclavicular nerve

18. All *except* which of the following lie superficial to the prevertebral layer of cervical fascia?

a. Esophagus
b. Sternocleidomastoid muscle
c. Accessory nerve
d. Vagus nerve
e. Roots of the brachial plexus

19. All *except* which of the following drain into the internal jugular vein?

a. Posterior auricular vein
b. Inferior petrosal sinus
c. Superior thyroid vein
d. Common facial vein
e. Lingual vein

20. All *except* which of the following muscles are innervated by branches of the cervical plexus?

a. Geniohyoid
b. Mylohyoid
c. Omohyoid
d. Thyrohyoid
e. Sternohyoid

Answers and Explanations to Multiple Choice Review Questions

CHAPTER 1: BASIC STRUCTURES AND CONCEPTS

1. **Answer c:**

    Functional components designated "special" (SVE, SVA, and SSA) are found only in cranial nerves and not in spinal nerves.

    a: Every spinal nerve contains GSA fibers.
    b: Every spinal nerve contains GSE fibers.
    d: Every spinal nerve contains GVE (sympathetic postganglionic) fibers.

2. **Answer d:**

    The gray ramus communicans contains only postganglionic sympathetic fibers. The neurons of the autonomic nervous system (both sympathetic and parasympathetic components) are designated GVE.

    a: The gray ramus communicans does not contain preganglionic sympathetic fibers.
    b: Every spinal nerve receives at least one gray ramus communicans.
    c: The gray ramus communicans contains postganglionic sympathetic fibers from neuron cell bodies in the sympathetic chain (paravertebral) ganglion.
    e: The gray ramus communicans does not contain GVA fibers.

3. **Answer b:**

    Abduction is movement away from the midline.

    a: Adduction is movement toward the midline.
    c: Pronation is a movement restricted to the forearm in which the palm is turned to face posteriorly.

    d: Flexion decreases the angle between bones at a joint.
    e: Extension increases the angle between bones at a joint.

4. **Answer d:**

    A ligament crosses a joint to bind two bones together.

    a: A tendon connects a muscle to bone.
    b: An aponeurosis is a flattened tendon that provides attachment for a flat muscle.
    c: A raphe is a union between two flat muscles.
    e: A retinaculum is a thickening of deep fascia that binds tendons as they cross joints.

5. **Answer a:**

    The thoracic duct receives most lymph from the body below the diaphragm and from the left half of the body above the diaphragm.

    b: Lymph from the right upper extremity, the right side of the thorax, and the head and neck drains to the right lymphatic duct.
    c: Lymph from the left side of the head and neck drains via the left jugular lymph trunk to the thoracic duct near its termination. Lymph from the right side of the head and neck drains via the right jugular lymph trunk to the right lymphatic duct.
    d: The thoracic duct receives most lymph from the left side of the thorax and all of the abdomen but also the left side of the head and the upper and lower extremity.
    e: The thoracic duct receives most lymph from the body below the diaphragm and

from the left half of the body above the diaphragm.

6. **Answer c:**

The cell bodies of GSE neurons in spinal nerves are located in the ventral horn of the spinal cord.

a: The dorsal root ganglion contains the cell bodies of the GSA and GVA neurons.

b: The paravertebral (sympathetic chain) ganglion contains the cell bodies of postganglionic sympathetic neurons (GVE).

d: The dorsal horn of the spinal cord contains neurons intrinsic to the central nervous system that do not contribute axons to the spinal nerve. The dorsal horn receives the terminations of the central axons of GVA and GSA neurons located in the dorsal root ganglion.

e: Preganglionic sympathetic neuron cell bodies (GVE) are found in the intermediolateral cell column of the spinal cord at T1-L2.

7. **Answer e:**

Elastic arteries are able to expand and recoil with the contraction of the heart because they contain numerous layers of elastic fibers and relatively little smooth muscle.

a: Elastic arteries contain numerous layers of elastic fibers and relatively little smooth muscle.

b: Elastic arteries are also called conducting arteries because they carry blood from the heart to the muscular distributing arteries.

c: The blood flow into the capillary bed is regulated by the terminal part of the arteriole known as the precapillary sphincter.

d: Most of the arteries of the body are muscular, or distributing, arteries.

8. **Answer c:**

Synchondroses include the epiphyseal plates that serve as growth zones for adjoining bone segments, particularly in long bones.

a: Synchondroses allow no movement.

b: Synchondroses occur in the epiphyseal plates of growing long bone, as well as in the sphenooccipital synchondroses of the skull base.

d: Synchondroses are primary cartilaginous joints and not synovial joints.

e: Synchondroses are joined by a plate of hyaline cartilage.

9. **Answer d:**

Cardiac muscle undergoes involuntary spontaneous and rhythmic contraction that is modulated by the function of the autonomic nervous system.

a: Cardiac muscle is striated like skeletal muscle but differs in that it is not under voluntary control.

b: Cardiac muscle consists of branching cells that have end-to-end connections with neighboring cells.

c: The function of cardiac muscle is modulated by the action of the autonomic nervous system at the sinoatrial (SA) node rather than by direct innervation.

e: The muscular wall of blood vessels, including the coronary arteries, is composed of smooth muscle.

10. **Answer a:**

The patella is a sesamoid bone that develops in the tendon of the quadriceps femoris muscle.

b: Flat bones include the ribs, sternum, scapula, and calvaria, but not the patella.

c: Irregular bones include vertebrae, hip bones, and bones of the skull base and face.

d: Short bones include the carpal bones of the hand and the tarsal bones of the foot.

e: Long bones include the bones of the extremities excluding the carpals and tarsals, which are short bones.

CHAPTER 2: UPPER EXTREMITY

1. **Answer c:**

The deltoid muscle is innervated by the axillary nerve, a terminal branch of the posterior cord of the brachial plexus.

a: The long thoracic nerve that supplies the

serratus anterior muscle arises from the C5, C6, and C7 roots of the brachial plexus.

b: The pronator teres muscle is supplied by the median nerve, which is formed by contributions from the medial and lateral cords.

d: The biceps brachii muscle is innervated by the musculocutaneous nerve from the lateral cord of the brachial plexus.

e: The infraspinatus muscle is supplied by the suprascapular nerve, which arises from the upper trunk of the brachial plexus.

2. **Answer c:**

The ability to elevate the point of the shoulder (as in a "shrug") is a function of the trapezius muscle, which attaches superiorly to the occipital bone of the skull and ligamentum nuchae and inferiorly and laterally to the clavicle, acromion, and spine of the scapula. The trapezius is innervated by the accessory nerve, and damage to this nerve may result in a "drooped" shoulder.

a: The suprascapular nerve supplies the supraspinatus and infraspinatus muscles which are functionally a part of the rotator cuff of the shoulder. Neither muscle elevates the shoulder.

b: The axillary nerve innervates the deltoid and teres minor muscles, neither of which elevates the shoulder.

d: The dorsal scapular nerve supplies the rhomboid major and minor muscles, which attach to the medial border of the scapula and stabilize the shoulder girdle but do not elevate the shoulder.

e: The medial pectoral nerve innervates the pectoralis major and minor muscles. The pectoralis major flexes and adducts the humerus, and the pectoralis minor stabilizes the pectoral girdle by pulling the scapula forward and downward. Neither muscle elevates the scapula.

3. **Answer e:**

The medial cord of the brachial plexus is formed from the anterior division of the lower trunk, which contains fibers from C8 and T1 only.

a: The medial cord is named according to its medial relationship to the second part of the axillary artery.

b: The medial cord gives fibers to the ulnar and median nerves but not to the radial nerve.

c: The medial cord gives rise to the medial pectoral nerve, but the lateral pectoral nerve arises from the lateral cord.

d: The medial cord lies medial to the second part of the axillary artery.

4. **Answer d:**

The biceps brachii flexes the elbow joint and supinates the forearm. It can compensate for loss of supinator muscle function.

a: The brachialis is a strong flexor of the elbow but cannot supinate the forearm.

b: The brachioradialis is a weak flexor of the elbow but cannot supinate the forearm.

c: The flexor carpi ulnaris flexes and adducts the hand at the wrist joint.

e: The anconeus is an extensor of the elbow joint only.

5. **Answer a:**

The radial nerve spirals around the shaft of the humerus posteriorly and is commonly injured in mid-shaft fractures as it lies against the bone. Damage to the radial nerve will affect innervation of the extensors of the wrist (the muscles of the posterior forearm), resulting in a "wrist drop."

b: Damage to the ulnar nerve, usually as it passes behind the medial epicondyle at the elbow, may result in a deformity known as "claw hand."

c: "Headwaiter's tip hand" is a term that describes the position of the upper extremity in Erb-Duchenne palsy, which results from damage to the upper roots of the brachial plexus.

d: Erb-Duchenne palsy results from damage to the upper roots of the brachial plexus and may produce a condition known as "headwaiter's tip hand."

e: Klumpke's paralysis is associated with injury to the lower roots.

6. **Answer a:**

The teres major muscle adducts and medially rotates the arm, but it is not considered a part of the rotator cuff. Its tendon does not reinforce the capsule of the shoulder joint because its insertion into the humerus is distal to the shoulder joint.

b: The teres minor muscle laterally rotates the arm. Its tendon forms part of the rotator cuff, blending with and reinforcing the posterior part of the capsule of the shoulder joint.

c: The subscapularis muscle medially rotates the arm. Its tendon forms part of the rotator cuff, blending with and reinforcing the anterior part of the capsule of the shoulder joint.

d: The supraspinatus muscle assists in abduction of the arm and pulls the head of the humerus upward into the glenoid cavity. Its tendon forms part of the rotator cuff and reinforces the upper part of the capsule of the shoulder joint.

e: The infraspinatus muscle laterally rotates the arm and, as a part of the rotator cuff, stabilizes the shoulder joint.

7. **Answer a:**

All of the thenar muscles, including the opponens pollicis, are innervated by the median nerve and not the ulnar nerve.

b: All of the hypothenar muscles, including the flexor digiti minimi, are innervated by the ulnar nerve and would be affected.

c: The third and fourth lumbrical muscles are innervated by the ulnar nerve and would be affected. (The first and second lumbrical are innervated by the median nerve and would not be affected.)

d: All of the interosseus muscles, including the first palmar interosseus, are innervated by the ulnar nerve and would be affected.

e: All of the interosseus muscles, including the first dorsal interosseus, are innervated by the ulnar nerve and would be affected.

8. **Answer d:**

The superficial branch of the radial nerve has a cutaneous distribution over the lateral half of the dorsum of the hand.

(The ulnar nerve supplies the medial half of the dorsum of the hand and all of the little finger.) Damage to the radial nerve at or above the elbow could also result in a sensory loss over this area, but it would likely be accompanied by wrist drop.

a: The median nerve has no cutaneous distribution on the dorsum of the hand.

b: The lateral antebrachial cutaneous nerve has no cutaneous distribution on the dorsum of the hand.

c: The posterior antebrachial cutaneous nerve has no cutaneous distribution on the dorsum of the hand.

e: The deep branch of the radial nerve has no cutaneous distribution on the dorsum of the hand.

Answers to matching questions 9 through 11

9. **Answer c:**

The ulnar artery gives rise to the common interosseus artery in the distal cubital fossa close to the proximal end of the interosseus membrane.

10. **Answer a:**

The brachial artery ends in the cubital fossa by dividing into the radial and ulnar arteries.

11. **Answer b:**

The radial artery passes from the dorsum of the hand to the palm between the two heads of the first dorsal interosseus muscle. In the palm it anastomoses with the deep palmar branch of the ulnar artery to form the deep palmar arch.

CHAPTER 3: LOWER EXTREMITY

1. **Answer b:**

All of the intrinsic muscles of the foot, except the extensor hallucis brevis and extensor digitorum brevis, are innervated by the tibial nerve. Damage to the tibial nerve would affect all of the muscles that abduct and adduct the toes, including the abductor hallucis, the abductor digiti mimimi, the adductor hallucis, and the dorsal and plantar interossei.

a: Most of the cutaneous innervation of the

dorsum of the foot is derived from the superficial and deep peroneal nerves, not by branches of the tibial nerve.

c: Dorsiflexion of the foot is a function of the muscles of the anterior compartment of the leg, all of which are innervated by the deep peroneal nerve.

d: Eversion of the foot is a function of the muscles of the lateral compartment of the leg, which are innervated by the superficial peroneal nerve.

e: Extension of the knee is a function of the quadriceps femoris muscle of the anterior thigh, which is innervated by the femoral nerve.

2. **Answer d:**

The femoral sheath is a downward extension of the transversalis fascia and iliacus fascia that line the abdominal cavity. It invests the femoral artery, femoral vein, and femoral canal as they pass from the abdomen into the thigh.

a: Scarpa's fascia is the fibrous layer of superficial fascia over the lower abdominal wall. It fuses with the fascia lata below the inguinal ligament.

b: The external oblique aponeurosis does not extend into the thigh. Its inferior limit is the inguinal ligament, which is the boundary between the abdominal wall and the thigh.

c: The superficial perineal fascia (Colles' fascia) is an extension into the perineum of the deep layer of the superficial abdominal fascia (Scarpa's fascia).

e: The peritoneum does not normally extend into the thigh.

3. **Answer b:**

The great saphenous vein lies within the superficial fascia as it ascends on the medial side of the leg and thigh and does not lie in the adductor canal at any point.

a: The saphenous nerve descends through the thigh in the adductor canal and becomes cutaneous at the knee.

c: The femoral vein forms at the adductor hiatus as an upward continuation of the popliteal vein and ascends in the adductor canal and femoral triangle medial to the femoral artery.

d: The femoral artery descends in the thigh through the femoral triangle and adductor canal to end at the adductor hiatus as the popliteal artery.

e: The nerve to the vastus medialis descends in the adductor canal lateral to the saphenous nerve.

4. **Answer e:**

The gastrocnemius muscle is primarily a plantar flexor of the foot at the ankle joint, but it may also assist in flexion of the knee joint since its origin lies above the knee joint.

a: The tibialis posterior muscle plantar flexes and inverts the foot but is unable to flex the knee because it does not cross the knee joint.

b: The flexor digitorum longus muscle flexes the toes and plantar flexes the foot but is unable to flex the knee because it does not cross the knee joint.

c: The peroneus longus is an evertor of the foot and does not act across the knee joint.

d: The soleus muscle plantar flexes the foot but is unable to flex the knee because it does not cross the knee joint.

5. **Answer e:**

The plantar arterial arch is formed from the lateral plantar artery (from the posterior tibial artery) and is completed medially by anastomosis with the deep plantar artery from the dorsalis pedis.

a: The anterior tibial artery becomes the dorsalis pedis artery as it crosses the ankle joint.

b: The posterior tibial artery terminates behind the medial malleolus by dividing into the medial and lateral plantar arteries.

c: The medial plantar artery supplies the medial side of the great toe and anastomoses with the plantar metatarsal arteries but does not contribute directly to the plantar arch.

d: The peroneal artery supplies the posterior and lateral compartments of the leg and normally ends at the ankle. Its perforating branch may give rise to the dorsalis pedis artery, but it does not contribute directly to the plantar arch.

6. **Answer b:**

   The superior gluteal nerve and artery enter the gluteal region through the greater sciatic foramen above the piriformis muscle.

   a: The internal pudendal artery and the pudendal nerve enter the gluteal region through the greater sciatic foramen below the piriformis muscle.

   c: The sciatic nerve enters the gluteal region through the greater sciatic foramen below the piriformis muscle.

   d: The obturator artery does not traverse the greater sciatic foramen or enter the gluteal region.

   e: The tendon of the obturator internus muscle enters the gluteal region through the lesser sciatic foramen.

7. **Answer a:**

   The iliofemoral ligament is the strongest and most important ligament of the hip joint. It reinforces the capsule of the hip joint anteriorly and strongly resists hyperextension and medial rotation.

   b: The ischiofemoral ligament is a thin ligament that reinforces the hip joint posteriorly. It does limit extension and medial rotation of the joint, but not as effectively as the iliofemoral ligament.

   c: The pubofemoral ligament reinforces the hip joint anteriorly and inferiorly and resists excessive abduction of the hip joint.

   d: The ligament of the head of the femur may function to resist adduction of the hip joint in children but does not restrict movement of the joint in adults.

   e: The transverse acetabular ligament is the part of the labrum acetabulare that bridges the acetabular notch. It does not limit movement of the hip joint.

8. **Answer c:**

   The common peroneal nerve is vulnerable to direct trauma as it passes superficially around the neck of the fibula.

   a: The saphenous nerve becomes cutaneous on the medial side of the knee and descends on the medial leg with the great saphenous vein. It is not related to the neck of the fibula.

   b: The tibial nerve crosses the knee joint in the popliteal fossa and is not related to the neck of the fibula.

   d: The deep peroneal nerve arises from the common peroneal nerve within the peroneus longus muscle of the lateral compartment. Here it lies away from the neck of the fibula protected by muscle and is less vulnerable to injury than is the common peroneal nerve.

   e: The femoral nerve divides into its terminal branches in the upper anterior thigh and only its saphenous branch extends below the knee.

9. **Answer a:**

   The gluteus medius muscle abducts and medially rotates the thigh.

   b: The gluteus maximus muscle extends and laterally rotates the thigh.

   c: The obturator internus muscle laterally rotates the thigh.

   d: The obturator externus muscle laterally rotates the thigh.

   e: The quadratus femoris muscle laterally rotates the thigh.

10. **Answer b:**

    Anterior movement of the tibia on the femur is resisted by the anterior cruciate ligament that arises from the anterior intercondylar area of the tibia and runs upward posteriorly and laterally to attach to the medial surface of the lateral femoral condyle.

    a: The medial meniscus increases congruity between the medial tibial and femoral condyles but does not significantly restrict anterior or posterior sliding movements between the tibia and femur.

    c: The posterior cruciate ligament resists posterior movement of the tibia on the femur, but not anterior movement.

    d: The coronary ligament is the part of the fibrous capsule of the knee joint that anchors the menisci to the tibial condyles. It does not restrict anterior or posterior sliding movements between the tibia and femur.

e: The fibular collateral ligament is the longitudinal ligament that extends from the lateral femoral condyle to the head of the fibula. It does not restrict anterior or posterior sliding movements between the tibia and femur.

CHAPTER 4: THORAX

1. Answer b:

The sound from the left atrioventricular (mitral) valve is best heard over the apex of the heart in the left fifth intercostal space in the midclavicular line.

a: The valve of the inferior vena cava is a rudimentary valve and produces no discernible heart sound.

c: The right atrioventricular (tricuspid) valve is best heard over the medial ends of the fourth to sixth intercostal spaces on the right side.

d: The aortic semilunar valve is best heard over the right second intercostal space next to the sternum.

e: The sounds from the pulmonary semilunar valve are best heard over the medial ends of the first and second intercostal spaces on the left side.

2. Answer b:

The middle cardiac vein ascends in the posterior interventricular sulcus to empty directly into the coronary sinus.

a: The small cardiac vein accompanies the right coronary artery to the coronary sulcus where it empties into the termination of the coronary sinus.

c: The great cardiac vein ascends in the anterior interventricular sulcus to enter the coronary sulcus and become continuous with the coronary sinus.

d: The coronary sinus lies in the coronary sulcus, separating the left atrium and left ventricle.

e: The oblique vein of the left atrium drains the left side of the left atrium and passes to the coronary sulcus where it joins the great cardiac vein to form the coronary sinus.

3. Answer c:

The superior mediastinum lies posterior to the manubrium. It is limited above by the thoracic inlet and below by a line joining the manubriosternal joint to the lower border of the T4 vertebral body.

a: The arch of the aorta is one of the structures found within the superior mediastinum.

b: The heart and pericardium are contained in the middle mediastinum.

d: The paired first ribs, the body of the first thoracic vertebra, and the upper end of the manubrium sterni form the boundaries of the thoracic inlet, which marks the upper extent of the superior mediastinum.

e: The anterior mediastinum is the narrow space between the pericardial sac and the posterior surface of the body of the sternum.

4. Answer c:

Visceral afferent fibers conducting pain from the heart arise from cell bodies located in the dorsal root ganglia at T1-T4 and reach the heart via the cardiac branches of the cervical sympathetic ganglia.

a: The inferior vagal ganglion contains the cell bodies of visceral afferent fibers associated with the cardiac reflexes and not pain.

b: The intermediolateral cell column contains the cell bodies of preganglionic sympathetic neurons and not afferent neurons.

d: The cervical sympathetic ganglia contain the cell bodies of postganglionic sympathetic neurons, some of which are distributed to the heart via the cervical sympathetic cardiac nerves.

e: The sympathetic chain (paravertebral) ganglia at T1-T4 contain the cell bodies of postganglionic sympathetic neurons, which are distributed to the pulmonary and esophageal plexuses and the T1-T4 spinal nerves.

5. Answer b:

The transverse pericardial sinus is a passage from the left side to the right side of the pericardial cavity. It is related anteriorly to the ascending aorta on the right and the pulmonary trunk on the left.

a: The superior vena cava lies posterior to a finger placed into the transverse pericardial sinus from the right side.

c: The arch of the aorta lies outside the pericardial sac and is unrelated to the transverse pericardial sinus.

d: The pulmonary trunk lies anterior to a finger placed into the transverse pericardial sinus from the left side.

e: The right pulmonary artery lies outside the pericardial sac and is unrelated to the transverse pericardial sinus.

6. **Answer e:**

The superficial and deep lymphatic plexuses of the lung end in the bronchopulmonary nodes at the root of the lung.

a: The thoracic duct does not have an associated group of lymph nodes, and lymph from the lung does not drain directly to the thoracic duct.

b: The tracheobronchial nodes lie around the main bronchi and the bifurcation of the trachea. They receive the lymphatic drainage of the lung after it has first passed through the bronchopulmonary nodes.

c: The bronchomediastinal lymph trunk is formed in the superior mediastinum by efferent vessels from the tracheobronchial, parasternal, posterior mediastinal, and brachiocephalic nodes.

d: The parasternal nodes lie along the course of the internal thoracic artery. They receive lymph from the diaphragm and the thoracic and abdominal walls, but not from the lungs.

7. **Answer c:**

The thoracic duct ascends in the posterior mediastinum behind the esophagus and between the descending thoracic aorta and the azygous vein.

a: Neither the right nor the left recurrent laryngeal nerves lie in the posterior mediastinum. The right recurrent laryngeal nerve loops around the first part of the

right subclavian artery in the root of the neck. The left recurrent laryngeal nerve hooks around the arch of the aorta in the superior mediastinum.

b: The trachea passes from the neck into the superior mediastinum and ends at the level of the sternal angle by dividing into the two primary bronchi.

d: The phrenic nerve descends through the superior mediastinum and middle mediastinum, but not the posterior mediastinum.

e: The heart, including the left atrium, is found in the middle mediastinum.

8. **Answer d:**

The artery to the SA node (sinoatrial artery) is usually a branch of the right coronary artery.

a: The atrioventricular bundle begins as a continuation of the AV node, not the SA node.

b: The SA node does not lie in the interatrial septum but in the wall of the right atrium near the superior end of the sulcus terminalis.

c: The SA node lies in the wall of the right atrium within the pericardial sac.

e: The SA node receives direct innervation from parasympathetic fibers in the cardiac branches of the vagus nerves.

9. **Answer a:**

The circumflex artery lies in the posterior part of the coronary sulcus between the left atrium and left ventricle and mainly supplies these structures.

b: The right atrium and right ventricle are mainly supplied by the right coronary artery, not by the circumflex artery.

c: The distribution of the circumflex artery does not normally reach the apex, which is supplied variably by the anterior interventricular, posterior interventricular, and right marginal arteries.

d: The right ventricle is supplied mostly by the right coronary artery and is not typically supplied by the circumflex artery.

e: The circumflex artery supplies the left ventricle, but the posterior part of the interventricular septum is commonly supplied by branches of the right coronary artery.

10. **Answer e:**

The posterior intercostal arteries to the first two intercostal spaces arise from the supreme intercostal artery, a branch of the costocervical trunk.

a: The only branches of the ascending aorta are the right and left coronary arteries.

b: The descending thoracic aorta gives rise to paired posterior intercostal arteries that supply all of the intercostal spaces except the first two.

c: The right bronchial artery does not supply any intercostal spaces but commonly arises from the third posterior intercostal artery.

d: The internal thoracic artery supplies anterior intercostal arteries to the first five or six intercostal spaces.

CHAPTER 5: ABDOMEN

1. **Answer b:**

The hepatic portal vein receives most of the blood from the gastrointestinal tract through the superior mesenteric, inferior mesenteric, and splenic veins and their tributaries.

a: The hepatic portal vein forms from the union of the splenic and superior mesenteric veins. The inferior mesenteric vein ends in the splenic vein.

c: The hepatic portal vein reaches the liver through the hepatoduodenal ligament, not the falciform ligament.

d: The hepatic portal vein forms posterior to the neck of the pancreas.

e: The hepatic portal vein ends in the sinusoids of the liver, which are drained by the tributaries of the hepatic veins.

2. **Answer c:**

The spleen is supplied by the splenic artery, a branch of the celiac trunk.

a: The duodenum is supplied by branches of both the celiac trunk and the superior mesenteric artery.

b: The body and tail of the pancreas are typically supplied by branches of the splenic artery (from the celiac trunk). The head of the pancreas, however, is supplied by inferior pancreaticoduodenal arteries from the superior mesenteric artery, as well as by superior pancreaticoduodenal arteries from the gastroduodenal artery.

d: The appendicular artery arises from the posterior cecal branch of the ileocolic artery (a branch of the superior mesenteric artery).

e: The transverse colon is supplied mostly by the middle colic artery from the superior mesenteric artery.

3. **Answer d:**

The deep inguinal ring transmits the round ligament of the uterus in the female and the spermatic cord in the male.

a: The deep inguinal ring is the mouth of a tubular evagination of the transversalis fascia that lines the peritoneal cavity.

b: An indirect inguinal hernia traverses the deep inguinal ring, the inguinal canal, and the superficial ring. A direct inguinal hernia reaches the superficial inguinal ring directly through the abdominal wall.

c: The deep inguinal ring lies lateral to the inferior epigastric artery as it passes upward to enter the rectus sheath.

e: The deep inguinal ring lies just above the inguinal ligament midway between the anterior superior iliac spine and the pubic tubercle.

4. **Answer d:**

The conjoint tendon is formed from a fusion of the lower parts of the transversus abdominis aponeurosis and the internal oblique aponeurosis.

a: The inguinal ligament is the thickened lower border of the external oblique aponeurosis.

b: The superficial inguinal ring is a defect in the aponeurosis of the external oblique aponeurosis.

c: The anterior wall of the inguinal canal is formed medially by the inner surface of the external oblique aponeurosis and laterally by the fibers of the internal abdominal oblique muscle.

e: The aponeurosis of the external abdominal oblique muscle contributes to the anterior lamina of the rectus sheath throughout its length.

5. **Answer c:**

The free edge of the falciform ligament contains the ligamentum teres hepatis, the remnant of the left umbilical vein of the fetus.

a: The lesser omentum is the ventral mesentery of the stomach and includes the hepatogastric and hepatoduodenal ligaments.

b: The falciform ligament is a double layer of peritoneum.

d: The caudate and quadrate lobes of the liver are separated by the porta hepatis and the structures entering or leaving the liver.

e: The falciform ligament connects the liver to the anterior body wall above the umbilicus.

6. **Answer b:**

The epiploic foramen is limited superiorly by the caudate lobe of the liver.

a: The first part of the duodenum forms the inferior boundary of the epiploic foramen.

c: The head of the pancreas is separated from the epiploic foramen by the first part of the duodenum and is not one of its boundaries.

d: The common bile duct lies in the hepatoduodenal ligament, which is the anterior boundary of the epiploic foramen.

e: The hepatic veins do not form a boundary of the epiploic foramen.

7. **Answer b:**

The left gonadal vein typically ends in the left renal vein, whereas the right gonadal vein ends directly in the inferior vena cava.

a: The left renal vein is longer than the right renal vein because the inferior vena cava lies to the right of midline.

c: The renal veins lie anterior to the renal pelvis and renal arteries.

d: The renal veins end in the inferior vena cava and do not join the portal venous system.

e: The cysterna chyli is part of the lymphatic system and not the venous system.

8. **Answer d:**

The splenic artery supplies the spleen and pancreas but not the suprarenal glands.

a: The superior suprarenal arteries arise from the inferior phrenic artery.

b: The inferior suprarenal arteries arise from the renal artery.

c: The middle suprarenal artery arises directly from the abdominal aorta.

9. **Answer a:**

The duodenum begins at the pylorus of the stomach and ends at the jejunum.

b: The duodenum is formed from both the foregut and midgut, the junction between the two being in the second part of the duodenum.

c: The second part of the duodenum receives the terminations of the common bile duct and the main and accessory pancreatic ducts.

d: The most proximal and distal parts of the duodenum have mesenteries and are not retroperitoneal.

e: The horizontal third part of the duodenum crosses posterior to the superior mesenteric vessels.

10. **Answer c:**

The inferior mesenteric artery is said to be the artery of the hindgut. It supplies the descending colon, sigmoid colon, rectum, and upper half of the anal canal, all derived from the embryonic hindgut.

a: The celiac artery is said to be the artery of the foregut. It supplies the structures derived from the caudal part of the embryonic foregut (and the spleen).

b: The superior mesenteric artery is said to be the artery of the midgut. It supplies the head of the pancreas and the intestines from the second part of the duodenum to the left colic flexure.

d: The internal iliac artery supplies the pelvis, the perineum, and the gluteal region of the lower extremity.

e: The external iliac artery supplies the lower extremity.

CHAPTER 6: PELVIS AND PERINEUM

1. **Answer c:**

Colles' fascia is the superficial perineal fascia. It forms the superficial boundary of the superficial perineal pouch and is not part of the urogenital diaphragm.

a: The deep transverse perineal muscle is one of the muscles included in the urogenital diaphragm.

b: The sphincter urethrae muscle is one of the muscles included in the urogenital diaphragm.

d: The perineal membrane is the inferior fascia of the urogenital diaphragm. It covers the superficial surface of the deep transverse perineal and sphincter urethrae muscles and is part of the urogenital diaphragm.

e: The superior fascia of the urogenital diaphragm covers the deep surface of the deep transverse perineal and sphincter urethrae muscles and is part of the urogenital diaphragm.

2. **Answer a:**

The coccygeus muscle extends from the sacrum and coccyx to the ischial spine and does not attach to the perineal body.

b: The anterior component of the pubococcygeus muscle is anchored to the perineal body, forming the levator prostatae muscle in the male and the pubovaginalis muscle in the female.

c: The perineal body serves as a central attachment for numerous structures, including the external anal sphincter.

d: The superficial transverse perineal muscle arises from the ischial ramus and inserts into the perineal body.

e: The perineal body serves as a central attachment for numerous structures, including the superior and inferior fascia of the urogenital diaphragm.

3. **Answer c:**

The peritoneum on the superior surface of the bladder reflects onto the anterior surface of the uterus, forming the uterovesical pouch, which does not contact the anterior vaginal wall.

a: The urethra is directly related to the anterior wall of the vagina.

b: The base of the bladder is directly related to the anterior wall of the vagina.

d: The wall of the posterior fornix of the vagina is directly related to the rectouterine pouch (of Douglas).

e: The rectum is directly related to the posterior wall of the vagina.

4. **Answer e:**

The lymphatic drainage from the ovary is along the ovarian vessels directly to the aortic nodes.

a: Most of the lymphatic drainage of the pelvis follows the internal iliac arteries to the internal iliac nodes.

b: The external iliac nodes receive most of the lymphatic drainage from the lower extremity.

c: The superficial inguinal nodes receive lymph from the superficial thigh and leg, perineum, anterior abdominal wall, and buttock.

d: The inferior mesenteric nodes lie along the course of the inferior mesenteric artery and receive lymph from structures supplied by the inferior mesenteric artery.

5. **Answer b:**

The pelvic viscera receive parasympathetic innervation from the sacral parasympathetic outflow (via the pelvic splanchnic nerves), not from the vagus nerve.

a: The hypogastric nerves are direct continuations of the superior hypogastric plexus. They end in the inferior hypogastric plexus.

c: There is no associated prevertebral ganglion because the sympathetic fibers in the hypogastric nerves are postganglionic, arising from cell bodies in the lower lumbar sympathetic chain ganglia.

d: The hypogastric nerves are direct continuations of the superior hypogastric plexus.

e: The parasympathetic innervation to the descending and sigmoid colon ascends from the inferior hypogastric plexus through the hypogastric nerves to the superior hypogastric plexus, and it is distributed in the inferior mesenteric plexus along the inferior mesenteric artery.

6. **Answer a:**

The uterine artery does not cross the pelvic brim because it arises from the internal iliac artery and supplies the uterus, both of which lie in the lesser pelvis.

b: The ovarian artery arises from the abdominal aorta and descends across the pelvic brim to enter the lesser pelvis and supply the ovary and uterine tube.

c: The superior rectal artery is a direct continuation of the inferior mesenteric artery, which arises from the abdominal aorta. It descends into the lesser pelvis to supply the rectum and upper half of the anal canal.

d: The round ligament of the uterus attaches to the uterus in the lesser pelvis and crosses the pelvic brim to enter the deep inguinal ring on the anterior abdominal wall.

e: The ureter arises from the pelvis of the kidney on the posterior abdominal wall and crosses the pelvic brim to reach the urinary bladder in the minor pelvis.

7. **Answer e:**

The perineal nerve terminates in the ischiorectal fossa by dividing into the deep perineal nerve and the posterior scrotal nerves.

a: The bulbourethral glands are located in the deep perineal pouch on either side of the membranous urethra embedded in the deep transverse perineal and sphincter urethrae muscles.

b: The deep transverse perineal muscle forms part of the urogenital diaphragm and is contained within the deep perineal pouch.

c: The sphincter urethrae muscle forms part of the urogenital diaphragm and is contained within the deep perineal pouch.

d: The membranous urethra penetrates the urogenital diaphragm and the deep perineal pouch.

8. **Answer b:**

The duct of the seminal vesicle unites with the ductus deferens near the base of the prostate to form the ejaculatory duct, which opens onto the colliculus seminalis.

a: The prostatic utricle is a blind pouch on the colliculus seminalis.

c: The 25 to 30 prostatic ducts open independently into the prostatic sinus.

d: The ducts of the bulbourethral glands open independently into the spongy urethra.

e: The ejaculatory ducts are paired ducts that form on each side by union of the duct of the seminal vesicle with the ductus deferens.

9. **Answer c:**

The sacral plexus is a somatic plexus formed from the ventral rami of the sacral spinal nerves and does not contain parasympathetic fibers.

a: Parasympathetic innervation to the pelvis arises from the sacral parasympathetic outflow via the nervi erigentes (pelvic splanchnic nerves).

b: Parasympathetic fibers from the nervi erigentes enter the inferior hypogastric plexus, and many synapse on terminal ganglia there.

d: The vesical plexus is an extension of the inferior hypogastric plexus around the bladder. It contains parasympathetic fibers destined for the urinary bladder.

e: The pelvic plexus is another name for the inferior hypogastric plexus.

10. **Answer d:**

The pectinate line marks the divide between visceral and somatic innervation, blood supply, venous drainage, and lymphatic drainage.

a: The pectinate line joins the lower margins of the anal valves.

b: The anocutaneous (white) line lies below the pectinate line.

c: The junction of the internal and external anal sphincters is marked by the white line.

CHAPTER 7: BACK

1. Answer d:

The first cervical vertebra, the atlas, is unique in that it has no body or spinous process. Its body has fused with the superior surface of the body of the second cervical vertebra, the axis, to form the peglike dens (odontoid process).

a: The first cervical vertebra has a superior articular facet on its lateral mass for articulation with the occipital bone of the skull.

b: All cervical vertebrae have a transverse foramen in the transverse process.

c: The atlas has paired transverse processes.

e: The vertebral arch of the atlas is its posterior arch, which with the anterior arch and paired lateral masses forms its vertebral foramen.

2. Answer c:

The typical thoracic vertebra has a costal facet on each transverse process for articulation with the tubercle of the rib of the same number.

a: The head of the rib articulates with demifacets on the bodies of the vertebra of the same number and the vertebra above.

b: The neck of the rib has no articulation with the vertebra.

d: No articulation exists between the transverse processes of adjacent vertebrae.

e: No articulation exists between the spinous processes of adjacent vertebrae.

3. Answer d:

All of the suboccipital muscles, including the obliquus capitis inferior, are innervated by the suboccipital nerve (the dorsal ramus of the first cervical spinal nerve).

a: The lesser occipital nerve is a cutaneous

branch of the cervical plexus and is derived from the ventral ramus of the second cervical spinal nerve.

b: The greater occipital nerve (the dorsal ramus of the second cervical spinal nerve) supplies cutaneous innervation to the back of the scalp.

c: The least occipital nerve is the dorsal ramus of the third cervical spinal nerve. It provides cutaneous innervation to the scalp of the occipital region.

e: The dorsal ramus of C2 is the greater occipital nerve. It provides cutaneous innervation to the scalp.

4. Answer e:

The ligamentum flavum connects the laminae of adjacent vertebrae.

a: The ligamentum nuchae is an extension of the supraspinous ligament into the cervical region.

b: The supraspinous ligament connects the tips of the spinous processes.

c: The interspinous ligament connects adjacent spinous processes.

d: The posterior longitudinal ligament runs on the posterior surfaces of the vertebral bodies and intervertebral discs.

5. Answer c:

The internal vertebral venous plexus lies in the epidural space within the vertebral canal.

a: Neither the external or internal venous plexus lies within the substance of the spinal cord.

b: The subdural space is a potential space formed only by the tearing of the arachnoid away from the inner surface of the overlying dura. It has no contents.

d: The subarachnoid space contains only cerebrospinal fluid.

e: The internal vertebral venous plexus lies outside the dural sac but within the vertebral canal.

6. Answer d:

The secondary curvature of the spine is found in the cervical and lumbar regions and is concave posteriorly.

a: The secondary curvature of the spine is

not present before birth. It becomes apparent in the lumbar region when the infant begins to walk.

b: The lumbar curvature develops when the infant begins to walk and is present throughout life.

c: The primary curvature of the spine is convex posteriorly (or concave anteriorly), not the secondary curvature.

7. **Answer b:**

The spinalis muscles form the medial column of the erector spinae group. Individual bundles arise from and insert into vertebral spinous processes.

a: The spinalis muscles form the medial column of the erector spinae group.

c: The spinalis muscle inserts into spinous processes, not transverse processes.

d: The erector spinae group is an extensor of the vertebral column.

e: The intrinsic muscles of the back are innervated by the dorsal primary rami of spinal nerves and not by ventral rami.

8. **Answer d:**

The subarachnoid space extends caudally to the level of the second sacral vertebra.

a: At the level of T12 the spinal cord is surrounded by all layers of the meninges.

b: The spinal cord ends at the lower border of L1, and below this level lies the lumbar cistern of the subarachnoid space.

c: The subarachnoid space at the level of L4 contains the cauda equina.

e: The dural sac and the coextensive subarachnoid space end at the level of S2.

9. **Answer a:**

The cauda equina consists of the ventral and dorsal roots of the lower lumbar and sacral spinal nerves.

b: The ventral and dorsal rami are branches of the spinal nerve and arise outside the vertebral canal.

c: A spinal nerve forms from the union of the dorsal root and the ventral root as they exit the vertebral canal through the intervertebral foramen.

d: Both ventral roots and dorsal roots are found in the cauda equina.

10. **Answer b:**

The transversospinalis muscle group includes the semispinalis, multifidus, and rotator muscles.

a: The splenius capitis muscle belongs to the splenius group, which is also called the spinotransverse group.

c: The rectus capitis posterior major belongs to the suboccipital group of muscles.

d: The serratus posterior superior muscle is considered an extrinsic back muscle. It functions to elevate the ribs.

e: The iliocostalis lumborum muscle belongs to the erector spinae (sacrospinalis) muscle group.

CHAPTER 8: HEAD AND NECK

1. **Answer c:**

The isthmus of the thyroid gland lies over the second and third tracheal rings.

a: The cricothyroid membrane lies in the midline between the upper poles of the thyroid lobes and superior to the isthmus of thyroid.

b: The thyroid lobes and the isthmus lies caudal to the laminae of the thyroid cartilage.

d: The cricoid cartilage lies between the upper poles of the thyroid lobes and superior to the isthmus of thyroid.

e: The isthmus of the thyroid gland usually lies superior to the level of the jugular notch.

2. **Answer e:**

The superior thyroid artery is commonly the first branch of the external carotid artery.

a: The branches of the costocervical trunk are the deep cervical artery and the superior intercostal artery.

b: The thyrocervical trunk gives rise to the inferior thyroid artery but not the superior thyroid artery.

c: The branches of the common carotid artery are the internal and external carotid arteries.

d: The internal carotid artery usually has no branches in the neck.

3. **Answer e:**

The posterior cricoarytenoid abducts the vocal fold (opens the rima glottidis) by laterally rotating the arytenoid cartilage.

a: The thyroarytenoid muscle decreases the tension and length of the vocal ligament by tilting the thyroid cartilage posteriorly.

b: The vocalis muscle varies the length, thickness, and tension of the vocal ligament.

c: The cricothyroid muscle tenses and lengthens the vocal ligament by tilting the thyroid cartilage forward.

d: The lateral cricoarytenoid muscle adducts (closes the rima glottidis) the vocal fold by medially rotating the arytenoid cartilage.

4. **Answer e:**

The subclavian artery passes between the anterior and middle scalene muscles as it crosses the first rib and is divided into three parts by the anterior scalene muscle.

a: The internal thoracic artery arises from the first part of the subclavian artery and descends on the inside of the anterior thoracic wall.

b: The vertebral artery arises from the first part of the subclavian artery and ascends in the groove between the longus colli and anterior scalene muscles.

c: The thyrocervical trunk is a short trunk that arises from the first part of the subclavian artery at the medial border of the anterior scalene muscle.

d: The common carotid artery ascends in the neck within the carotid sheath on the anterior surfaces of the anterior scalene and longus colli muscles.

5. **Answer d:**

The inferior oblique muscle depresses the pupil when the pupil is fully adducted.

a: The superior rectus muscle elevates the abducted pupil but not the adducted pupil.

b: The inferior rectus muscle depresses the abducted pupil but not the adducted pupil.

c: The only function of the medial rectus muscle is to adduct the pupil.

e: The superior oblique muscle elevates the pupil when the pupil is fully adducted.

6. **Answer e:**

The facial nerve innervates the orbicularis oculi muscle, which functions to close the eye.

a: The buccal branch of the mandibular nerve is a sensory nerve and innervates no muscles.

b: The infraorbital nerve is a sensory nerve and innervates no muscles.

c: The ophthalmic nerve is a sensory nerve and innervates no muscles.

d: The oculomotor nerve supplies the extrinsic muscles of the eye except the lateral rectus and superior oblique muscles. None of these muscles functions to close the eye.

7. **Answer d:**

Preganglionic parasympathetic fibers from the superior salivatory nucleus join the facial nerve and pass to the submandibular and pterygopalatine ganglia.

a: The geniculate ganglion is the sensory ganglion of the facial nerve and contains no parasympathetic neuron cell bodies.

b: The otic ganglion contains the cell bodies of postganglionic parasympathetic neurons that supply the parotid gland.

c: The superior cervical sympathetic ganglion contains the cell bodies of postganglionic sympathetic neurons.

e: Pregnaglionic parasympathetic fibers from the inferior salivatory nucleus join the glossopharyngeal nerve and pass to the otic ganglion.

8. **Answer a:**

The skin of the temporal region overlying the pterion is supplied by the auriculotemporal nerve.

b: The great auricular nerve (from the ventral rami of C2 and C3 via the cervical plexus) supplies the skin over the auricle, the parotid gland, and the angle of the jaw.

c: The lesser occipital nerve (from the ventral ramus of C2 via the cervical plexus) supplies the skin of the neck and the scalp behind the ear.

d: The greater occipital nerve (from the dorsal ramus of C2) supplies the posterior scalp as far anteriorly as the vertex.

e: The supraorbital nerve (from the ophthalmic nerve) supplies the upper eyelid and the forehead and scalp as far posteriorly as the vertex.

9. **Answer d:**

The infratemporal fossa communicates medially with the pterygopalatine fossa via the pterygomaxillary fissure.

a: The superior orbital opens from the middle cranial fossa into the orbit.

b: The inferior orbital fissure opens from the orbit into the pterygopalatine fossa posteriorly and into the infratemporal and temporal fossae anteriorly.

c: The foramen spinosum opens from the infratemporal fossa into the middle cranial fossa.

e: The sphenopalatine foramen opens from the pterygopalatine fossa into the nasal cavity.

10. **Answer c:**

The upper eyelid is supplied largely by terminal branches of the ophthalmic artery, including the supraorbital, the supratrochlear, and the lacrimal.

a: The nasal cavity is supplied mostly by branches of the sphenopalatine artery, a terminal branch of the maxillary.

b: The dura is supplied in part by the middle meningeal and accessory meningeal arteries from the maxillary artery.

d: The upper teeth are supplied by the posterior superior alveolar artery from the maxillary artery and by the middle and anterior superior alveolar arteries from the infraorbital artery, a branch of the maxillary.

e: The palate is supplied in part by the greater and lesser palatine arteries from the descending palatine branch of the maxillary artery.

11. **Answer c:**

The intrinsic muscles of the larynx are innervated by the inferior laryngeal nerve via the recurrent laryngeal nerve; neither is found in the posterior triangle of the neck.

a: The ability to shrug the shoulder is a function of the trapezius muscle, which is supplied by the accessory nerve. The accessory nerve is vulnerable as it crosses the posterior triangle.

b: The rhomboid major and minor muscles are supplied by the dorsal scapular nerve. The dorsal scapular nerve crosses the floor of the posterior triangle.

d: The supraspinatus muscle initiates abduction of the shoulder. It is innervated by the suprascapular nerve, which is found in the posterior triangle.

e: The supraclavicular nerves provide sensation over the upper pectoral region. They emerge posterior to the sternocleidomastoid muscle to cross the posterior triangle.

12. **Answer c:**

The glossopharyngeal nerve has no meningeal branch.

a: The meningeal branch of the ophthalmic nerve supplies the tentorium cerebelli and the falx cerebri. The dura of the anterior cranial fossa is supplied by meningeal branches of the anterior and posterior ethmoidal nerves.

b: The meningeal branch of the mandibular nerve enters the cranial cavity through the foramen spinosum and is distributed along the course of the middle meningeal artery.

d: The meningeal branch of the vagus nerve enters the cranial cavity through the jugular foramen and supplies the dura of the posterior cranial fossa.

e: Meningeal branches of the upper cervical spinal nerves pass along the hypoglossal nerve to enter the cranial cavity through the hypoglossal canal and supply dura of the posterior cranial fossa.

13. **Answer a:**

Parasympathetic innervation to the parotid gland begins in the glossopharyngeal nerve and traverses the tympanic nerve and plexus, the lesser petrosal nerve, the otic ganglion, and the auriculotemporal nerve.

b: Parasympathetic innervation to the submandibular gland begins in the facial nerve and traverses the chorda tympani, the lingual nerve, the submandibular ganglion, and the submandibular branches of the ganglion.

c: Parasympathetic innervation to the lacrimal gland begins in the facial nerve and traverses the greater petrosal nerve, the nerve of the pterygoid canal, the pterygopalatine ganglion, the maxillary nerve, the zygomatic and zygomaticotemporal nerves, and the lacrimal nerve.

d: Parasympathetic innervation to the sublingual gland begins in the facial nerve and traverses the chorda tympani, the lingual nerve, the submandibular ganglion, and the sublingual branches of the lingual nerve.

e: Parasympathetic innervation to the glands of the nasal mucosa begins in the facial nerve and traverses the greater petrosal nerve, the nerve of the pterygoid canal, the pterygopalatine ganglion, and the nasal branches of the ganglion.

14. **Answer c:**

The buccinator muscle is a facial muscle and is supplied by the buccal branch of the facial nerve.

a: The tensor veli palatini is innervated by the nerve to the tensor veli palatini from the trunk of the mandibular nerve.

b: The anterior belly of the digastric muscle is supplied by the nerve to the mylohyoid (from the inferior alveolar branch of the mandibular nerve).

d: The lateral pterygoid muscle is supplied by the nerve to the lateral pterygoid (from the anterior division of the mandibular nerve).

e: The masseter muscle is supplied by the masseteric nerve (from the anterior division of the mandibular nerve).

15. **Answer a:**

The cricothyroid muscle is innervated by the external laryngeal nerve (from the superior laryngeal branch of the vagus nerve).

b: The thyroarytenoid muscle is supplied by the inferior laryngeal nerve (from the recurrent laryngeal branch of the vagus nerve).

c: The lateral cricoarytenoid muscle is supplied by the inferior laryngeal nerve (from the recurrent laryngeal branch of the vagus nerve).

d: The posterior cricoarytenoid muscle is supplied by the inferior laryngeal nerve (from the recurrent laryngeal branch of the vagus nerve).

e: The transverse arytenoid muscle is supplied by the inferior laryngeal nerve (from the recurrent laryngeal branch of the vagus nerve).

16. **Answer b:**

The second cranial nerve is the optic nerve, the nerve of vision. The neurons of the optic nerve are classified as special somatic afferent (SSA).

a: The first cranial nerve is the olfactory nerve, the nerve of smell. The neurons of the olfactory nerve are classified as special visceral afferent (SVA).

c: The seventh cranial nerve, the facial nerve, contains taste fibers that are classified as special visceral afferent (SVA).

d: The ninth cranial nerve, the glossopharyngeal nerve, contains taste fibers that are classified as special visceral afferent (SVA).

e: The tenth cranial nerve, the vagus nerve, contains taste fibers that are classified as special visceral afferent (SVA).

17. **Answer b:**

The greater occipital nerve is derived from the dorsal ramus of the second cervical spinal nerve.

a: The great auricular nerve is derived from the ventral rami of C2 and C3 via the cervical plexus.

c: The lesser occipital nerve is derived from the ventral ramus of the second cervical spinal nerve.

d: The transverse cervical nerve is derived

from the ventral rami of C2 and C3 via the cervical plexus.

e: The supraclavicular nerve is derived from the ventral rami of C3 and C4 via the cervical plexus.

18. **Answer e:**

The prevertebral fascia ensheaths the prevertebral muscles, the scalene muscles, and the intrinsic back muscles. The roots of the brachial plexus are covered by the prevertebral fascia as they emerge between the anterior and middle scalene muscles.

a: The esophagus lies in front of the prevertebral fascia.

b: The sternocleidomastoid muscle is invested by the superficial layer of deep cervical fascia and lies superficial to the prevertebral fascia.

c: The accessory nerve lies superficial to the prevertebral fascia as it pierces the sternocleidomastoid muscle and crosses the posterior cervical triangle to reach the deep surface of the trapezius muscle.

d: The vagus lies within the carotid sheath anterior to the prevertebral fascia.

19. **Answer a:**

The posterior auricular vein joins the posterior division of the retromandibular vein to form the external jugular vein.

b: The inferior petrosal venous sinus exits the skull through the jugular foramen to end in the internal jugular vein.

c: The superior thyroid vein ends in the internal jugular vein.

d: The common facial vein ends in the internal jugular vein.

e: The lingual vein ends in the internal jugular vein.

20. **Answer b:**

The mylohyoid muscle is innervated by the mylohyoid nerve from the mandibular division of the trigeminal nerve.

a: The geniohyoid muscle is supplied by fibers from C1 that travel with the hypoglossal nerve.

c: The omohyoid muscle is innervated by the cervical plexus via the ansa cervicalis.

d: The thyrohyoid muscle is supplied by fibers from C1 that travel with the hypoglossal nerve.

e: The sternohyoid muscle is innervated by the cervical plexus via the ansa cervicalis.

INDEX

Mosby's Reviews Series
Copyright © 1997,
Mosby–Year Book, Inc.

How to install this program—Windows users

1. Place the disk in Drive A: (or B:)
2. From Program Manager, select File, then Run, then enter:
   A:SETUP (or B:SETUP if your disk drive is B:)
3. Follow the instructions on screen.

How to run this program—Windows users

Open the MOSBY Program Group and select the Mosby's Reviews Series icon.

How to install this program—Macintosh users

1. Insert the disk into the disk drive. Double-click on the disk icon.
2. Double-click on the install icon. The program will be saved to your hard drive.

How to run this program—Macintosh users

Open the MOSBY folder and select the Mosby's Reviews Series icon.

For complete instructions on using the program, please read the "How to use this Program" file.

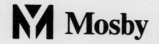
Mosby

Dedicated to Publishing Excellence

WE WANT TO HEAR FROM YOU!

To help us publish the most useful materials for students, we would appreciate your comments on this book.   Please take a few moments to complete the form below, and then tear it out and mail to us. Thank you for your input.

Mosby's reviews: ANATOMY

1. What courses are you using this book for?

__medical school   __1st year
__osteopathic school   __2nd year
__dental school   __3rd year
__pharmacy school   __4th year
__physician assistant program   __other _____
__nursing school
__undergrad
__other_____

2. Was this book useful for your course? Why or why not?

__yes __no_____

_____

_____

3. What features of textbooks are important to you? (*check all that apply*)

__color figures   __text summaries
__summary tables and boxes   __self-assessment questions
__price
__other_____

_____

4. What influenced your decision to buy this text? (*check all that apply*)
__required/recommended by instructor   __bookstore display   __journal advertisement
__recommended by student   ---other _____

5. What other instructional materials did/would you find useful in this course?

__computer-assisted instruction   __slides
__other_____

Are you interested in doing in-depth reviews of our textooks?   ___yes ___no

NAME:_____

ADDRESS:_____

_____

TELEPHONE: _____

THANK YOU!

A Times Mirror
Company

NO POSTAGE
NECESSARY
IF MAILED
IN THE
UNITED STATES

BUSINESS REPLY MAIL
FIRST CLASS MAIL   PERMIT No. 135   St. Louis, MO.

POSTAGE WILL BE PAID BY ADDRESSEE

CHRIS REID
MEDICAL EDITORIAL
MOSBY–YEAR BOOK, INC.
11830 WESTLINE INDUSTRIAL DRIVE
ST.LOUIS, MO 63146-9987

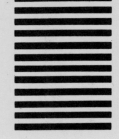